Baillière's
CLINICAL ENDOCRINOLOGY AND METABOLISM

INTERNATIONAL PRACTICE AND RESEARCH

Baillière's

CLINICAL ENDOCRINOLOGY AND METABOLISM

INTERNATIONAL PRACTICE AND RESEARCH

Volume 3/Number 1
May 1989

Imaging Endocrine Disorders

F.-L. CHAN MB, BS, FRCR
C. WANG MD, FRCP
Guest Editors

Baillière Tindall
London Philadelphia Sydney Tokyo Toronto

Baillière Tindall 24–28 Oval Road
W.B. Saunders   London NW1 7DX, UK

The Curtis Center, Independence Square West,
Philadelphia, PA 19106–3399, USA

1 Goldthorne Avenue
Toronto, Ontario M8Z 5T9, Canada

Harcourt Brace Jovanovich Group (Australia) Pty Ltd,
32–52 Smidmore Street, Marrickville, NSW 2204, Australia

Exclusive Agent in Japan:
Maruzen Co. Ltd. (Journals Division)
3–10 Nihonbashi 2-chome, Chuo-ku, Tokyo 103, Japan

ISSN 0950–351X

ISBN 0–7020–1345–5 (single copy)

Baillière's Clinical Endocrinology and Metabolism is published three times each year by
Baillière Tindall. Annual subscription prices are:

TERRITORY	ANNUAL SUBSCRIPTION	SINGLE ISSUE
1. UK	£35.00 post free	£18.50 post free
2. Europe	£45.00 post free	£18.50 post free
3. All other countries	Consult your local Harcourt Brace Jovanovich office for dollar price	

The editor of this publication is Katharine Hinton, Baillière Tindall,
24–28 Oval Road, London NW1 7DX, UK.

Baillière's Clinical Endocrinology and Metabolism was published from 1972 to 1986 as
Clinics in Endocrinology and Metabolism.

Typeset by Phoenix Photosetting, Chatham.
Printed and bound in Great Britain by Mackays of Chatham PLC, Chatham, Kent.

Contributors to this issue

JAFFER AJANI MD, Assistant Professor and Associate Intern, Department of Medical Oncology, The University of Texas, M.D. Anderson Cancer Center, 1515 Holcombe Boulevard, Houston, TX 77030, USA.

JEAN FRANÇOIS BONNEVILLE MD, Professor of Medicine, Chief of the Department of Neuroradiology, University Hospital of Besancon, 25030 Besancon, France.

C. HUMBERTO CARRASCO MD, Associate Professor of Radiology, Department of Diagnostic Radiology, The University of Texas, M.D. Anderson Cancer Center, 1515 Holcombe Boulevard, Box 57, Houston, TX 77030, USA.

FRANÇOISE CATTIN MD, Department of Neuroradiology, University Hospital of Besancon, 25030 Besancon, France.

FU LUK CHAN MB, BS, FRCR, Consultant Radiologist in Charge, Diagnostic Radiology Division, Institute of Radiology and Oncology, Queen Mary Hospital, Pokfulam Road, Hong Kong.

CHUSILP CHARNSANGAVEJ MD, Radiologist, M.D. Anderson Cancer Center; Professor of Radiology, M.D. Anderson Cancer Center, 1515 Holcombe Boulevard, Box 57, Houston, TX 77030, USA.

JULIAN C. CHEN MD, Research Fellow, Tri-Hospital Magnetic Resonance Centre, 200 Elizabeth Street, Toronto, Ontario, Canada.

KENNETH M. COOKE MBBS, FRACR, Department of Radiology, The Children's Hospital, Pyrmont Bridge Road, Camperdown, Sydney 2050, Australia.

CHRISTOPHER COWELL MBBS, FRCP(C), FRACP, Department of Endocrinology, The Children's Hospital, Pyrmont Bridge Road, Camperdown, Sydney 2050, Australia.

JEAN LOUIS DIETEMANN MD, Professor of Medicine, Department of Neuroradiology, University Hospital of Strasbourg, 67000 Strasbourg, France.

GERALD D. DODD JR MD, Professor and Chairman, Department of Diagnostic Radiology, The University of Texas, M.D. Anderson Cancer Center, 1515 Holcombe Boulevard, Houston, TX 77030, USA.

KIM DONAGHUE MBBS, FRACR, Department of Endocrinology, The Children's Hospital, Pyrmont Bridge Road, Camperdown, Sydney 2050, Australia.

J. T. HALL BS, MD, Department of Radiology, St. Alphonsus Regional Medical Center, Boise, ID 83706, USA.

ROBERT HOWMAN-GILES MBBS, FRACP, DDU, Department of Nuclear Medicine, The Children's Hospital, Pyrmont Bridge Road, Camperdown, Sydney 2050, Australia.

WALTER KUCHARCZYK MD, FRCP(C), Assistant Professor, University of Toronto; Director, Tri-Hospital Magnetic Resonance Centre, 200 Elizabeth Street, Toronto, Ontario, Canada.

ALBERT H. LAM MBBS, FRACR, DDU, Department of Radiology, The Children's Hospital, Pyrmont Bridge Road, Camperdown, Sydney 2050, Australia.

T. JOHN MARTIN MD, DSc, FRACP, Professor of Medicine, St. Vincent's Hospital; Director, St. Vincent's Institute of Medical Research, Melbourne 3065, Australia.

BARRY M. McCOOK MD, Instructor of Radiology, Vanderbilt University Medical Center, Twentyfirst and Garland Avenues, Nashville, TN 37232, USA.

JAMES A. PATTON PhD, Professor of Radiology, Associate Director, Nuclear Medicine, Vanderbilt University Medical Center, Twentyfirst and Garland Avenues, Nashville, TN 37232, USA.

WILLIAM R. RICHLI MD, Assistant Professor and Assistant Radiologist, Department of Diagnostic Radiology, The University of Texas, M.D. Anderson Cancer Center, 1515 Holcombe Boulevard, Houston, TX 77030, USA.

NAGUIB A. SAMAAN MD, Professor and Deputy Department Chairman, Medical Specialities Department, Chief, Section of Endocrinology, The University of Texas, M.D. Anderson Cancer Center, 1515 Holcombe Boulevard, Houston, TX 77030, USA.

MARTIN P. SANDLER MD, Associate Professor, Radiology and Medicine, Director of Nuclear Medicine, Vanderbilt University Medical Center, Twentyfirst and Garland Avenues, Nashville, TN 37232, USA.

EGO SEEMAN BSc, MBBS, FRACP, Senior Lecturer in Medicine, University of Melbourne; Consultant Endocrinologist, Austin Repatriation General and Box Hill Hospitals, Heidelberg 3084, Melbourne, Australia.

MERL DE SILVA MBBS, FRACR, Director, Department of Radiology, The Children's Hospital, Pyrmont Bridge Road, Camperdown, Sydney 2050, Australia.

SIDNEY WALLACE MD, Professor and Radiologist, Deputy Department Chairman, Department of Diagnostic Radiology, The University of Texas, M.D. Anderson Cancer Center, 1515 Holcombe Boulevard, Houston, TX 77030, USA.

CHRISTINA WANG MD, FRACP, Professor in Medicine, Department of Medicine, University of Hong Kong, Queen Mary Hospital, Pokfulam Road, Hong Kong.

Table of contents

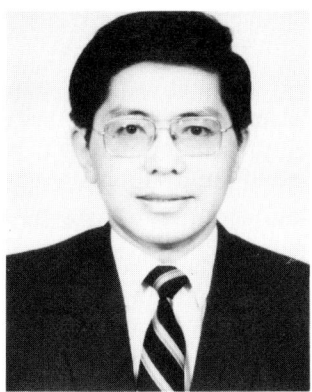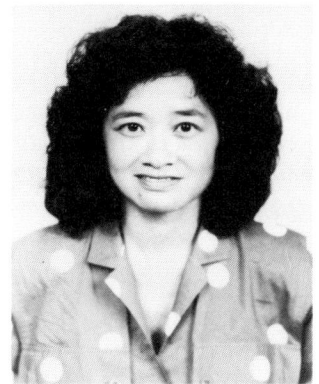

Foreword

Technological advances in diagnostic imaging have served enormous impact on the practice of clinical medicine. With the evolution of computed tomography (CT) and magnetic resonance imaging (MRI), sophistication in instrumentation for ultrasonography, improvement in nuclear medicine procedures and progress in interventional radiology, the last ten years have witnessed dramatic and exciting improvements in our ability to image the endocrine system. This issue presents an opportunity for clinicians to enjoy an overview of the role of state-of-the-art diagnostic imaging in a wide range of endocrine disorders. Our goal is to discuss and illustrate the complementary applications and strategy of multiple imaging procedures used in the approach to the clinical problem.

The major portion of the book is organized into gland-related chapters. There are five articles on medical imaging in the localization and characterization of the causative pathologies in disorders of individual endocrine glands. Two of these are devoted to the hypothalamic–pituitary region: one on the more commonly available CT modality; one on the application of MRI which advances rapidly with the promise of the technique of choice for this region. The role of MRI in other endocrine glands is less clear, and therefore is incorporated into the discussion on the imaging management, utilizing, where applicable, CT, ultrasonography, scintigraphy, vascular studies and interventional methods, on the thyroid, parathyroid, adrenal, pancreatic and gastrointestinal endocrine systems in the respective chapters. These chapters aim to underscore the choice of imaging modalities when facing a particular clinical problem. A chapter on 'Parathyroid Imaging' originally planned to be contributed by Professor Okerlund of San Francisco is, however, sadly missing owing to his sudden untimely death. The application of hepatic artery embolization for hepatic metastases is also addressed in the chapter on the endocrine pancreas. In addition, one article critically discusses the use of bone densitometry in the clinical management of metabolic bone diseases. Finally, an overview of diagnostic imaging in paediatric endocrinology is provided with discussion on selected topics such as precocious puberty, bone age assessment, pituitary, thyroid and parathyroid disorders in children.

We extend our heartfelt thanks to our colleagues for generously contributing their time and expertise to make this issue a possibility, and to the publisher for patience and guidance. We sincerely hope that the sharing of experiences of the authors will provide readers with a valuable reference guide that will enhance the care of their patients.

F. L. CHAN
C. WANG

1

Non-invasive techniques for the measurement of bone mineral

EGO SEEMAN
T. JOHN MARTIN

The past two decades have seen the development of precise, reproducible, non-invasive and safe techniques for measuring bone density of the axial and appendicular skeleton. These techniques have provided important clinical information about the behaviour of the skeleton in health and disease. The purpose of this chapter is to acquaint the general reader with the value, and limitations, of this information and to describe the clinical applications of the methods. Only those techniques currently in use and readily available in most large centres will be discussed. More detailed information can be obtained from two excellent reviews (Genant et al, 1988; Mazess and Wahner, 1988).

The most important application of these techniques is in the detection, prevention and treatment of osteoporosis in women, the commonest metabolic bone disease encountered in clinical practice. Almost 15% of all women over 65 years of age will suffer a fracture in their lifetime and up to 33% of women and 17% of men reaching 90 years of age will fracture their hip. Hip fracture is associated with a 12–20% reduction in expected survival. The economic burden of hip fractures is over 6 billion dollars annually in the United States. By the year 2050, people aged over 65 years will comprise 22% and people aged over 85 years 5%, of the population compared with 11% and 1% respectively in 1980. The magnitude of the morbidity, mortality and cost make osteoporosis an important public health problem (Melton, 1988).

THE RELEVANCE OF BONE DENSITY TO BONE STRENGTH

The prevention of fractures would be more effective if information regarding the relative importance of bone quantity and bone quality to bone strength were known. Our ability to measure bone quality and the degree of trauma is limited. However, in vitro, 90% of the variance of bone strength is attributable to bone quantity (Smith CB and Smith, 1976; Carter and Hayes, 1977). There is a linear relationship, in vitro, between the breaking strength of bone and its density (Figure 1): the breaking strength of bone is pro-

portional to the square of its density; the elastic modulus of bone is proportional to the cube of its density. Thus, small changes in density will be
associated with large changes in bone strength and stiffness. This relationship between bone strength and density has been found using samples of
vertebrae, proximal femur or iliac crest (Bell et al, 1967; Dalen et al, 1976;
Mosekilde et al, 1987).

For these techniques to have clinical value, bone mineral density must be
an important determinant of bone strength in vivo, and must be an
independent predictor of fracture risk. In a 6-year prospective study of 521
Caucasian women, Hui et al (1988) showed that age and bone mineral
content of the radius, measured using single photon absorptiometry, were
independent predictors of risk for facture (Figure 2). For any given bone
mineral density, the risk of fracture increased as age increased. For any
given age, the risk of fracture increased as bone mineral content decreased.
This instructive study will be referred to in more detail later. Wasnich et al

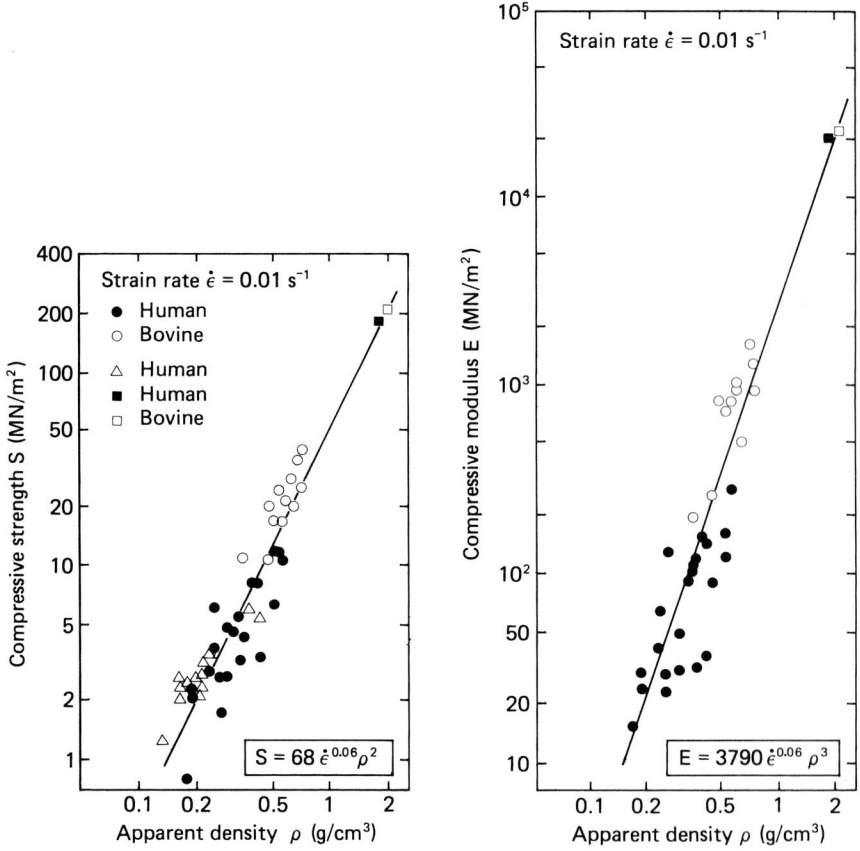

Figure 1. Influence of apparent density on the compressive strength and modulus of bone.
Human and bovine cortical and trabecular bone tested in compression. From Carter and Hayes
(1977), with permission.

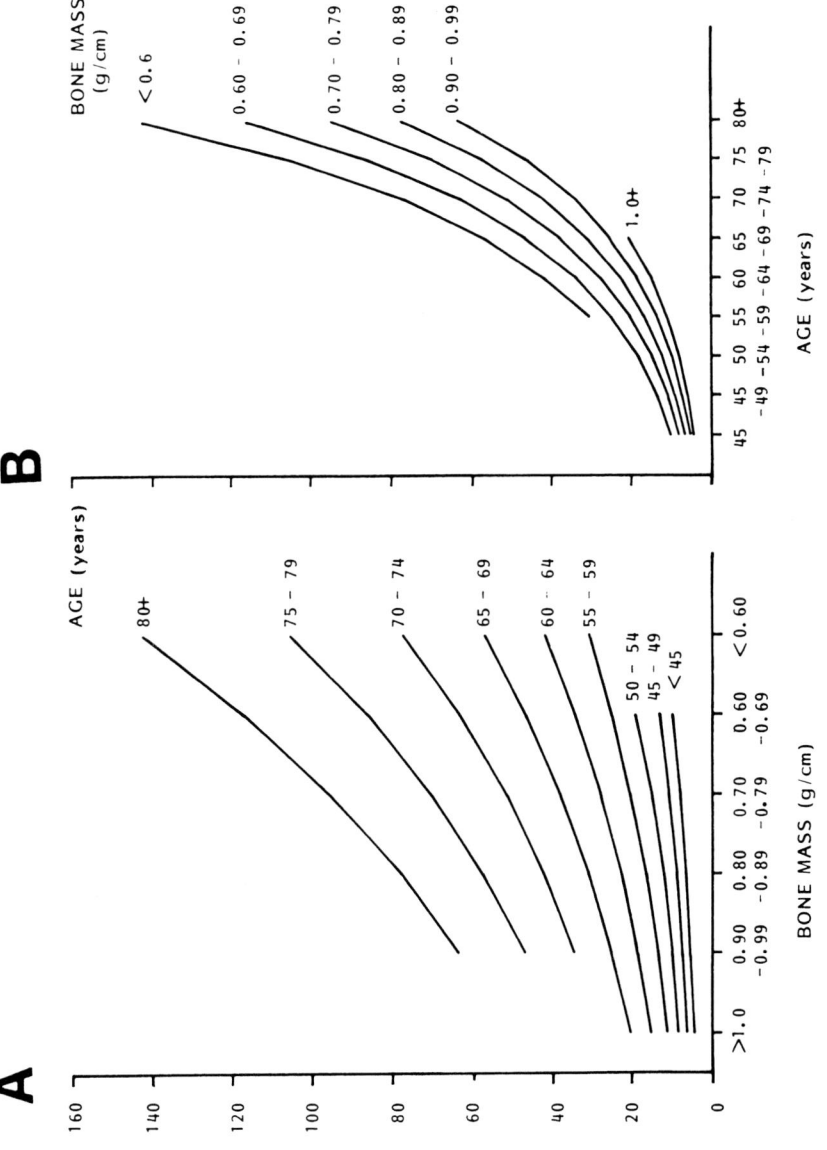

Figure 2. The incidence of fracture as a function of bone mass (A) and age (B). From Hui et al (1988), with permission.

(1985) have shown that the risk of both spinal and non-spinal fractures increased as bone mineral density decreased. This was found using measurements of bone mineral density of the proximal and distal radius, lumbar spine or os calcis.

Melton (1988) have shown that the incidence and prevalence of hip fractures and the prevalence of vertebral fractures increased as bone mineral density decreased (Figure 3). In a random sample of women in the

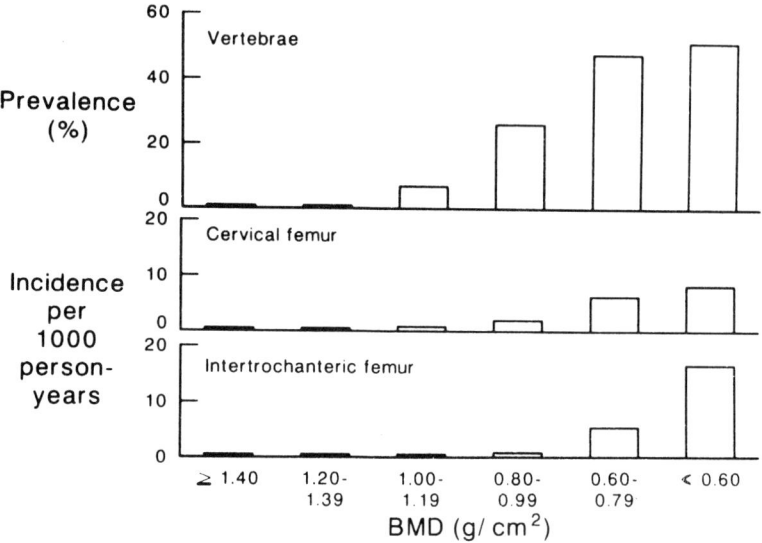

Figure 3. Occurrence of vertebral and proximal femoral fractures at various levels of vertebral and proximal femoral bone mineral density. From Riggs and Melton (1986), with permission.

population of Rochester, Minnesota, the prevalence of fractures was 4% in the 60% with spinal bone mineral density $>1.0\,\text{g/cm}^2$. In the 40% with spinal bone mineral density $<1.0\,\text{g/cm}^2$, the prevalence was 32%. Almost half the 10% of women with bone mineral density $<0.8\,\text{g/cm}^2$ had fractures. With respect to hip fractures, the incidence of cervical or intertrochanteric fractures (per 1000 persons per year) was approximately 4.0 for women with a bone mineral density of $>1.0\,\text{g/cm}^2$, 8.3 cervical fractures for women with a cervical bone mineral density of $<0.6\,\text{g/cm}^2$ and 16.6 intertrochanteric fractures for women with a intertrochanteric bone mineral density of $<0.6\,\text{g/cm}^2$. These studies confirm the importance of bone mineral density as an independent predictor of fracture risk and the value of these non-invasive techniques in estimating this risk.

THE LIMITED CLINICAL UTILITY OF FRACTURES

Currently, bone densitometry is the only method of assessing the effectiveness of a treatment or the fracture risk conferred by a disease. In an individual, fractures are too uncommon to be a sensitive measure of whether or not a treatment is effective. This can only be determined by large clinical trials (Kanis, 1984). For example, the incidence of new vertebral fractures in untreated patients with postmenopausal osteoporosis is about one fracture per patient per year (Riggs et al, 1982a). Iskrant and Smith (1969) reported an incidence of 7 patients with new fractures per 100 subjects per year in radiologically osteoporotic women. The incidence of vertebral fractures in the US is about 1.5 per 100 women per year (Holbrook et al, 1984). The highest incidence of hip fractures occurs in women over 85 years of age and is 3–4 per 100 persons per year (Melton, 1988). In contrast, bone densitometry provides a quantitative estimate of fracture risk and a measureable response to ageing, disease and medical treatment, in an individual.

METHODS FOR MEASURING BONE MINERAL DENSITY

The techniques for measuring bone mineral density that are widely accessible and well established include single photon absorptiometry (SPA), dual photon absorptiometry (DPA), and single or dual energy quantitative computed tomography (QCT). Dual energy X-ray absorptiometry (DEXA) is a new technique with potentially important practical advantages.

The principles of measurement for each of the techniques are similar and involve the passage of a beam of radiation over the region of interest. The attenuation of the incident beam of radiation, represented by the area under the curve, is proportional to the amount of intervening tissue (Figure 4).

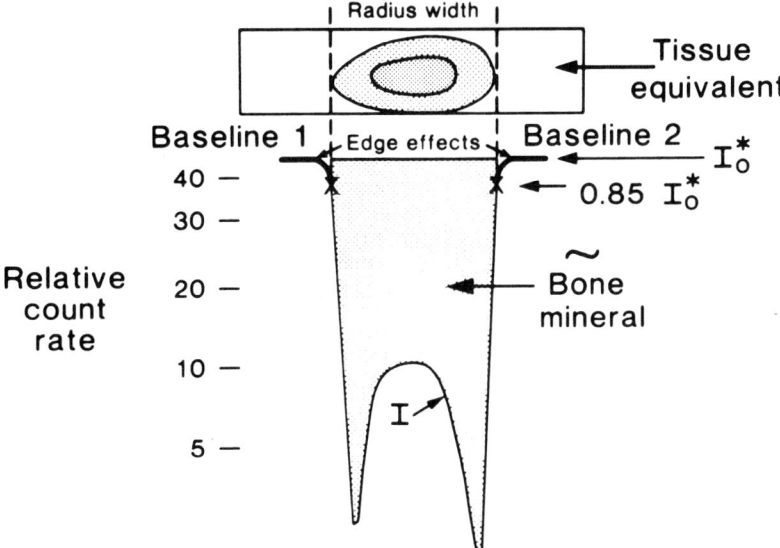

Figure 4. Single photon absorptiometry. Plot of the radiation beam intensity as a function of position across the bone sample. The area under the curve gives a value proportional to the bone mineral content. I, attenuated; I*, unattenuated. From Wahner et al (1983), with permission.

This attenuation is quantified by using reference standards of known mineral density. The number of energy levels required for measurement of bone density is determined by the number of intervening tissues. For example, in the forearm, the skin thickness is minimal and only a single energy is needed (*single* photon absorptiometry). At the spine, proximal femur or when total body measurement is undertaken, the soft tissue contribution to the attenuation must be resolved to obtain a measure of bone mineral density. This is achieved by using two energy sources (*dual* photon absorptiometry or *dual* energy QCT). If these energies come from a single isotope this is referred to as dual *photon* absorptiometry. If two isotopes are used and each provides one photon energy this is called dual *beam* absorptiometry. Each of these methods quantifies bone mineral differently. Only QCT provides an estimate of density (mass per unit volume). For consistency, the term bone mineral density will be used throughout.

Single photon absorptiometry (SPA)

SPA has been in use for many years and was first described by Cameron and Sorenson (1963). A rectilinear scanning system with a source and detector moves over the region of interest (mid-, distal or ultra-distal radius, or os calcis). The limb being measured is surrounded by a tissue equivalent (water or gel) to ensure the region being measured has a constant thickness. A monoenergetic beam of photons, usually from I-125 (27 keV) is transmitted across the region of interest. The attenuated beam intensity is compared to the transmission in soft tissue and this relationship is described mathematically (Mazess and Wahner, 1988). The value obtained is standardized using a reference of known mineral content. Using SPA, a measure of bone mineral content of the region scanned is obtained (g). When this value is divided by the bone width, a measure of mineral content per unit length (g/cm) is obtained. If the measurement is divided by the estimate of the cross-sectional area of the region scanned a measurement referred to as the linear density (g/cm^2) is obtained. SPA has a precision of 1–3%.

Dual photon absorptiometry (DPA)

DPA is an important technique because bone mineral density can be measured at the spine and proximal femur, the common sites of fracture in osteoporosis. The principle of the technique involves radiation transmission of photons from a radioactive source placed beneath the patient (Figure 5). The source is mechanically linked to a collimated radiation detector above the patient. The source and detector move in a raster pattern over the region to be measured; the 2nd, 3rd and 4th lumbar vertebrae, proximal femur (femoral neck, trochanter and Wards triangle) or the total body. Using DPA, a measure of bone mineral content (g) of the region scanned is thus obtained. When divided by the area scanned a measure of *areal* bone mineral density (g/cm^2) is obtained.

Measurements at the lumbar spine are taken in the anteroposterior position with the legs elevated to reduce the lumbar lordosis. The

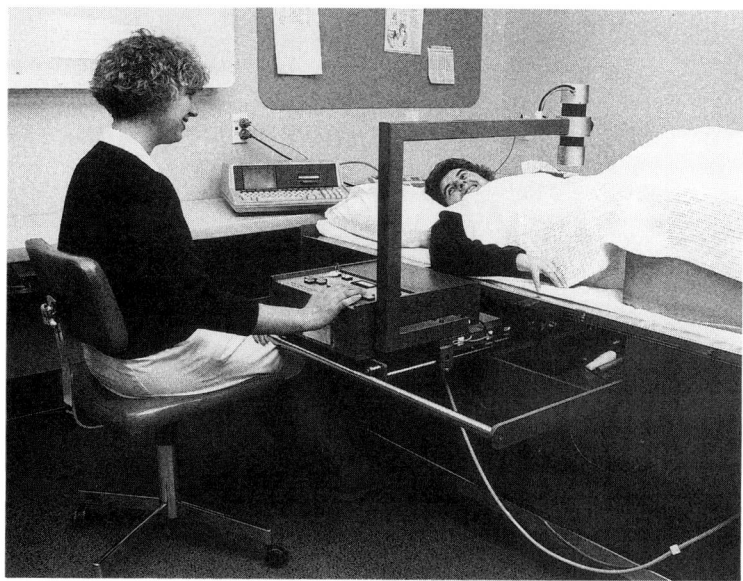

Figure 5. Dual photon absorptiometry. Scanning table with detector apparatus.

measurements include the vertebral body, arches, spinous processes. Aortic calcification or osteophytes may adversely influence the result. Measurement of the femoral neck, trochanter and Wards triangle, the region most sensitive to loss of trabecular bone (Kerr et al, 1986) is done by scanning the whole region of the proximal femur. A region of interest is chosen manually or with computer assistance. Alternatively, the direction of scanning can be fixed at 53 degrees to scan perpendicular and across the femoral neck. The femoral anteversion is corrected by having the foot internally rotated during scanning.

DPA is also used for measuring total body mineral. The procedure involves rectilinear scanning of the whole body. The duration of scanning is 60 min but has been shortened by modification of scanning speeds over regions of soft tissue. Scanning takes approximately 20 min per region. Precision is 1–3% for repeat measurements at the spine, 2–4% at the proximal femur and <1.5% for total body calcium determinations. The radiation exposure is 1–3 mrem.

Quantitative computed tomography (QCT)

QCT can selectively measure the trabecular centrum or spongiosum of the vertebral body, the cortical shell or both (Figure 6). The contribution of other mineralized tissues such as the vertebral arches, spinous processes, aortic calcification or osteophytes can be excluded using this method. Precise relocalization of the section of the vertebrae measured is needed for acceptable reproducibility. A slice 2–10 mm thick is taken through the centre of the 2nd, 3rd and 4th lumbar vertebra parallel to the endplate in the

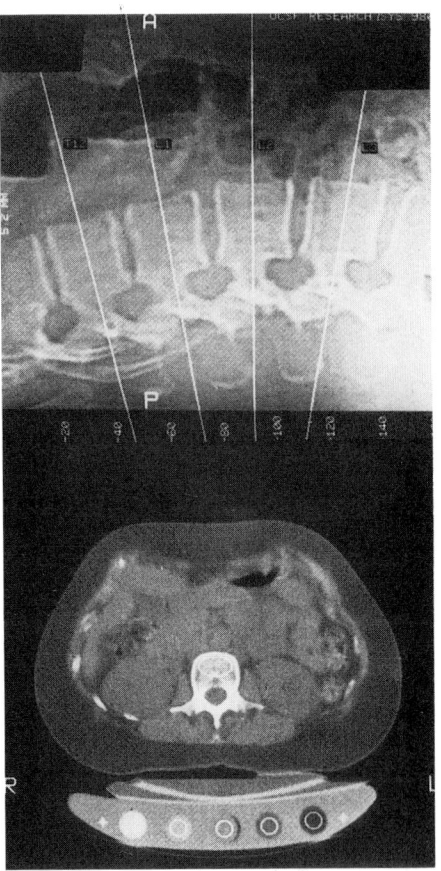

Figure 6. Lateral scout views permit localization of the mid plane of vertebral bodies. An oval region of interest is used to determine bone mineral density. A circular region of interest in the standards is used for calibration. From Genant et al (1988), with permission.

lateral position. An elliptical region of interest in the anterior part of the vertebral body is then chosen as shown in Figure 6. Scanning is done with reference solutions of known mineral concentration. The Hounsfield units, a measure of attenuation, of the reference solutions are plotted against their known concentration providing a standard curve (Genant et al, 1988). Bone mineral density, mass (mg) per unit volume (ml or cm^3) is thus obtained.

Dual energy QCT is used to correct for the effect marrow fat has on the measurement of bone mineral density obtained using single energy QCT. The attenuation of the incident beam is due to mineral and fat tissue. The contribution of the fat tissue may be substantial as marrow fat increases as age increases. Dual energy QCT is used to adjust for this effect. Lower values, by 20–30 mg/ml, for bone density may be obtained using single energy QCT (Genant et al, 1983; Cann et al, 1985; Laval-Jeantet et al, 1986). This may be reduced using correction methods (Genant et al, 1988).

The dual energy technique improves this error but at the price of a lower precision and higher radiation exposure. For dual energy measurement, a second scan is obtained through the same region using a second energy to resolve the soft tissue (marrow fat) contribution to the attenuation. Scanning takes 10 min. The radiation exposure is 100–300 mrem but may be up to 500 mrem (Cann, 1981). The precision is 2–3% (single energy QCT) and 3–5% (dual energy QCT).

Dual energy X-ray absorptiometry (DEXA)

This technique (Mazess et al, 1988; Stein et al, 1988; Wahner et al, 1988) is similar in principle to DPA. Scanning is done in a rectilinear fashion with pixel by pixel recording of the two different energy intensities. The whole vertebra is measured; the body, arches and spinous processes and an areal density measurement (g/cm^2) is obtained. There have been a number of important advances. An X-ray source of radiation is used. Even at a current of 1 mA, an X-ray tube emits a photon flux equivalent to about a 500 Ci radio-active source. The cost of replacing the expensive 1 Ci radionucleotide source every 18 months is eliminated. The absence of source decay eliminates problems with decreasing count rates over the lifetime of the source. The precision has a coefficient of variation of <1–2%. Beam size is 2 mm compared with 8 mm for DPA improving resolution (Figure 7).

Difficulties with soft tissue determination and edge detection are elimi-

(a)　　　　　　　　　　　　　　　　　(b)

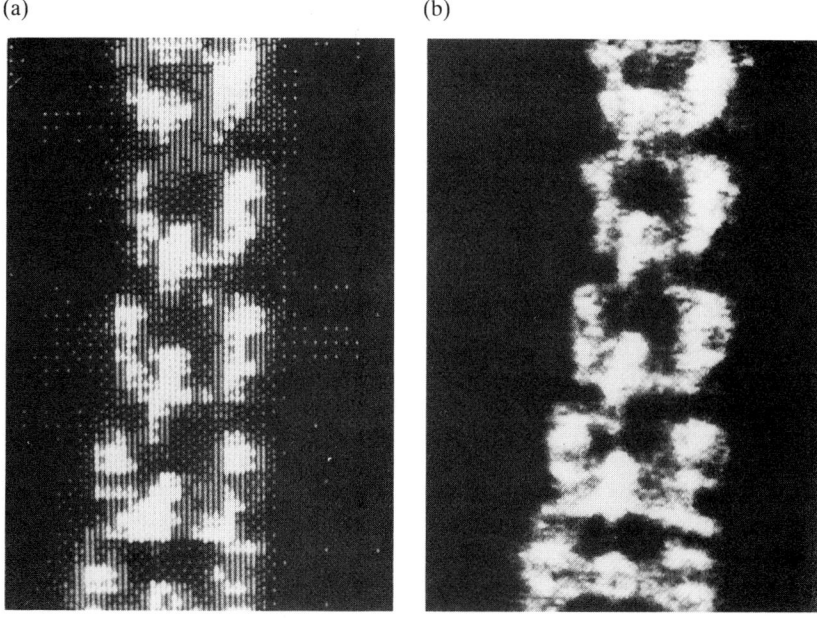

Figure 7. Comparison of the video display image of the lumbar spine using DPA (a) and quantitative digital radiography (QDR) (b). Note the superior resolution and smaller effect of 'noise' in the QDR image. From Kelly et al (1988), with permission.

nated, the high photon flux allows a faster scanning speed with more scan passes per unit area. The operator can display the previous image and superimpose it on the current image for better relocalization in longitudinal studies. The low radiation exposure (<2 mrem) and short scanning time (<5 min) allows duplicate measurements to be done. The technique is versatile; measurement of the spine, proximal femur, forearm and total body can be performed as well as other regions such as the knee or wrist. The correlation between DEXA and DPA measurements is 0.98. The long-term reproducibility assessed over 180 days using a phantom is better than DPA, having a coefficient of variation of 0.23% compared with 0.73%. The smallest change not attributable to measurement error is 0.025 g/cm^2 (Kelly et al, 1988). These improvements probably make this technique the method of choice.

Other methods

Other methods for measuring bone density include peripheral QCT, metacarpal morphometry (radiogrammetry), ultrasound transmission, Compton scattering, neutron activation analysis, technetium-diphosphonate uptake measurement, use of the Singh index and others. These techniques will not be dealt with because they are limited by being available in few centres. Many are experimental, time consuming or difficult to perform. The reader is referred to a well referenced and concise review by Mazess (1983).

WHICH METHOD SHOULD BE USED?

There is considerable controversy regarding which method is the 'best' for assessing bone mineral density. The decision depends on the question being asked and recognition of the heterogeneity of the skeleton.

Regional specificity

The skeleton is not a uniformly functioning entity. The skeletal response to ageing, loss of gonadal function, illness and medical treatment varies in magnitude and even direction. For example, fluoride therapy may increase bone mineral density of the axial skeleton while having no effect or decreasing bone mineral density in the appendicular skeleton (Riggs, 1984). Similar observations have been made using other forms of therapy (Reeve et al, 1980). Following oophorectomy or spontaneous menopause, early bone loss from the spine is substantial, whereas changes at the radius are smaller or undetectable (Genant et al, 1982). The effects of endocrine diseases on the skeleton exhibit regional specificity (Seeman et al, 1982).

As shown in Figure 8, a variety of diseases of hormonal deficiency or excess result in changes in the axial and appendicular skeleton which are generally in the same direction but may be greater in magnitude at the axial site. For example, the patients with glucocorticosteroid excess had signifi-cantly decreased bone mineral density at the spine but not at the

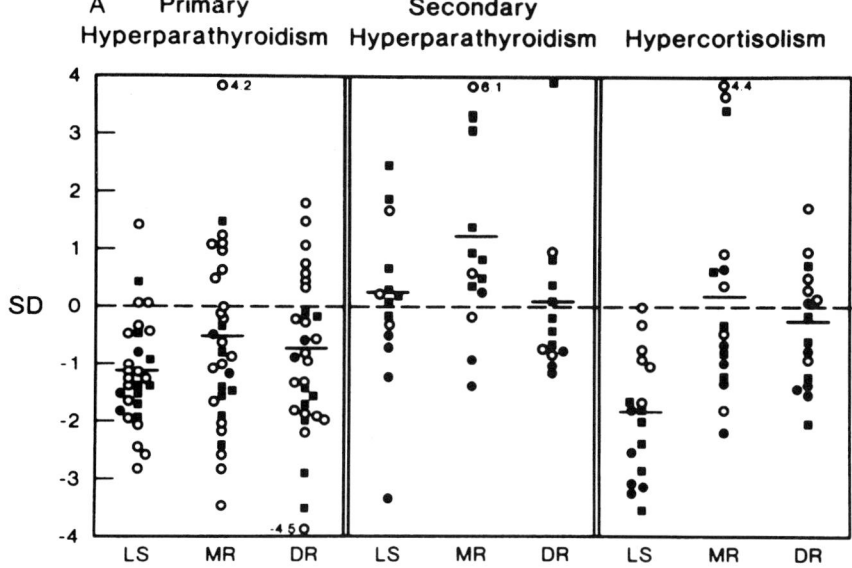

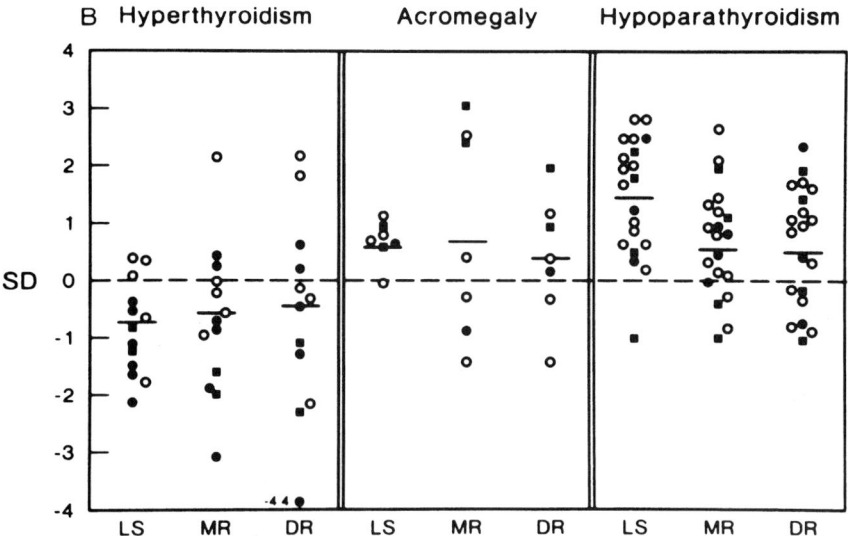

Figure 8. Values (expressed as z-scores) for bone mineral density of the lumbar spine (LS), mid radius (MR) and distal radius (DR) in six endocrine disorders. Scanning sites for males (■) and premenopausal (●) and postmenopausal (○) females. From Seeman et al (1982), with permission.

appendicular sites. Had only one skeletal region been examined in these examples, quite different conclusions regarding the effect of treatment or disease would have been made. This heterogeneity of skeletal responses suggests that measurements of more than one region of the skeleton are preferable when addressing the effect of disease, ageing or treatment on bone mineral density.

If measurement of more than one site is not feasible, it is preferable to measure the region of interest; the spine, if questions about vertebral bone mineral density are being addressed, or the hip, if questions regarding femoral neck bone mineral density are being addressed. In general, there are statistically significant correlations between regions of about 0.3–0.7. These moderate correlations, reflect the wide dispersion of measurements around the regression line. They are not high enough for a value or a rate of change at one site to predict a value or rate of change at another. Moreover, measurements of the same site using different techniques correlate weakly unless care is taken to ensure that the results are expressed in similar units (Mazess and Vetter, 1985; Sambrook et al, 1985).

Cortical and trabecular bone

There is probably more than one reason for the regional specificity seen in health and disease. One of the most commonly cited reasons is the differing proportions of trabecular and cortical bone in the axial and appendicular skeleton. The skeleton consists of 75% cortical bone and 25% trabecular bone. Trabecular bone is found mainly in the axial skeleton and in the metaphyses of long bones. Trabecular bone has a more rapid turnover and a greater surface to volume ratio than cortical bone (Parfitt, 1988). The common regions which fracture in osteoporosis, the distal radius, vertebrae, proximal femur, pelvis and proximal humerus contain substantial amounts of trabecular bone. There is uncertainty regarding what proportions of each type of bone are present in a given region. Based on dissection of post mortem specimens of human vertebrae, the mean trabecular content of whole vertebra was 25%, ranging 20–30%. The mean trabecular content of the vertebral body was 40%, ranging 35–50% (Nottestad et al, 1987). The trabecular content of the radius may vary markedly along its length. Based on serial sectioning and ashing of specimens from four subjects of differing age, Schlenker and VonSeggen (1976) found that the trabecular bone of the distal radius comprised 38–50% of the total mineral present. Differing blood supply, marrow content, proximity to articular surfaces and biomechanical factors may influence the behaviour of a region. Thus, changes in bone mineral density in a region may not be readily interpreted as being due to a change in either cortical bone or trabecular bone. Axial and trabecular, appendicular and cortical are not interchangeable terms.

THE NORMAL RANGE

Accurate non-invasive techniques for measuring the spine and proximal femur have been available for about 10 years. Thus, of necessity, few long-term prospective studies have examined the natural history of the earlier gain and later loss of bone at these sites. A substantial amount of the available information is based on cross-sectional and retrospective studies. This information is used to make inferences about the longitudinal behaviour of the skeleton in individuals. Some of the controversies in the literature may be explained by the constraints imposed by the use of cross-sectional data. The age and the rate of attainment of peak bone mineral density, the age at which bone loss begins, the rate of loss, the duration of loss and the age when bone loss slows or ceases may be erroneously determined. Small numbers of subjects within adjacent decades may be insufficient to detect small real changes across those decades (Mazess, 1982; Sambrook et al, 1987).

Working within these constraints, the available data suggests that bone mineral density increases during growth and maturation to reach its adult

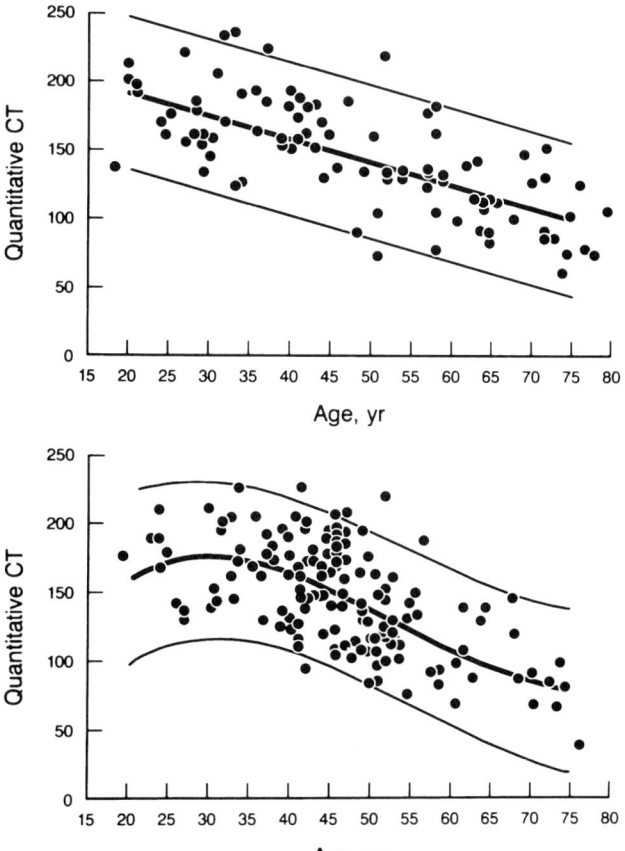

Figure 9. Normal values for vertebral trabecular bone measured by QCT showing a linear diminution in men and curvilinear diminution in women. From Genant et al (1988), with permission.

peak in the fourth decade of life. Thereafter, irrespective of the method used, the site examined, or the population studied, bone mineral density decreases in women and men. The age of onset, rate of decline and magnitude of this decrease varies according to the method of measurement, the site measured, and the race and sex of the population studied (Riggs and Melton, 1986).

In women, after attaining peak bone mineral density at about 30–35 years of age, there is a diminution* (according to DPA data) in bone mineral density from maturity to old age at the spine (47%), femoral neck (58%), femoral trochanter (53%), distal radius (39%), and mid radius (30%) (Riggs et al, 1981, 1982b). As shown in Figure 9, a diminution of similar magnitude, 50% or 1.2% per year is found using QCT (Genant et al, 1988).

In men, the observations are less consistent. Using QCT, the diminution was 40% or 0.72% per year (Genant et al, 1988). Meier et al (1984) reported the diminution of over 50%, or 1.2% per year, from maturity to old age but did not report their observations in women. A diminution of 27% in men and 43% in women in the trabecular bone volume of the iliac crest has been reported using histomorphometry (Meunier et al, 1973). These observations differ from those using DPA where a diminution of 14% was found (Riggs et al, 1981).

It is difficult to reconcile the 10:1 difference in vertebral fracture incidence between men and women with the similar diminution in trabecular bone in both sexes. Men have 10–15% greater bone mineral *density* than women. In the studies by Genant et al (1988) peak bone mineral density at the spine was about 175 mg/ml in both sexes, by old age the value was 110 mg/ml in men and 90 mg/ml in women. Differences in vertebral *mass* and vertebral dimensions may contribute to the difference in fracture incidence (Mazess, 1982).

Age-related bone loss

The diminution in bone mineral density is ascribed to age-related bone loss which is the same in both sexes and menopause-related bone loss superimposed upon the age-related bone loss in women. Age-related bone loss may begin between the ages of 40–50 years in both sexes at the spine and a decade later at the appendicular sites such as the radius. This bone loss may be linear and occurs at a similar rate in both sexes, 0.3–0.6% per year at appendicular sites, 0.8–1.2% per year in the axial skeleton. There is evidence, based on cross-sectional studies (Riggs et al, 1981; Marcus et al, 1983; Buchanan et al, 1988), for the occurrence of spinal but not radial bone loss before menopause. In a longitudinal study, Riggs et al (1986) found substantial spinal, but not radial, bone loss prior to the menopause. Hormonal measurements confirmed that these subjects were premenopausal. An understanding of the pathogenesis of this premenopausal bone loss is important if half the total spinal bone loss seen during ageing occurs before menopause as has been suggested (Riggs et al, 1986).

---

* The term diminution is used to denote that the lower value, being based on cross-sectional data, may not be due to bone *loss*.

This age-related bone loss may continue throughout life but may slow in the last two decades of life. Indeed, bone mineral density may increase late in life due to continued periosteal bone deposition (Garn et al, 1967; Hui et al, 1982). Hui et al (1982) conducted a prospective study of 268 caucasian women aged 50–95 years and found that age-related bone loss at the radius was best defined by a quadratic function which predicted an increase of bone mineral density after the age of 86 years. This was confirmed in 42 women aged 73–95 with a mean of 86.8 years followed for over 6 years with repeat bone mineral density measurements. These data are consistent with a slowing of the endosteal bone loss and accretion of bone on the periosteal surface resulting in an increase in bone width which was observed in a significant proportion of the women. There is little longitudinal data available to confirm or refute whether persons aged over 75 years lose bone from the spine or proximal femur. It is difficult to infer longitudinal bone *loss* based on a *diminution* in bone mass observed in a cross-sectional sample of persons in the last two decades of life. There are usually only small numbers of persons used to obtain this information and these subjects are highly selected by virtue of having survived to extreme old age.

Menopause-related bone loss

Superimposed on the age-related component is the effect of menopause. We are not aware of any studies of premenopausal women having been followed into the postmenopausal state to provide information regarding the pattern of bone loss during these 5–10 perimenopausal years. The information is based on cross-sectional studies in women with natural menopause and prospective studies in oophorectomized women. Most cross-sectional studies suggest that bone loss associated with menopause is non-linear with a midlife 'accelerated' diminution in spinal bone mineral density consistent with a menopausal effect. To distinguish linearity or non-linearity at midlife in cross-sectional data requires large sample sizes as does detection of small changes at the extremes of life (Mazess, 1982; Sambrook et al, 1987).

Riggs et al (1981) found the diminution in spinal bone mineral density was linear in a cross-sectional study but there was evidence of accelerated bone loss in the persons who were studied around midlife compared to those studied at the extremes of life. Only two women were followed transmenopausally. In a prospective study involving 75 women who were no more than three years postmenopausal, Ettinger et al (1985) showed that loss of vertebral bone density measured by QCT was 9% during the two years of the study. Slemenda et al (1987) conducted a prospective study in 84 women classified into early and late peri- or postmenopausal groups. No significant radial bone loss was present in the early perimenopausal subjects with irregular menstruation but no consistent elevation of gonadotrophins. Combined analysis of late perimenopausal women (with irregular menstrual cycles and elevated gonadotrophins) and postmenopausal women, showed bone loss of 0.93% per year (radial midshaft) and 1.19% per year (distal radius) and significantly lower oestradiol, oestrone and androstenedione compared to the early perimenopausal group. Rates of bone loss correlated with oestrogen concentrations. The strength of the relationship between bone loss and oestrogen levels decreased when serum osteocalcin, a circulating marker of bone formation (Delmas et al, 1983), was included in the analysis. This suggests that increased bone turnover may be involved in the pathogenesis of the bone loss. High levels of osteocalcin and low oestrogen may be markers of rapid bone loss (Riis et al, 1984).

There is more information available regarding the effect of menopause-related bone loss from studies in oophorectomized subjects. In general, following oophorectomy, the rate of loss at the spine is twice that of appendicular sites such as the radius and is greater when QCT is used. The loss of bone follows an exponential decline. Spinal bone loss using DPA was 4–5% per year; using QCT the rate was approximately twice this value. In the prospective study by Ettinger et al (1985), bone loss at the radius was not detected following spontaneous menopause but was detectable following oophorectomy (Genant et al, 1982).

Thus, it is likely that spontaneous menopause does cause accelerated bone loss throughout the skeleton but the rate and duration of this bone loss varies. The differences in pattern of bone loss may explain some of the disparate clinical observations sited above. Accelerated bone loss at the spine may be more readily measureable in prospective studies than the slow and prolonged effect seen at appendicular sites such as the radius. The absolute amount of bone lost at the axial and appendicular skeleton may not differ as the more rapid spinal bone loss may cease more promptly than the slower appendicular bone loss. More time may be needed for the full expression of the menopausal effect on bone at appendicular sites.

It is uncertain how long this accelerated phase lasts and what the mechanisms are that determine when this bone loss ceases. It is generally stated that the perimenopausal loss lasts 5–10 years (Riggs and Melton, 1986). Stepan et al (1987) measured bone mineral density and parameters of bone turnover in 185 oophorectomized women assessed cross-sectionally at different times since oophorectomy. The imbalance between biochemical parameters of bone resorption and bone formation was greatest in those women studied within the first two years after surgery and then diminished exponentially but persisted for 10–12 years. The magnitude and duration of the imbalance between parameters of bone resorption and formation following spontaneous menopause is uncertain, but it may be smaller than after oophorectomy but persist longer.

It is likely that the bone loss due to menopause accounts for the majority of the total bone lost within the first 15–20 years after menopause (Richelson et al, 1984). After this, age-related bone loss may account for an increasing proportion of the total (Nordin, personal communication). This has important therapeutic implications. Oestrogen replacement therapy may protect against vertebral fractures but may be less protective against hip fractures which occur 15–30 years after menopause and about 10–15 years after the end of menopause-related bone loss. In the long-term prospective studies by Lindsay et al (1980), bone loss became measureable about 8–10 years after in the treated group despite continued oestrogen replacement (Figure 10). This may be non-oestrogen dependent, age-related bone loss.

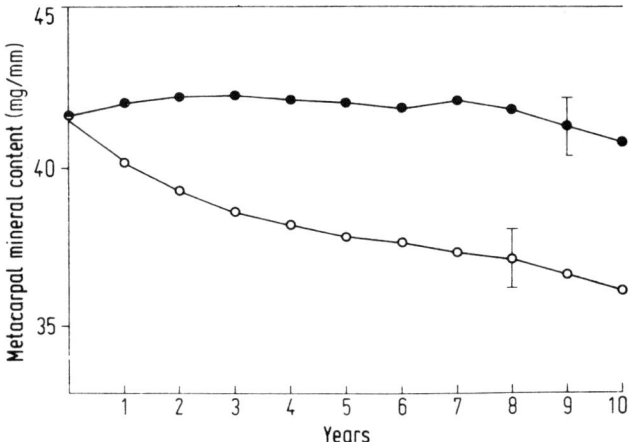

Figure 10. Metacarpal mineral content in patients receiving oestrogens (●) compared to placebo controls (○) showing a decrease in bone mineral content despite continued oestrogen treatment. x-axis, years after surgically induced menopause. From Lindsay et al (1980), with permission.

THE CLINICAL DEFINITION OF OSTEOPOROSIS

The clinical definition of Type 1 or postmenopausal osteoporosis is the presence of one or more nontraumatic (or spontaneous) vertebral crush fractures. The clinical definition of Type 2 or senile osteoporosis is the occurrence of hip fracture associated with a fall from no greater than the standing position. These definitions, like hypertension defined by the presence of stroke, defeat the purpose of the health initiative for which they are intended. They have been expedient and used because there have been no methods available for accurately measuring bone mineral density.

In general, patients who incur fractures in the manner described above, whether they are vertebral, hip or other fractures, have lower bone mineral density than the controls. Lower bone mineral density is found irrespective of the region examined or the method used to measure bone mineral density. It is the degree of overlap with controls that varies. The older the fracture group being studied, the greater the overlap with controls. Controls are usually chosen by comparability of age and the absence of fractures or diseases known to affect bone mineral density. However, it is the bone mineral density (or blood pressure) not the presence or absence of a fracture (or stroke) which should be used to define normality. The term 'normal' should not be used because persons of comparable age have lost bone.

The role of peak bone mineral density and excessive bone loss

It is frequently assumed that the lower bone mineral density found in patients with fractures is due to excessive bone loss. However, bone mineral density in adulthood is determined by the amount of bone attained during growth and maturation and the amount lost during ageing and following menopause. Thus, the low bone mineral density in patients with osteoporosis may be the result of attaining a low peak bone mineral density at maturity. Alternatively, bone loss, in excess of that seen in the rest of the population, may be responsible. This excessive bone loss may result from changes in the rate or the duration of the menopause-related or age-related bone loss. Which of these alternatives or combination of mechanisms is responsible for the lower bone mineral density found in patients with fractures is not known. Indeed, a portion of the lower bone mineral density may be the consequence rather than a cause of the fracture.

There is no convincing evidence that patients with Type 1 or Type 2 osteoporosis lose bone more rapidly than controls of comparable age. In normal subjects, rates of bone loss are normally distributed with no evidence of a separate group of fast bone losers (Smith et al, 1975). Rapid bone loss follows oophorectomy. However, oophorectomized patients do not have lower bone mineral density than women with spontaneous menopause of comparable duration (Meema et al, 1965; Nordin et al, 1968; Richelson et al, 1984). Thus, the rapid phase of bone loss following oophorectomy may be shorter in duration than the more protracted phase of bone loss following spontaneous menopause. This inverse relationship between the rate and duration of bone loss suggests that persons who lose bone rapidly may not necessarily be destined for lower bone mineral density than persons who lose bone more slowly. Consequently, rate of bone loss may not be a marker for increased risk of fracture (Seeman and Cooper, 1987).

Whether patients with either type of fracture come from a population of normal subjects with low peak bone mineral density and undergo age-related and menopause-related bone loss at the same rate and for the same duration as the rest of the population is uncertain (Johnston et al, 1968; Newton-John and Morgan, 1970). There is evidence to support this possibility in Type 1 osteoporosis. Women with Type 1 osteoporosis have daughters with bone mineral density at the spine which is lower than age-matched controls (Seeman et al, 1989). The magnitude of this diminution, relative to their controls, is about half the diminution seen in their osteoporotic mothers, relative to their controls. This is consistent with the view that the variability of bone mineral density in the population is genetically determined (Smith et al, 1973; Pocock et al, 1987). At least in Type 1 osteoporosis, the attainment of a low peak bone mineral density may be a sufficient explanation for the lower bone mineral density. This information has bearing on the role of screening in the prevention of osteoporosis.

Postmenopausal (Type 1) osteoporosis: vertebral fractures

Patients with vertebral fractures have a mean age of 65 years with a range of 55–75 years and have lower bone mineral density than controls of comparable age. If excessive trabecular bone loss were involved in the pathogenesis, the overlap with controls would be less in regions of the skeleton containing substantial amounts of trabecular bone such as the spine. The overlap is considerable when radial bone mineral density is

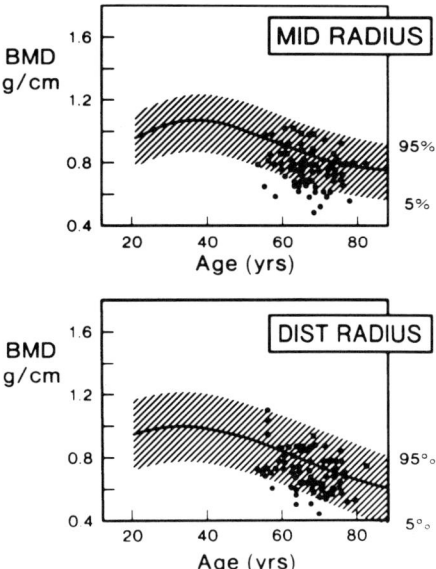

Figure 11. Values for the normal range (shaded) for bone mineral density at the mid radius and distal radius and values for 76 women with spinal fractures. From Wahner et al (1983), with permission.

measured (Figure 11). Better discrimination would be expected using QCT to measure the trabecular centrum of the vertebral body than would be found using QCT to measure the cortical shell of the vertebral body. Jones et al (1987) used QCT to demonstrate this in a group of six controls and seven patients aged 60–70 years with osteoporosis. A 63% difference between the patients (35 ± 30 mg/ml) and controls (95 ± 27 mg/ml) was found when the bone mineral densities of the trabecular centrum was compared. An 18% difference between the patients (170 ± 27 mg/ml) and controls (192 ± 25 mg/ml) was found when the bone mineral densities of the cortical shell were compared. Similar observations were made in six younger patients with osteoporosis and six controls of comparable age. These interesting observations have not been examined with larger numbers of subjects.

This preferential diminution of spinal trabecular bone has been found by comparing QCT and DPA measurements. Patients with osteoporosis had lower spinal values relative to controls using QCT than was found using DPA. For example, the percentage diminution relative to control, comparing QCT and DPA, was 65% vs. 16%, 54% vs. 23%, and 35.6% vs. 13.7% (Gallagher et al, 1985; Sambrook et al, 1985; Reinbold et al, 1986). These studies were all cross-sectional. It cannot be assumed that the deficit of bone mineral density at the trabecular sites is due to more bone loss than occurred in controls. These patients may have had a lower peak bone mineral density at maturity (Johnston et al, 1968; Newton-John and Morgan, 1970).

Senile (Type 2) osteoporosis: hip fractures

Patients with hip fractures are usually older than patients with Type 1 osteoporosis having a mean age of 75 years or more (Riggs and Melton, 1983). The extent of overlap is greater in patients with hip fractures because they are compared with controls who are also older. Patients with hip fractures do not have lower spinal bone mineral density than controls. The standardized deviation relative to controls, or z-score*, being $+0.24$ (Riggs et al, 1982b). At the femoral sites, bone mineral density is lower than controls of comparable age with a z-score of -0.31 (femoral neck) and -0.53 (intertrochanteric region). Similarly, and as can be discerned from Figure 12, older patients with vertebral fractures have spinal bone mineral

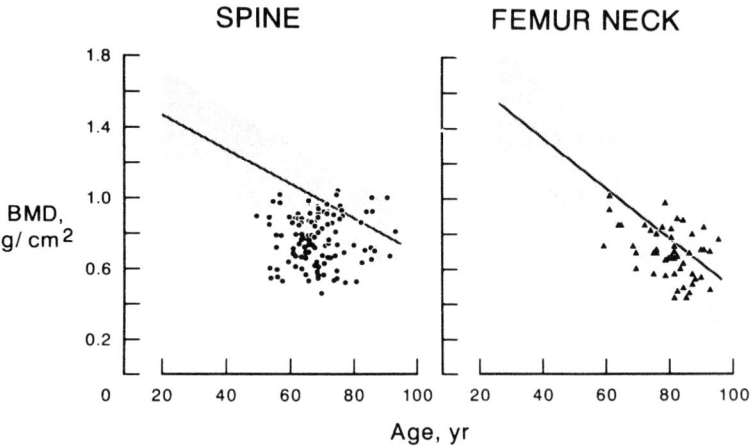

Figure 12. Bone mineral density at the lumbar spine in normal women (shaded) and 111 patients with spinal fractures and at the femoral neck in normal subjects (shaded) and 49 patients with hip fractures. From Riggs and Melton (1986), with permission.

density that overlaps more within the reference range. For example, expressed as a z-score, the deviations from the normal age-adjusted mean for women with vertebral fractures aged 51–65, 66–75 and >75 years were -1.92, -1.27 and -0.50 respectively. The same is found with measurements at the mid radius (-1.03, -0.59, -0.48) and distal radius (-0.75, -0.38, -0.30). At each site, the deviation was significant for the patients 51–65 and 66–75 years of age. This point is further illustrated by Mazess et al (1988). Patients with Type 1 and Type 2 osteoporosis were compared with young controls and controls of comparable age. Both fracture groups had a similar diminution of bone mineral density relative to young controls. However, the diminution of bone mineral density in the hip fracture patients, relative to their age-matched controls, was greater than the diminution found in the patients with vertebral fractures relative to their

---

* The z-score is the number of standard deviations by which an individual or group value differs from the mean of the population.

age-matched controls. This may be because the patients with vertebral fractures were slightly older than the groups usually reported and the patients with hip fractures were slightly younger than is usually reported.

Hip fractures are associated with trauma and occur 10–15 years later in life than vertebral fractures and often 20–30 years after menopause. During this time, bone loss due to menopause has probably expressed itself fully at trabecular bone and stopped or declined substantially at cortical bone. Age-related bone loss continues at about 1% or less. Thus, it is likely that age-related bone loss makes an important contribution to the pathogenesis of hip fractures. Cortical and trabecular bone loss may contribute more equally to this loss. In men, the diminution in femoral bone mineral density is 39%, or two thirds that seen in women. At the spine, there is a 14% diminution across age found in men which is one quarter that found in women. This may explain why the female to male ratio for hip fractures is only 2:1 but 10:1 for vertebral fractures (Riggs et al, 1982b).

The other important contrasting feature in the pathogenesis of hip fractures is the occurrence of falls. Tinetti et al (1988) in a 1-year prospective study found that 108 of 336 persons > 75 years (32%) fell at least once. Fractures occurred in 6%. The risk for falls increased from 8% in those with no risk factors, to 78% in those with more than four risk factors. The odds ratio for use of sedatives, cognitive impairment, lower extremity disability and palmo-mental reflex were 28.3, 5.0, 3.8, and 3.0 respectively. The exponential increase in incidence of hip fractures after the age of 65–75 years is likely to be the result of an increasing proportion of the population having low bone mass (Newton-John and Morgan, 1970) and the increasing frequency and severity of falls occurring in this population at risk as a result of 20–30 years of bone loss.

The fracture threshold

Patients with either type of fracture have values for bone mineral density which overlap minimally with the values found in young persons. As a working principle, the lower limit in young persons (5th percentile or the mean minus 2 standard deviations) represents the level separating the patients with fractures from young normals. This level is referred to as the 'fracture threshold'. Up to 50% of women in the 6th and 7th decade of life have bone mineral density below this level and virtually all women over ~ 75 years of age have bone mass falling within the range where fractures occur (Figure 12). Should all of these women be regarded as having a disorder called 'osteoporosis'?

The term 'fracture threshold' has practical utility in its ease of delineation, but the term is misleading in that there is no level of zero risk. Bone density is a continuous variable which provides information concerning the *risk* of fracture not the *certainty* of fracture. Standard radiographs provide the latter information. For a given stress, the risk of fracture increases as bone mineral density decreases. This applies to all women, whether they are pre- or postmenopausal, and to men as well. The magnitude of this risk is small above the 'fracture threshold' and increases markedly below the threshold.

What is the relationship between the amount of bone loss and the increase in fracture risk? In vitro bone strength decreases threefold with a 10% change in the mineral content (Vose and Kubala, 1959; Currey, 1969). The study by Hui et al (1988) provides fascinating insight into the relationship between age, changing bone mineral density and fracture risk in vivo. As shown in Figure 2, age and bone mineral density were independent predictors of fracture risk. A decrease of bone density by $0.1 \, g/cm^3$ about 10% over 10 years (1% loss per year) conferred an increase in risk of eight fractures per 1000 person-years. A change in age of 10 years conferred an increase risk of 21 fractures per 1000 patient-years. That is, the increase in risk as age increased was 2.5 times the increase in risk conferred by decreasing bone density. The absolute increase in risk associated with falling bone mineral density was greater in older women. In the study by Melton et al (1986), as bone mineral density decreased, the incidence rate increased quadratically for cervical and cubically for intertrochanteric fractures. This relationship between bone density and fracture in vivo is non-linear as described between bone strength and bone density in vitro. Age and bone density were independent predictors of fracture, a 10-year increase in age was associated with a 1.94-fold increase in risk, a 10-year loss, (equivalent to about $0.1 \, g/cm^2$ or a 10% reduction in bone mineral density), was associated with a 1.44-fold increase in risk (Melton et al, 1989b).

Frequency of the measurements

How many measurements are needed to observe an effect if there is one? If no change is observed, has no change occurred? Longitudinal measurements in individuals have wide confidence intervals around them and changes of under 4% are difficult to detect. For example, using techniques with a coefficient of variation of 2%, if 100 persons with no change in bone mineral density were measured twice, 15 persons would be found to be losing bone when they were not (Heaney, 1986). The confidence interval about a rate of loss of 4% is $+1.5\%$ and -9.5% (Cummings and Black, 1986). Newer methods should circumvent some of these difficulties.

INDICATIONS FOR BONE MINERAL DENSITY MEASUREMENT

Treatment of established osteoporosis

Like the sphygmomanometer for treatment of hypertension, these techniques for measuring bone mineral density are invaluable, if not indispensable, clinical tools for assessing the efficacy of treatment of established osteoporosis. The aim of treatment is to prevent further bone loss and to increase bone mass. Measurement of bone density is essential for determining whether a response to treatment or lack of response is present. Many forms of treatment have been studied and offer considerable promise in the treatment of osteoporosis. Discussion of the results of these studies is beyond the brief of this review.

Prevention of bone loss

The selection of persons for preventive therapy rests on the assumption that low peak bone mineral density is a risk factor for fracture and that any further increase in risk due to bone loss should be prevented.

Oestrogen

Pending the results of further studies, it would be reasonable to assume that women in the upper third of the young normal range of bone mineral density do not require replacement therapy as the amount of bone they will lose will not result in them approaching the fracture threshold. Bone mineral density measurement could be repeated once within the next 3 years. Bone loss within this time may be reversible (Lindsay, 1988). Women in the lower third of the normal range probably should be considered for oestrogen replacement therapy. Women in the middle third of the normal range could have repeat measurements done annually during the next 3 years and a decision made according to the changes observed. This applies to women presenting at the time of menopause.

Women often present for counselling some years after menopause. The guidelines quoted above can be modified in accordance with the number of years since menopause. For example, a woman in the mid-range of normal for bone mineral density and >6 years postmenopausal will probably have gone through the accelerated phase of bone loss and the decision not to treat can be made with greater confidence. A woman in the low range and 3–6 years postmenopausal may achieve some restoration of bone mineral density when oestrogen is commenced.

Leanness is a risk factor for osteoporosis. Obesity is a protective partly because adipose tissue contains aromatase enzymes which convert androgens of adrenal origin to weak oestrogens. Obesity may militate against using oestrogen in view of the increased risk for endometrial carcinoma and the protection obesity confers against perimenopausal bone loss. Ribot et al (1988) found that obese postmenopausal women had higher bone mineral density at the spine than lean postmenopausal women of comparable age. Moreover, bone mineral density was no lower than that of premenopausal subjects.

Oestrogens have generally not been recommended in women over 60–65 years of age. In Lindsay's study (Lindsay et al, 1980), women taking oestrogen started to lose bone after the 8–10th year despite continued oestrogen therapy suggesting that this represented non-oestrogen dependent bone loss (see Figure 10). However, there are data suggesting that bone mineral density can be increased in elderly postmenopausal women (Quigley et al, 1987). In addition, if the imbalance between parameters of bone resorption and bone formation persists longer than the 10–12 years found following oophorectomy (Stepan et al, 1987) this would support using oestrogens at this time. These disparities need to be resolved before guidelines can be provided.

Exercise

Immobilization causes bone loss and physical activity may have an important role in the attainment of peak bone mineral density, the prevention of perimenopausal bone loss and the restoration of bone already lost in healthy postmenopausal women and women with established osteoporosis (Dalsky, 1987). The available evidence suggests that bone mineral density can be increased with supervised exercise in postmenopausal women, but the increase is small. Increases in the order of 2–6% have been found in studies of 6–18 months duration. Whether exercise can restore the 30–50% diminution found with ageing and following menopause is unknown. Virtually nothing is known about the effect of exercise on peak bone mineral density, in preventing perimenopausal bone loss or in treating patients with osteoporosis. Despite the paucity of information, weight-bearing exercise should be recommended. Activities of varying types should be encouraged to maintain components of fitness such as muscle strength, mobility, flexibility and agility which may reduce the frequency and severity of falls.

Calcium

Matkovic et al (1979) showed that dietary calcium intake may be important in the attainment of peak bone mineral density. Matkovic et al (1988) remeasured metacarpal bone mineral content in 432 men and 573 women of the original cross-sectional study and found no difference in the amount of bone loss that had occurred in the intervening 10 years in the subjects with high calcium intake compared to the amount of bone loss that occurred in subjects with a low calcium intake. Dietary calcium supplementation has been shown to slow the rate of bone loss measured at the radius or using total body calcium measurements (Riis et al, 1986). This has not been confirmed at the spine or examined at the proximal femur. Information regarding the efficacy of dietary calcium in preventing bone loss at the proximal femur would be particularly important because the age-related decrease in intestinal calcium absorption and secondary hyperparathyroidism have been implicated in the pathogenesis of age-related bone loss.

Assessment of persons at risk

The following clinical risk factors have been described:

1. Historical
    (a) Caucasian or Asian origin.
    (b) Gynaecological factors: late menarche; episodic amenorrhoea or oligomenorrhoea suggesting anovulatory cycles or prolongation of the luteal phase; early menopause; unilateral or bilateral oophorectomy; no oestrogen contraception; no postmenopausal oestrogen replacement therapy; nulliparity; prolonged lactation.
    (c) Excessive ethanol use and/or tobacco consumption.
    (d) Use of glucocorticosteroids, dilantin, heparin; excessive thyroxine, antacids.
    (e) Dietary calcium deficiency; excessive protein, salt, phosphate consumption.
    (f) Illnesses such as anorexia nervosa, amenorrhoea athletica, hyper-

prolactinaemia, primary hyperparathyroidism, Cushing's syndrome, malabsorption, liver disease, thyrotoxicosis.
(g)   A family history of fractures.
(h)   Non-traumatic fractures; loss of height.
2.   Examination—Caucasian, Asian, dentures, low body weight, thin skin, short stature
3.   Radiological—Radiolucency on a routine X-ray may be due to technical factors and accurate quantification may be advisable. Presence of asymptomatic fractures may be due to early clinical disease or due to epiphysitis (Scheurmann's disease) which is not associated with low bone mineral density.

The predictive strength of risk factors

The usefulness of these historical risk factors in predicting whether a person has a low bone mineral density has not been confirmed. Nor have these risk factors proven useful in discriminating persons with fractures from those without fractures. van Hermert et al (1987) studied 1167 women aged 45–65 years to evaluate the predictive strength of 17 risk factors (including age, tobacco, knee diameter, forearm diameter, height, weight, menopausal and menarcheal age, parity, lactation and amenorrhoea). During the 9 years of observation, 16% of the subjects had fractures. The estimated fracture incidence was 22 per 1000 women-years. Dividing the subjects into low and high quintiles according to numbers if risk factors did not distinguish those with fractures from those without fractures. For example, the highest risk quintile had a 38% sensitivity (correctly identifying those with fractures) and 84% specificity (correctly identifying those without fractures).

Johnston and Slemenda (1988) evaluated the use of risk factors in predicting bone mineral density. The risk factors evaluated were height, weight, body mass index, tobacco, alcohol, serum oestrogen, osteocalcin and androgens. These risk factors accounted for 34.7% (mid radius), 16.6% (distal radius) and 24.7% (lumbar spine) of the variance of bone mineral density at these sites. Less than 50% of persons with low bone mineral density were correctly classified using these historical risk factors.

SCREENING

Broad based screening of a large population of persons is different from the use of densitometric methods in clinical practise. The two are often confused because a decision involving an individual follows both. There are important differences. There are a number of criteria to be fulfilled before screening can be recommended.

Does the morbidity and mortality justify screening?

The morbidity, mortality and economic cost of hip fractures is well recognized and was summarized in the introduction. By contrast, vertebral fractures may not constitute a public health problem. Vertebral fractures are frequently asymptomatic (Gershon-Cohen et al, 1953) and vertebral crush fractures may be considerably less common than is assumed. Data from a population based random sample of women in Rochester, Minnesota, suggest that few of the women in the community have symptomatic crush fractures. Although the prevalence in the community studied was large, most of these fractures were asymptomatic wedge fractures (Melton et al, 1989a). Of 200 women > 50 years of age, 56 (28%) were assessed as having one or more fractures after allowing for normal anatomical variations in the vertebrae. The prevalence rose from 6.1% in 50–54-year-old women to 51.7% in > 85 year olds and reached 78% in women over 90 years of age. It was estimated that 18% of women > 50 years and 27% of women > 65 years had one or more fractures. The calculated incidence was 5/1000 person-years in 50–54 year olds and 29.6/1000 person-years in the elderly. The majority however were wedge fractures. Although bone mineral density was lower, there was substantial overlap within the normal range. Screening would not identify those persons at risk for wedge fractures.

Jensen et al (1982) examined 75% of 285 70-year-old subjects. The 18% with wedge fractures had normal appendicular bone mineral density. Five percent had crush fractures and low bone mineral density. Harma et al (1986) studied 57 440 subjects. In those < 65 years of age, there were 19/3698 persons with fractures (0.5%). In those < 75 years of age, there were 31/2028 persons with fractures (1.5%) and in those > 85 years of age, there were 16/551 persons with fractures (3%). The incidence (number with new fractures/year/100 000 persons) determined by repeating the radiographs 5 years later was 49 in < 65 year olds and 183 in < 75 year olds. Pogrund et al (1977) examined the incidence of fractures in 3600 persons identified from the electoral role and found 1%, 3% and 7% of < 65, < 75 and > 85 years of age, respectively, had fractures. Most subjects had asymptomatic wedge fractures. Thus, crush fractures may be relatively common in specialist clinics, but less commonly in the community. Although debilitating and often crippling, vertebral fractures have a low mortality.

Would screening prevent fractures?

There must be an effective treatment available to justify screening and oestrogen therapy has been shown to prevent bone loss effectively (Lindsay et al, 1980). There is no need to screen if a decision to use oestrogen is made for reasons other than those related to the prevention of bone disease. However, if this is not the case, it is likely that the incidence of vertebral fractures would be substantially reduced by identifying persons with low bone mineral density at the age of 50 years for two reasons. First, most of the bone lost during the subsequent 10–15 years is probably menopause-related bone loss. Second, it is plausible that patients with Type 1 osteoporosis may come from a population of women who attain a low bone mineral density at maturity (Vose and Kubala, 1959; Johnston et al, 1968; Newton-John and Morgan, 1970; Seeman et al, 1989).

The issue with respect to hip fractures is different. Falls have an important role in the pathogenesis of hip fracture. Hip fractures occur because a demineralized skeleton incurs trauma following a fall. If the bone loss associated with ageing and menopause were prevented that same fall would have less likelihood of resulting in fracture. The question is whether a measure of bone mineral density at the age of 50 years predicts the risk of hip fracture better than the predictive value of age itself. As was shown in Figure 2, Hui et al (1988) found that increasing age was a better predictor than decreasing bone mineral density for fracture. The data was based on radial bone mineral measurements, not femoral neck measurements so that there may have been better predictive strength using measurements of the femoral neck. There were wide confidence intervals around the risk estimates because of the small number of hip fractures. The relative risk between the lowest and highest bone mineral density values was > 2. However, as shown in panel B, the increase in risk at the age 50–54 years between the highest and lowest bone mineral measurement is slight compared to the increase in risk in older persons. These are the measurements that would be obtained if screening were done. Melton and colleagues have approached the question of how current bone mineral density predicts future fracture risk theoretically (Melton et al, 1989b). Based on estimates of life expectancy, age-specific rates of bone loss and bone mineral density-specific fracture incidence rates, the estimated lifetime risk for a 40-year-old woman with a high bone mineral density was negligible and increased to 9.2% (cervical) and 5.1% (intertrochanteric) with a bone density of $1.0 \, g/cm^2$ and to 25% for a bone mineral density of $0.6 \, g/cm^2$.

It is uncertain whether persons who will fracture their hip come from the lower quartile of values at the age of 50 years. This may be more likely in the case of vertebral fractures where the variability in peak bone mineral density is much greater than the rate and duration of bone loss that will ensue over the 10–15 years. As discussed in relation to the fracture threshold on page 22, the 2.5-fold greater risk conferred by increasing age over the increase in risk conferred by decreasing radial bone mineral density may not be measurable at the time of screening. Concomitants of age such as immobility, loss of sensory and motor skills contribute to the increased severity and frequency of falls. Ill health and immobility may lower bone mineral density during the latter decades of life in a person with values in the mid or upper normal range at the time when screening would be done.

Aitken (1987) measured cortical bone mineral density using metacarpal morphometry in 233 women with a mean age of 80 years on admission to hospital following femoral neck fracture. During follow-up, 18 of 36 patients with bone density < 30th percentile on admission died whereas three of 28 with bone density > 70th percentile died. These data suggest that low bone density was a marker for illness and reduced survival. Cooper et al (1987) studied over 700 patients attending a casualty department for X-ray of the hip after a fall. Bone mineral density, assessed using the Singh Index, was lower in the young persons who fractured their hip than in young persons who fell but did not fracture their hip. By contrast, in elderly persons, no difference in Singh Index was found comparing persons who fractured their hip with persons who did not. These data suggest that the severity of the fall contributed to the fracture.

Oestrogen replacement therapy reduces the relative risk of hip fracture by 50%; it does *not* abolish the risk. Therapy must probably be given permanently. The protective effect is lost unless treatment is current and reduced when treatment is less than 6 years (Hutchinson et al, 1979). In the long-term prospective studies by Lindsay et al (1980), bone mineral density at the spine was 25% higher than the placebo in the group but 12% higher at the femoral neck (Lindsay et al, 1987). One interpretation of this data is that oestrogen may be less effective in preventing bone loss at the hip.

What is the best method of screening?

There must be a safe and cost-effective method of screening. Are measurements at the radius or os calcis equally as sensitive and specific for predicting vertebral or hip fractures as measurements at the actual sites of fracture? The answer to this question is not known. Newer techniques, such as DEXA may contribute to resolving some of the problems associated with the economic aspects of screening. The improved speed of scanning and ability to measure a variety of sites at low radiation exposure will reduce cost. Thus, taken together, these and other concerns suggest that mass screening should not be implemented at this time.

SUMMARY

Non-invasive, safe and precise techniques for measuring bone mineral density are available and have an important role in the detection, prevention and treatment of bone loss associated with ageing, menopause and many illnesses affecting women and men. The three most widely accessible and established techniques for measuring regional bone mineral density are single and dual photon absorptiometry and quantitative computed tomography. A technique of greater accuracy, dual energy X-ray absorptiometry, has only recently become available. These techniques have made it possible to measure the magnitude, time course and regional specificity of the skeleton's response to ageing, menopause and illness. A better understanding of the clinical epidemiology of fractures and the mechanisms responsible for bone loss has been obtained.

Practical information has been obtained about the dose, duration and efficacy of oestrogen replacement therapy in preventing perimenopausal bone loss and the benefits and limitations of different forms of exercise on bone mineral density in healthy postmenopausal women. The beneficial effect of dietary calcium on peak bone mineral density and in decreasing bone loss in cortical bone has been documented. Information regarding the prevention and treatment of bone loss in exogenous hypercortisolism and the magnitude and reversibility of bone loss associated with many diseases which affect bone has been obtained. One of the most important clinical applications of these techniques is the assessment of the efficacy of treatment of patients with postmenopausal osteoporosis. As antifracture efficacy is not readily measurable, considerable information is being obtained about many potentially useful forms of therapy that may prevent bone loss and increase bone mineral density.

The role of these non-invasive methods in the assessment of fracture risk and the need for oestrogen or other therapy in an individual who has attained a low peak bone mass or has risk factors predisposing to excessive bone loss, differs from broader public health initiatives of population screening. There are concerns regarding the safety, efficacy and limited number of treatment regimens available for persons found by screening to be at risk. The most economic and convenient methods for predicting fracture risk with high sensitivity and specificity are not established. There are uncertainties regarding the relative importance of bone mineral density measured at the time of screening, the amount of bone lost in the subsequent years and risk factors predisposing to falls in the pathogenesis of hip fractures. These, and other concerns, suggest that broad-based screening should not be implemented at this time.

Like the sphygmomanometer's contribution to the investigation, prevention and treatment of hypertensive vascular disease, the techniques discussed in this chapter may prove to reduce measurably the burden of bone disease on the growing number of elderly persons in our community.

REFERENCES

Aitken JM (1987) Relationship between mortality after femoral neck fracture and osteoporosis. In Christiansen C, Johansen JS & Riis BJ (eds) *Osteoporosis*, vol. 1, pp. 45–48. Kobenhavn K, Denmark: Osteopress ApS.

Bell GH, Dunbar O & Beck JS (1967) Variations in strength of vertebra with age and their relation to osteoporosis. *Calcified Tissue Research* 1: 75–86.

Buchanan JR, Myers C, Lloyd T & Greer RB III (1988) Early vertebral trabecular bone loss in normal pre-menopausal women. *Journal of Bone and Mineral Research* 3: 583–586.

Cameron JR & Sorenson J (1963) Measurement of bone mineral *in vivo*: an improved method. *Science* 142: 230–232.

Cann CE (1981) Low-dose CT scanning for quantitative spinal mineral analysis. *Radiology* 140: 813–815.

Cann CE, Genant HK, Kolb FO & Ettinger B (1985) Quantitative computed tomography for prediction of vertebral fracture risk. *Metabolic Bone Disease and Related Research* 6: 1–7.

Carter DR & Hayes HC (1977) The compressive behaviour of bone as a two-phase porous structure. *Journal of Bone and Joint Surgery* 59A: 954–962.

Cooper C, Barker DJP, Morris J & Briggs SJ (1987) Osteoporosis, falls and age in fracture of the proximal femur. *British Medical Journal* 295: 13–15.

Cummings SR & Black D (1986) Should peri-menopausal women be screened for osteoporosis? *Annals of Internal Medicine* 104: 817–823.

Currey JD (1969) The mechanical consequences of the variation in the mineral content of bone. *Journal of Biomechanics* 2: 1–11.

Dalen N, Hellstrom LG & Jacobson B (1976) Bone mineral content and mechanical strength of the femoral neck. *Acta Orthopaedica Scandinavica* 47: 503–508.

Dalsky GP (1987) Exercise: Its effect on bone mineral content. *Clinical Obstetrics and Gynecology* 30: 820–832.

Delmas PD, Stenner D, Wahner HW, Mann KG & Riggs BL (1983) Increase in serum bone-carboxyglutamic acid protein with aging in women. *Journal of Clinical Investigation* **71:** 1316–1321.

Ettinger B, Cann CE & Genant HK (1985) Menopausal bone loss can be prevented by low dose oestrogen with calcium supplements. *Journal of Computer Assisted Tomography* **9:** 633–634.

Gallagher C, Golgar D, Mahoney P & McGill J (1985) Measurement of spine density in normal and osteoporotic subjects using computed tomography: relationship of spinal density to fracture threshold and fracture index. *Journal of Computer Assisted Tomography* **9:** 634–635.

Garn SM, Rohmann CG, Wagner B & Ascoli W (1967) Continuing bone growth throughout life. A general phenomena. *American Journal of Physiological Anthropology* **26:** 313–318.

Genant HK, Cann CE, Ettinger B & Gordan GS (1982) Quantitative computed tomography of vertebral spongiosa: A sensitive method for detecting early bone loss after oophorectomy. *Annals of Internal Medicine* **97:** 699–705.

Genant HK, Cann CE, Boyd DP et al (1983) Quantitative computed tomography for vertebral mineral determination. In Frame B & Potts JT (eds) *Clinical Disorders of Bone and Mineral Metabolism*, pp 40–47. Amsterdam, Oxford, Princeton: Excerpta Medica.

Genant HK, Ettinger B, Harris ST, Block JE & Steiger P (1988) Quantitative computed tomography in assessment of osteoporosis. In Riggs BL & Melton LJ III (eds) *Osteoporosis: aetiology, diagnosis and management*, pp 221–250. New York: Raven Press.

Gershon-Cohen J, Rechtman AM & Schraer H (1953) Asymptomatic fractures in osteoporotic spines of the aged. *Journal of the American Medical Association* **153:** 625–627.

Harma M, Heliovaara M, Aromaa A & Knekt P (1986) Thoracic spine compression fractures in Finland. *Clinical Orthopaedics* **205:** 188–194.

Heaney RP (1986) En recherche de la difference. *Bone and Mineral* **1:** 99–114.

Holbrook TL, Grazier K, Kelsey JL & Stauffer RN (1984) *The frequency of occurrence, impact and cost of selected musculoskeletal conditions in the United States*. Chicago: American Academy of Orthopaedic Surgeons.

Hui SL, Wiske PS, Norton JA & Johnston CC Jr (1982) A prospective study of change in bone mass in post-menopausal women. *Journal of Chronic Disease* **35:** 715–725.

Hui SL, Slemenda CW & Johnston CC Jr (1988) Age and bone mass as predictors of fracture in a prospective study. *Journal of Clinical Investigation* **81:** 1804–1809.

Hutchinson TA, Polansky JM & Feinstein AR (1979) Post-menopausal oestrogens protect against fracture of hip and distal radius. *Lancet* **ii:** 705–709.

Iskrant AP & Smith RW (1969) Osteoporosis in women 45 years and over related to subsequent fracture. *Public Health Report* **84:** 33–38.

Jensen GF, Christianson C, Boese NJ et al (1982) Epidemiology of post-menopausal spinal and long bone fractures: A unifying approach to post-menopausal osteoporosis. *Clinical Orthopaedics* **166:** 75–81.

Johnston CC Jr & Slemenda CW (1988) Screening for osteoporosis. In Dequeker JV, Geusens P & Wahner HW (eds) *Bone Mineral Measurements by Photon Absorptiometry: Methodological Problems*. Leuven, Belgium: Leuven University Press.

Johnston CC Jr, Smith DM, Yu P-L & Deiss WP Jr (1968) In vitro measurement of bone mass in the radius. *Metabolism, Clinical and Experimental* **17:** 1140–1153.

Jones CD, Laval-Jeantet AM, Laval-Jeantet MH & Genant HK (1987) Importance of measurement of spongious vertebral bone mineral density in the assessment of osteoporosis. *Bone* **8:** 201–206.

Kanis JA (1984) Treatment of osteoporotic fracture. *Lancet* **i:** 27–33.

Kelly TL, Slovik DM, Schoenfeld DA & Meer RM (1988) Quantitative digital radiography versus dual photon absorptiometry of the lumbar spine. *Journal of Clinical Endocrinology and Metabolism* **67:** 839–844.

Kerr R, Resnick D, Sartoris DJ et al (1986) Computerized tomography of proximal femoral trabecular patterns. *Journal of Orthopaedic Research* **4:** 45–56.

Laval-Jeantet M, Roger B, Bouysse S, Bergot C & Mazess RB (1986) Influence of vertebral fat content upon quantitative CT density. *Radiology* **159:** 463–466.

Lindsay R (1988) Sex steroids in the pathogenesis and prevention of osteoporosis. In Riggs BL & Melton LJ III (eds) *Osteoporosis: aetiology, diagnosis and management*, pp 333–358. New York: Raven Press.

Lindsay R, Hart DM, Forrest C & Baird C (1980) Prevention of spinal osteoporosis in oophorectomized women. *Lancet* **ii:** 1151–1153.

Lindsay R, Hart DM & Abdallah Al-Azzawi F (1987) Inter-relationship of bone loss and its prevention and fracture expression. In Christiansen C, Johansen JS & Riis BJ (eds) *Osteoporosis*. Kobenhavn K, Denmark: Osteopress ApS.

Marcus R, Kosek J, Pfefferbaum A & Horning S (1983) Age-related loss of trabecular bone in pre-menopausal women: A biopsy study. *Calcified Tissue International* **35:** 406–409.

Matkovic V, Kostial K, Simonovic I et al (1979) Bone status and fracture rates in two regions of Yugoslavia. *American Journal of Clinical Nutrition* **32:** 540–549.

Matkovic V, Dekanic D & Koshal K (1988) The rate of cortical bone loss according to age, sex & calcium intake. Tenth Annual Scientific Meeting American Society for Bone and Mineral Research. *Journal of Bone and Mineral Research* **3**(supplement 1): S88 (abstract 80).

Mazess RB (1982) On aging bone loss. *Clinical Orthopaedics* **165:** 239–252.

Mazess RB (1983) Non-invasive bone measurements. In *Skeletal Research*, Vol. 2, pp 277–343. Academic Press.

Mazess RB & Vetter J (1985) Comparison of Dual-Photon Absorptiometry and Dual-Energy Computed Tomography for Vertebral Mineral. *Journal of Computer Assisted Tomography* **9:** 624–625.

Mazess RB & Wahner HM (1988) Nuclear Medicine and Densitometry. In Riggs BL & Melton LJ III (eds) *Osteoporosis, aetiology, diagnosis and management*, pp 251–295. New York: Raven Press.

Mazess RB, Barden H, Ettinger M & Schultz E (1988) Bone density of the radius, spine and proximal femur in osteoporosis. *Journal of Bone and Mineral Research* **3:** 13–18.

Meema HE, Bunker ML & Meema S (1965) Loss of compact bone due to menopause. *Obstetrics and Gynecology* **26:** 333–343.

Meier DE, Orwoll ES & Jones JM (1984) Marked disparity between trabecular and cortical bone loss with age in healthy men. *Annals of Internal Medicine* **101:** 605–612.

Melton LJ (1988) Epidemiology of fractures. In Riggs BL & Melton LJ III (eds) *Osteoporosis: aetiology, diagnosis and management*, pp 133–154. New York: Raven Press.

Melton LJ III, Kann SH, Wahner HW & Riggs BL (1989b) Lifetime fracture risk: An approach to hip fracture risk assessment based on bone mineral density and age. *Journal of Clinical Epidemiology* **41**(10): 985–994.

Melton LJ III, Kann SH, Frye MA et al (1989a) Epidemiology of vertebral fractures in women. *American Journal of Epidemiology*, in press.

Melton LJ III, Wahner HW, Richelson LS, O'Fallon WM & Riggs BL (1986) Osteoporosis and the risk of hip fracture. *American Journal of Epidemiology* **124:** 254–261.

Meunier P, Coupron P, Edouard C et al (1973) Physiological senile evolution and pathological rarefaction of bone. *Clinics in Endocrinology and Metabolism* **2:** 239–256.

Mosekilde Li, Mosekilde Le & Danielsen CC (1987) Biomechanical competence of vertebral trabecular bone in relation to ash density and age in normal individuals. *Bone* **8:** 79–85.

Newton-John H & Morgan DB (1970) The loss of bone with age, osteoporosis and fracture. *Clinical Orthopaedic* **71:** 229–252.

Nordin BEC, Young MM, Bentley B, Ormondroyd P & Sykes J (1968) Lumbar spine densitometry, methodology and results in relation to the menopause. *Clinical Radiology* **19:** 459–464.

Nottestad SY, Baumel LJJ, Kimmel DB, Recker RR & Heaney RP (1987) The proportion of trabecular bone in human vertebrae. *Journal of Bone and Mineral Research* **2:** 221–229.

Parfitt AM (1988) Bone remodelling: relationship to the amount and structure of bone, and the pathogenesis and prevention of fractures. In Riggs BL & Melton LJ III (eds) *Osteoporosis: Aetiology, diagnosis and management*, pp 45–93. New York: Raven Press.

Pocock MA, Eisman JA, Hopper JL et al (1987) Genetic determinants of bone mass. *Journal of Clinical Investigation* **80:** 706–710.

Quigley MET, Martin PL, Burnier AM & Brooks P (1987) *American Journal of Obstetrics and Gynecology* **156:** 1516–1523.

Reeve J, Meunier PJ, Parsons JA et al (1980) Anabolic effect of human parathyroid hormone fragment on trabecular bone in involutional osteoporosis. *British Medical Journal* **280:** 1340–1344.

Reinbold WD, Reiser EJ, Harris ST, Ettinger B & Genant HK (1986) Measurement of bone and mineral content in early post-menopausal and post-menopausal osteoporotic women. A comparison of methods. *Radiology* **160:** 469–478.

Ribot C, Tremollieres F, Pouilles JM et al (1988) Obesity and postmenopausal bone loss. The influence of obesity on vertebral density and bone turnover in postmenopausal women. *Bone* **8:** 327–331.

Richelson LS, Wahner HJ, Melton LJ & Riggs BL (1984) Relative contributions of aging and oestrogen deficiency to post-menopausal bone loss. *New England Journal of Medicine* **311:** 1273–1275.

Riggs BL (1984) Treatment of osteoporosis with sodium fluoride: An appraisal. In Peck WA (ed.) *Bone and Mineral Research Annual*, vol. 2, pp 366–393. Amsterdam: Elsevier.

Riggs BL & Melton LJ III (1983) Evidence for two distinct syndromes of involutional osteoporosis. *American Journal of Medicine* **75:** 899–901.

Riggs BL & Melton LJ III (1986) Involutional osteoporosis. *New England Journal of Medicine* **314:** 1676–1686.

Riggs BL, Wahner HW, Dunn WL et al (1981) Differential changes in bone mineral density of the appendicular and axial skeleton with aging. *Journal of Clinical Investigation* **67:** 328–335.

Riggs BL, Seeman E, Hodgson SF, Taves DR & O'Fallon WM (1982a) Effect of the fluoride/ calcium regime on vertebral fracture occurrence in post-menopausal osteoporosis: Comparison with conventional therapy. *New England Journal of Medicine* **306:** 446–450.

Riggs BL, Wahner HW, Seeman E et al (1982b) Changes in bone mineral density of the proximal femur and spine with aging: differences between the post-menopausal and senile osteoporosis syndromes. *Journal of Clinical Investigation* **70:** 716–723.

Riggs BL, Wahner HW, Melton LJ III et al (1986) Rates of bone loss in the appendicular and axial skeletons of women. *Journal of Clinical Investigation* **77:** 1487–1491.

Riis BJ, Christiansen C, Deftos LJ & Catherwood BD (1984) The role of serum concentrations of oestrogens in post-menopausal osteoporosis and bone turnover. In Christiansen C, Arnaud CD, Nordin BEC et al (eds) *Osteoporosis*, pp 333–336. Glostrup: Department of Clinical Chemistry, Glostrup Hospital.

Riis B, Thomsen K & Christiansen C (1986) Does calcium supplementation prevent post-menopausal bone loss? *New England Journal of Medicine* **316:** 173–177.

Sambrook PN, Bartlett C, Evans R et al (1985) Measurement of lumbar spine bone mineral. A comparison of dual-photon absorptiometry and computed tomography. *British Journal of Radiology* **58:** 621–624.

Sambrook PN, Eisman JA, Furler SM & Pocock MA (1987) Computer monitoring and analysis of cross-matched section of bone density studies with respect to age and menopause. *Journal of Bone and Mineral Research* **2:** 109–114.

Schlenker RA & Von Seggen WW (1976) The distribution of cortical and trabecular bone mass along the lengths of the radius and ulna and the implications for in vivo bone mass measurements. *Calcified Tissue Research* **20:** 41–52.

Seeman E & Cooper M (1987) The effect of early and surgically induced menopause on bone mass. In Christiansen C, Johansen JS & Riis BJ (eds) *Osteoporosis*, vol. 1, pp 85–86. Kobenhavn K, Denmark: Osteopress ApS.

Seeman E, Wahner HW, Offord KP et al (1982) Differential effects of endocrine dysfunction on the axial and appendicular skeleton. *Journal of Clinical Investigation* **69:** 1302–1309.

Seeman E, Hopper JL, Bach LA et al (1989) Bone mass in daughters of women with osteoporosis. *New England Journal of Medicine* **320:** 554–558.

Slemenda C, Hui SL, Longcope C & Johnston CC Jr (1987) Sex, steroids and bone mass. A study of changes about the time of menopause. *Journal of Clinical Investigation* **80:** 1261–1269.

Smith CB & Smith DA (1976) Relations between age, mineral density and mechanical properties of human femoral compacta. *Acta Orthopaedica Scandinavica* **47:** 496–502.

Smith DM, Nance WE, Kang KW, Christian JC & Johnston CC Jr (1973) Genetic determinants of bone mass. *Journal of Clinical Investigation* **52:** 2800–2808.

Smith DM, Khairi MRA & Johnston CC Jr (1975) The loss of bone mineral with aging and its relationship to risk of fracture. *Journal of Clinical Investigation* **56:** 311–318.

Smith DM, Khairi MRA, Nordin JA Jr & Johnston CC Jr (1976) Age and activity effects on rate of bone mineral loss. *Journal of Clinical Investigation* **58:** 716–721.

Stein JA, Hochberg AM & Lazewatsky L (1988) Quantitative digital radiography for bone mineral analysis. In Dequeker J, Geusens P & Wahner HW (eds) *Bone Mineral Measurement by Photon Absorptiometry*, pp 412–414. Leuven, Belgium: Leuven University Press.

Stepan JJ, Pospichal J, Presel J & Pacovsky V (1987) Bone loss and biochemical indices of bone remodelling in surgically induced post-menopausal women. *Bone* **8:** 279–284.

Tinetti ME, Speechley M & Ginter SF (1988) Risk factors for falls among elderly persons living in the community. *New England Journal of Medicine* **319:** 1701–1707.

van Hemert AM, Vandenbroucke JP, Birkenhager JC & Valkenburg HA (1987) Osteoporotic fractures in the general population. In Christiansen C, Johansen JS & Riis BJ (eds) *Osteoporosis*, vol. 1, pp 85–86. Kobenhavn K, Denmark: Osteopress ApS.

Vose GP & Kubala AL Jr (1959) Bone strength: its relationship to x-ray determined ash content. *Human Biology* **31:** 261.

Wahner HW, Dunn WL & Riggs BL (1983) Noninvasive bone mineral measurement. *Seminars in Nuclear Medicine* **13:** 282–289.

Wahner HW, Dunn WL, Brown ML, Hauser MF & Morin R (1988) Comparison of quantitative digital radiography (QDR) and dual photon absorptiometry (DPA) for bone mineral measurements of the lumbar spine. In Dequeker J, Geusens P & Wahner HW (eds) *Bone Mineral Measurement by Photon Absorptiometry*, pp 419–426. Leuven, Belgium: Leuven University Press.

Wasnich RD, Ross PD, Heilbrun LK et al (1985) Prediction of post-menopausal fracture risk with bone mineral measurements. *American Journal of Obstetrics and Gynecology* **153:** 745–751.

2

Hypothalamic–pituitary region: computed tomography imaging

J. F. BONNEVILLE
F. CATTIN
J. L. DIETEMANN

Magnetic resonance imaging (MRI) is now the method of choice for imaging the hypothalamic–pituitary region, especially suprasellar tumours (which will only be briefly described here). It is our opinion, however, that computed tomography (CT) with dynamic scanning remains the optimal technique for imaging intrasellar pituitary tumours. Moreover dynamic CT allows perfect delineation of all cavernous sinus components.

Before discussing CT imaging of the sellar region, we would like to emphasize some important points:

1. The limits of sella turcica on plain films are well-known (Besser, 1976; Bruneton et al, 1979; Bonneville et al, 1983c): an adenoma less than 4–5 mm in size rarely deforms the sellar walls, and the presence of a normal sella does not exclude a microadenoma. In the presence of hyperprolactinaemia for instance, CT will be performed according to clinical and laboratory arguments, whether plain films are normal or not. Indeed, X-ray studies of the sella are carried out essentially to orientate the CT examination for the choice of projection, thickness of sections, etc. In a work-up for hyperprolactinaemia, we currently limit the plain film study to a magnified lateral view.

2. Tomography, even with complex motion, virtually never provides supplementary information. We have completely abandoned this technique. There is frequently no topographical correlation between an abnormality of the sellar floor and the site of the microadenoma (Swanson et al, 1979; Turski et al, 1981; Bonneville and Dietemann, 1981; Wortzman and Rewcastle, 1982). 'Thinning' of the sellar walls often corresponds to localized, physiological variability in bone thickness. A good understanding of the anatomy of the sella turcica and the radiologist's personal experience is of fundamental importance here.

3. Only high-resolution CT scanners of the latest generation yielding precise sections of 1.0–1.5 mm thickness allow reliable diagnosis of intrasellar adenomas (Syvertsen et al, 1979; Wolpert et al, 1979; Bonne-

ville et al, 1982c; Hemminghytt et al, 1983). The first CT descriptions of microadenomas were hindered by partial volume effect.

4. Direct coronal sections are virtually always superior in quality to reformatted images from axial sections, and should constitute the first line of approach (Mass et al, 1978). Axial complementary sections are necessary only when plain films suggest the presence of a very anterior or very posterior adenoma, or when coronal sections are not diagnostic.

5. Intrasellar adenomas are nearly always less enhanced by the iodinated contrast medium than the normal pituitary. Compression of pituitary cells at the periphery of the adenoma should explain this lesser enhancement.

6. Dynamic CT in coronal sections is essential for demonstration of small adenomas (Bonneville et al, 1983c). This technique allows visualization of (i) the delay in enhancement of the adenoma by comparison with the healthy pituitary tissue, (ii) the contralateral displacement of the secondary pituitary capillary bed, and (iii) the intracavernous cranial nerves and veins directly. Gadolinium DTPA-enhanced MRI will probably be just as useful as dynamic CT in the future.

CT ANATOMY OF THE SELLAR REGION

The normal CT pattern and the major anatomical variants of the different structures will be described here.

The pituitary gland—classical CT pattern

The pituitary is best studied by 1.0 or 1.5 mm direct coronal sections. Without contrast medium the gland is easily recognizable between the sellar floor and the chiasmatic cistern, with an attenuation value similar to that of the brain. Its superior pole is readily recognized and its height can be measured. After intravenous injection of contrast, enhancement begins with the pituitary capillary bed, gradually spreading to the periphery of the gland in a centrifugal fashion. Approximately 80 s after bolus injection the gland is homogeneous and appears less enhanced than the cavernous sinus (Figure 1). The lateral borders of the gland in contact with the cavernous sinus are clearly visualized. The superior pole is virtually always flat or slightly concave upwards, but normal convexity of the superior pole is seen in about 5% of cases, particularly in young women. A triangular rise in the superior pole at the point of passage of the pituitary stalk may be present. Anatomical variants in the sphenoid sinus can cause pituitary asymmetry: the superior pole, parallel to the sellar floor, can appear tilted or convex upwards; the pituitary can be almost completely asymmetric and displaced to one side of the mid-sagittal plane. Very occasionally, extensive upward pneumatization of the sphenoid sinus results in absence of sellar excavation: the pituitary appears to be quite simply set on the roof of the sphenoid sinus. The CT appearance can be misleading, especially in axial section, if the anatomical variant in the sphenoid sinus is not first identified on plain films.

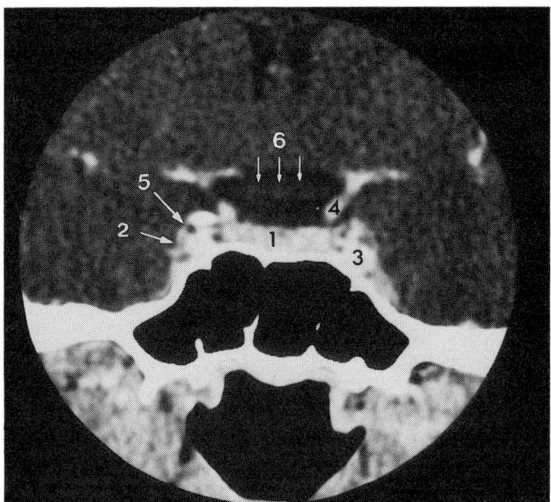

Figure 1. Normal coronal contrast-enhanced CT scan of the pituitary gland: 1. pituitary gland; 2, cavernous sinus; 3, intracavernous internal carotid artery; 4, supraclinoid internal carotid artery; 5, oculomotor nerve; 6, optic chiasm.

Shortness of the width of the sellar floor or intrasellar location of the carotid arteries may result in a convexity of the superior limit of the pituitary, frequently giving rise to an increased height of the gland simulating pathological patterns (Bonneville et al, 1986b) (Figure 2). The mean height of the gland is only slightly greater in women (4.4 ± 1.4 mm) than in men (4.4 ± 1.1 mm). However, Haughton et al (1980) reported a normal range of 1.4–6.7 mm. In view of this wide variability, measurement of pituitary height rarely provides significant diagnostic information. Nevertheless, it is considered highly suspicious when the height exceeds 8 mm. This is not an absolute rule: we have seen several cases where the pituitary height was

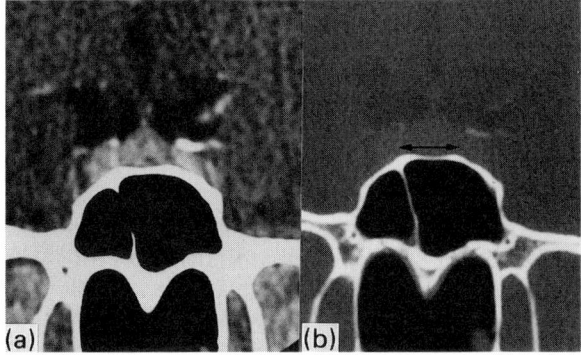

Figure 2. (a) Coronal enhanced CT scan. Bulging of the upper aspect of the pituitary gland. (b) Bone window demonstrates the short width of the sellar floor (less than 10 mm).

greater than 9 mm in young women in the absence of pregnancy or detectable endocrine disorders (Richmond and Wilson, 1978). Finally, as shown by Roppolo and Latchaw (1984), there is a slight decrease in pituitary height with advancing age. When the gland is small (2–3 mm), the superior pole is frequently concave upwards and there is thus free communication between supra- and intrasellar subarachnoid compartments. The posterior lobe of the pituitary is rarely seen on coronal scans.

In axial section, the anterior pituitary is virtually always less well-defined than in coronal section due to partial volume phenomenon in the vicinity of the sellar floor and the chiasmatic cistern. The posterior lobe of the pituitary is visible in more than 50% of cases, more frequently when the sella turcica is open. Following intravenous injection of contrast media, the posterior lobe generally appears in only a single section (never in more than two thin contiguous sections) as an oval zone, 4–5 mm in length and 2–3 mm thick, with less enhancement than the anterior lobe. The posterior lobe, sometimes pressed against a depression in the dorsum sellae which is not necessarily median, always shows a convex anterior border (Bonneville et al, 1985).

The pituitary gland—dynamic CT pattern

Dynamic pituitary CT is of major benefit for diagnosis of small pituitary lesions. Visualization of the pituitary capillary bed with this technique is today as fundamental for diagnosis of intrasellar lesions as was demonstration of the calcified pineal gland or internal cerebral vein for identification of the midline of the brain in the past.

Anatomy

A brief review of pituitary blood supply is necessary to understand the utility of dynamic CT. The various structures comprising the pituitary are directly or indirectly vascularized from two principal sources, the superior and inferior hypophyseal arteries. The inferior hypophyseal artery arises from each side of the intracavernous segment of the internal carotid artery; the superior hypophyseal artery, also paired, arises from the internal carotid immediately after its exit from the cavernous sinus following passage through the dura mater. There are transversal anastomoses between both superior hypophyseal and between both inferior hypophyseal arteries. Furthermore, the trabecular artery forms anastomoses with the superior and inferior pituitary network.

The anterior pituitary does not receive any direct arterial blood supply. At the superior part of the pituitary stalk, the hypophyseal arteries give rise to highly convoluted spiral capillary networks (referred to as 'gomitoli' by Fumagalli) which constitute the first capillary bed of the pituitary portal system (Xuereb et al, 1954). The first capillary bed is drained by the long portal vessels which descend the stalk and terminate in the second capillary bed, constituted by the anterior lobe sinusoids (Figure 3). These sinusoids, larger than the capillaries, are fed solely by portal vessels carrying blood

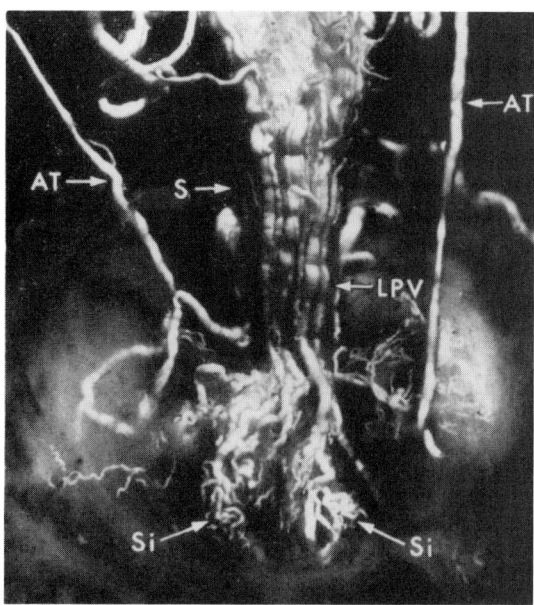

Figure 3. Anterosuperior view of the pituitary gland after partial removal of the central and upper portion of the pars distalis. On each side, a trabecular artery (AT) is seen entering the pars distalis. Note the prominent hypophyseal portal vessels (LPV) coursing down the stalk (S) and branching to form sinusoids (Si) in the pars distalis producing the pituitary 'tuft'. From Xuereb et al (1954), with permission.

which has already passed through the first capillary network in the pituitary stalk. There is an obviously functional significance to this vascular disposition: the capillary loops characteristic of the first vascular bed of the pituitary stalk are the site of nerve endings of certain hypothalamo–pituitary tract units; these release substances into the portal system which activate or suppress hormonal secretion by secretory cells of the anterior lobe. Popa and Fielding (1930), who first discovered the existence of the pituitary portal system, believed that this system functioned in an ascending fashion, i.e. from the pituitary to the hypothalamus. Proof that blood circulation actually occurs in the opposite direction, i.e. from the hypothalamus to the pituitary, was shown by subsequent morphological studies (Wislocki, 1938) and by in vivo observation in animals. Dynamic CT provides confirmation of the Wislocki hypothesis in living subjects, demonstrating that enhancement is progressive and clearly separated in time.

Unlike the anterior lobe, the posterior lobe has a conventional arterial–capillary–venous circulatory system, supplied by the right and left inferior hypophyseal arteries, with sinusoids far smaller than those of the anterior lobe. In the absence of a portal system, sinusoids of the posterior lobe appear to be enhanced far earlier than those of the anterior lobe. Finally, sinusoids of both lobes terminate in small venules in the periphery of the gland, draining into the venous sinus which surrounds the pituitary.

Technique

Dynamic scanning requires rapid injection of a bolus of 80 cm³ contrast medium at 15 cm³/s, pushed by 10 cm³ of saline solution. Six to eight 1.5 mm sections are taken, beginning at the time of the injection. With the General Electric 9800 CT/T system, scan time is 2 s, and the interscan delay time is 2.5 s.

Results

Dynamic CT (Figure 4) allows visualization of the intracavernous and supraclinoid internal carotid arteries, the central part of the secondary pituitary capillary bed (the pituitary tuft), the centrifugal contrast enhancement of the anterior pituitary, the posterior pituitary in axial section and the venous spaces of the cavernous sinus. The intracavernous internal carotid arteries and the branches of their intracranial division are perfectly opacified 10 s after the end of injection. The high quality of information thus available on the carotid siphons today renders carotid angiography superfluous prior to trans-sphenoidal surgery.

Approximately 10 s after optimal enhancement of internal carotid arteries, the secondary pituitary capillary bed is visualized as an unpaired median vascular structure, situated below the sellar diaphragm, as a prolongation in the direction of the pituitary stalk. Most frequently it appears as a vascular tuft, the surface of which covers approximately one quarter of the pituitary in the considered section (Figure 5a). Much less frequently, the pituitary tuft is far smaller appearing as a point of variable size (Figure 5b). The tuft is virtually always regular and symmetric; however, a moderate degree of asymmetry is possible in the absence of pathological changes. When the pituitary height is small, the pituitary capillary bed may be composed of a vascular band running immediately below the superior border of the gland (Figure 5c). Between 20 and 40 s after injection, there is a gradual, regular and symmetrical centrifugal enhancement of the anterior pituitary from the capillary bed. Sixty seconds after bolus injection, pituitary enhancement is homogeneous, and the pituitary capillary bed is no longer visible.

In dynamic axial sections posterior pituitary capillary enhancement occurs very soon after enhancement of the intracavernous carotid arteries due to the direct arterial blood supply. At some time after the bolus injection the posterior pituitary appears less enhanced than the anterior pituitary. Indeed, when contrast medium equilibrates between the intravascular and extravascular interstitial spaces, a lesser enhancement of the posterior lobe is seen, correlating with its lesser volume of the interstitial spaces (Figures 6a,b,c).

The capillary bed is regularly displaced or deformed (tuft sign) in cases of lateralized intrasellar microadenoma (Bonneville et al, 1983a). This sign is fundamental for the diagnosis of pituitary adenomas too small to deform the sellar floor or the superior pole of the pituitary. It is also essential for the diagnosis of isodense adenomas. When microadenomas are midline, the pituitary tuft is not displaced, but localized compression of its inferior part

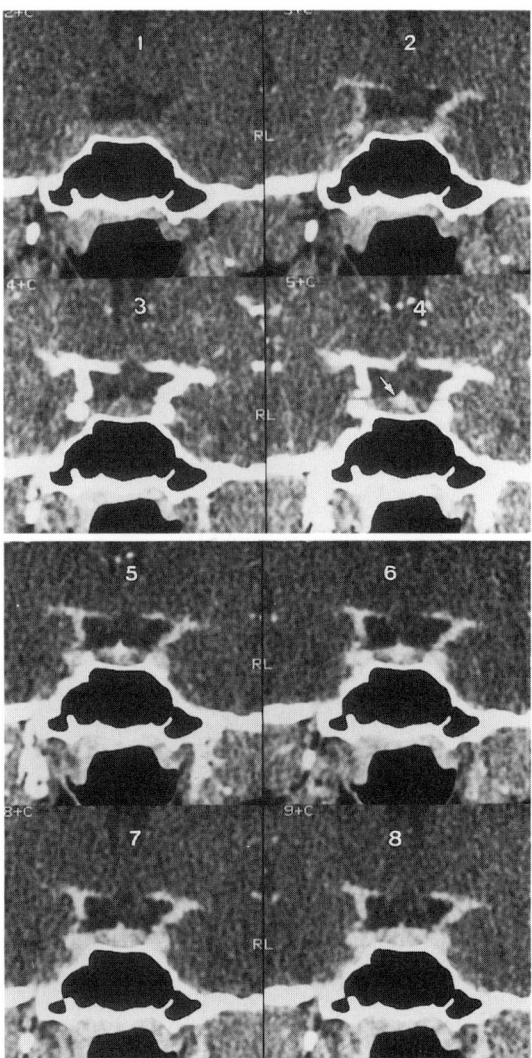

Figure 4. Normal dynamic coronal CT scan of the pituitary gland: 1, before bolus injection; 2, onset of enhancement of internal carotid arteries; 3, optimal visualization of internal carotid arteries; 4, opacification of the pituitary tuft (arrow); 5, 6, 7, centrifugal enhancement of the pituitary gland; 8, pituitary enhancement is almost homogeneous.

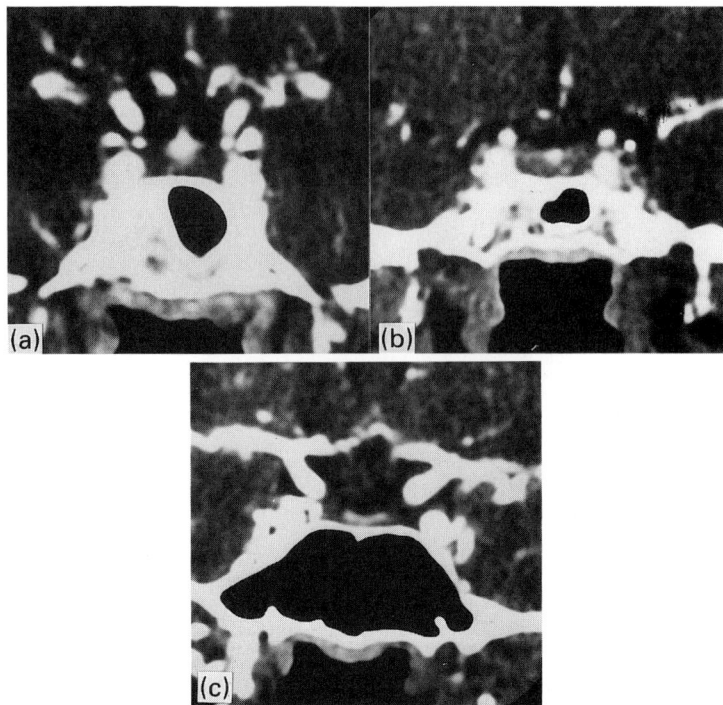

Figure 5. Variants of the secondary capillary bed: (a) tuft, (b) point-like, (c) band-like.

may occur. When the pituitary capillary bed is band-like, a localized absence of opacification has the same diagnostic significance as displacement of the tuft. Finally, after opacification of the pituitary bed, asymmetrical enhancement of the pituitary constitutes a further sign for the presence of an intrasellar lesion. In general, intrasellar microadenomas are enhanced more slowly and to a lesser extent than the healthy pituitary tissue.

The cavernous sinus

The cavernous sinuses are generally of symmetrical topography and volume (Rhoton et al, 1977, 1979). Under normal conditions the lateral dural wall is flat or slightly concave outwards in axial sections. The dural sheath at the lateral limit of the sinus frequently shows marked contrast enhancement. On the other hand, the sellar diaphragm itself, also constituted of a dural extension, rarely shows enhancement, probably due to a lesser degree of vascularization.

The internal carotid artery is well visualized within the cavernous sinus. Due to its sigmoidal form in both coronal and sagittal planes, it is virtually never completely visualized in a single plane. The artery occupies a medial position within the cavernous sinus, and is only 1 or 2 mm from the lateral

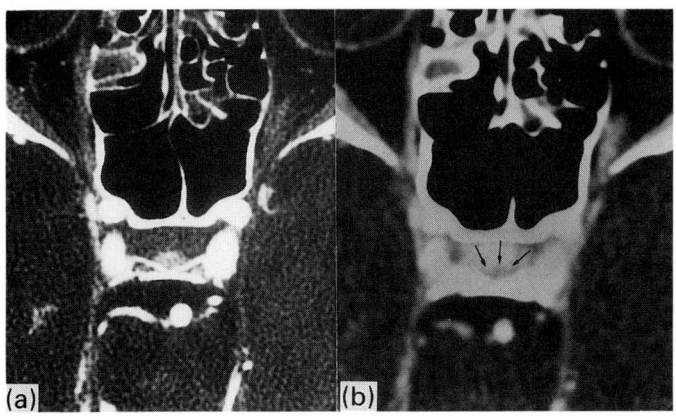

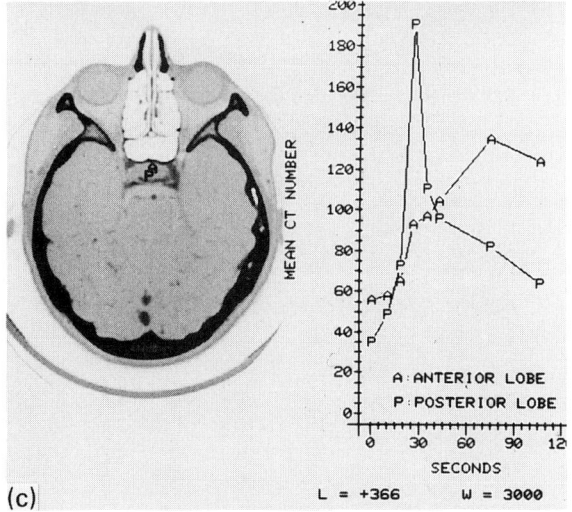

Figure 6. (a) Axial dynamic CT scan of the pituitary gland. Arterial phase. Enhancement of the posterior lobe contemporary of optimal opacification of the internal carotid arteries. (b) At the end of dynamic CT scan, the posterior pituitary appears less dense than the anterior pituitary. (c) Representative time/density curves for the anterior and posterior pituitaries.

pituitary border. In arteriosclerosis or in the elderly, or in cases of elongation of the carotid, the artery comes into direct contact with the gland and can change its shape. The laterosellar venous spaces can be perfectly defined with dynamic CT. They include a constant large space inferolateral to the horizontal portion of the cavernous carotid artery (Figure 7), a space often asymmetrical and inconsistently seen medial to the artery and a space between the artery and the sphenoid bone (i.e. vein of the carotid sulcus) when the artery does not touch the sphenoid bone (Figure 8).

Nervous structures crossing the cavernous sinus appear as round or oval

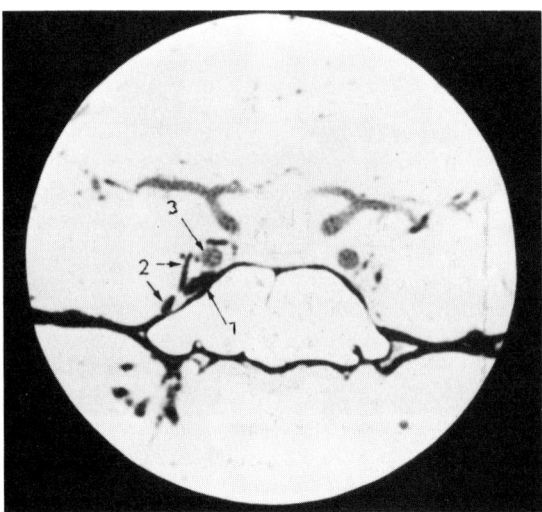

Figure 7. Normal coronal dynamic CT scan of the cavernous sinus, showing inferolateral vein (1), veins of the lateral wall of the cavernous sinus (2), and intracavernous internal carotid artery (3).

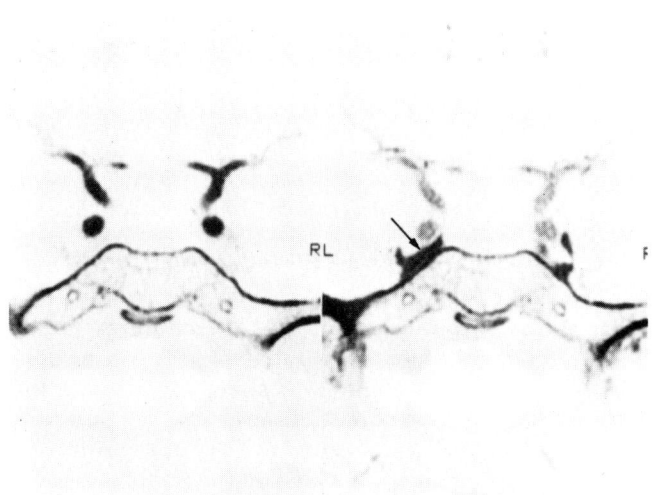

Figure 8. Normal coronal dynamic CT scan of the cavernous sinus. Prominent vein of the carotid sulcus (arrow), located between intracavernous internal carotid artery and sphenoid bone.

defects in coronal sections, axial sections or oblique reconstructions. The third (oculomotor) nerve is always seen in direct coronal sections on the anterior slices, immediately below the anterior clinoid processes. Size and attenuation value of the third nerve are variable. A voluminous third nerve presenting marked hypodensity can be mistaken for a fat nodule occupying the most anterior part of the sinus, and can also correspond to the presence of the third and fourth (trochlear) nerves in the same dural sheath. In the same anterior section, the sixth (abducens) nerve is frequently visible at the bottom of the cavernous sinus, immediately outside and in contact with the internal carotid artery. In the middle section of the sella, the third nerve is seen at the top, and the ophthalmic division of the trigeminal nerve at the inferior part, of the lateral wall of the sinus. Finally in the most posterior coronal sections parallel to the dorsum sellae, the Gasserian ganglion appears as an oval structure situated just in front of the tip of the petrous bone (Figure 9a). In axial sections, the entire course of the nerves can be visualized up to the entrance to the superior orbital fissure. The Gasserian ganglion is always readily visible in the Meckel cave, at the posteroinferior part of the cavernous sinus (Figure 9b). Fat deposits are normally seen in the anterior part of the sinus; but the presence of fat deposits in the middle or posterior part of the sinus, or between the pituitary and the cavernous sinus, is abnormal and is generally seen only in Cushing's disease.

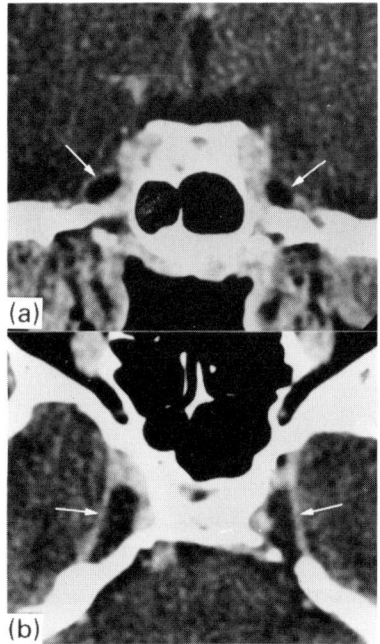

Figure 9. Gasserian ganglions: (a) coronal section; (b) axial section.

The suprasellar cistern

In coronal sections, the suprasellar cistern is roughly triangular with apex upwards, within which the chiasm is better visualized before enhancement. The superior pole of the pituitary is shaped by the bordering cistern. The sellar diaphragm *per se* is rarely visible. The pituitary stalk is seen between the gland and the infundibular recess of the third ventricle. The supraclinoid internal carotid arteries, their branches and the basilar artery are readily visible within the cistern.

In axial sections, the suprasellar cistern appears as a five- or six-branched star, depending on whether the section passes through the pons or through the interpeduncular fossa. From front to back, the six branches of the star corresponding to the extensions of the suprasellar cistern consist of the interhemispheric fissure, the sylvian fissures, the ambient cistern, and the interpeduncular cistern (Figure 10a). The optic nerves and chiasm are

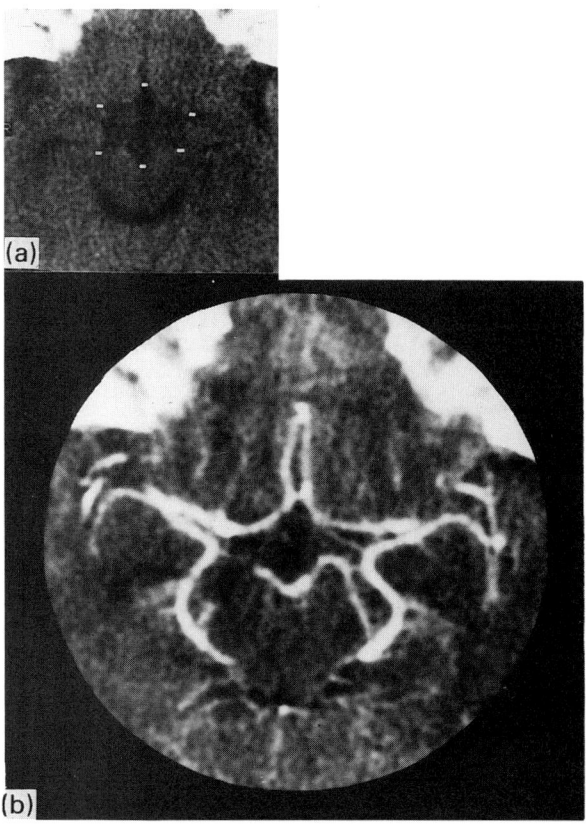

Figure 10. (a) Native CT scan demonstrating the typical six-branched star of the suprasellar cistern. (b) Dynamic CT scan at the same level: opacification of the circle of Willis and basilar veins.

situated at the anterior part of the suprasellar cistern, forming a mass the appearance of which varies with the angle of section. The circle of Willis is best studied by dynamic scans (Figure 10b).

COMPUTED TOMOGRAPHY OF PITUITARY ADENOMAS

Pituitary adenomas with extrasellar extension

Since the old category of 'chromophobe' adenomas has been abandoned, prolactinomas appear to be the most frequent adenomas with extrasellar extension. Non-secreting or non-functional adenomas are seen less commonly (Gold, 1981). A suprasellar extension can sometimes be found in mixed prolactinomas: growth hormone (GH)-secreting pituitary adenomas and gonadotropin-secreting adenomas. Pure GH-, thyroid stimulating hormone (TSH) and adrenocorticotrophin (ACTH) hormone-secreting pituitary adenomas demonstrate extension much less frequently. Radio-logical signs of adenomas with extension are generally identical, regardless of the type of tumour.

CT signs of pituitary adenomas with suprasellar extension

Plain films generally allow rough estimation of the amount and direction of extension of the adenoma thus permitting modification of the CT technique. Nevertheless even a normal sella does not exclude an adenoma with supra-sellar extension. Evaluation of these adenomas requires coronal sections with dynamic CT to delineate the relationship of the tumour with the internal carotid arteries and their branches, as well as other elements of the cavernous sinus. The secondary pituitary capillary bed is generally not identifiable unless the suprasellar extension of the adenoma is very moderate. Along with direct coronal sections, axial sections are taken for reformations.

Suprasellar extension is variable. The first stage is intermediate between strictly intrasellar adenomas and adenomas with true suprasellar extension. In direct coronal sections, these adenomas occupy the lower part of the chiasmatic cistern, their upper pole separated from the inferior surface of the optic chiasm by a variably thick layer of cerebrospinal fluid. Contrast between the opacity of the tumour and the hypodense cisterns allows precise anatomical definition of the adenoma, which extends superiorly most of the time vertically along the axis of the sella turcica. In axial sections, the perfectly round tumour occupies the central part of the chiasmatic cistern. At this stage, moderate dilatation of the crural and lateropeduncular cisterns is not uncommon.

Large pituitary adenomas with major superior extension completely fill the chiasmatic cistern in coronal sections (Figure 11a). The suprasellar extension can be median and symmetrical, or it can be lateralized. A dilatation of the cistern can still be seen. Stricture of the tumour at the sellar diaphragm level can yield an hourglass-like pattern. The inferior part of the

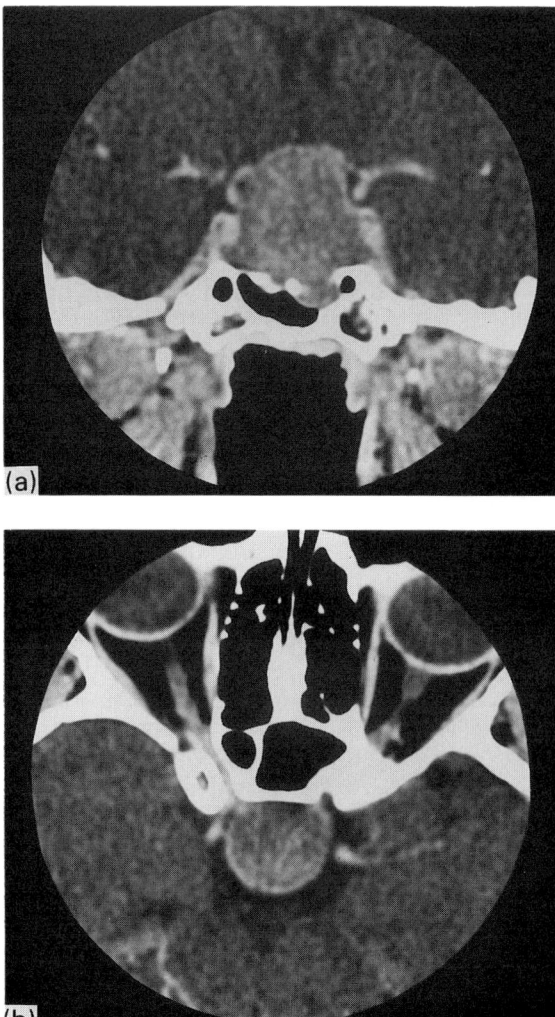

Figure 11. Pituitary adenoma with large suprasellar extension. (a) In coronal section the entire suprasellar cistern is filled by a homogeneously enhanced mass. Limited extension of the adenoma into the sphenoid sinus through the eroded sellar floor. (b) In axial section, the tumour occupies the anterior part of the suprasellar cistern.

third ventricle is amputated when the vertical diameter of the tumour reaches 3 cm. In axial sections, pituitary adenomas fill the anterior part of the suprasellar cistern. They are round or oval in shape, with a major anteroposterior axis (Figure 11b). At a later stage, the entire cistern is filled. Compression of the medial wall of the anterior horns of the lateral ventricles is possible. Posterior extension with compression of the cerebral peduncles is less common. When the adenoma is very large, it frequently presents polycyclic contours.

After intravenous injection of contrast medium, three principal types of enhancement can be seen:

1. Most frequently, enhancement is homogeneous and intense, but less than that seen with meningiomas.
2. Enhancement can be annular, with a central hypodensity not necessarily corresponding to a liquid content.
3. Rounded areas less dense than the adenoma are sometimes seen, corresponding to cysts when the hypodensity is close to that of cerebrospinal fluid (CSF), or more frequently, to areas of necrosis or old haemorrhage.

CT signs of pituitary adenomas with lateral extension

Lateral extension into the cavernous sinus may be encountered in prolactinomas as well as in GH-secreting pituitary adenomas. Invasion of the cavernous sinus causes enlargement of the sinus with convexity of the lateral wall (Figure 12). After intravenous contrast, enhancement of the sinus is less

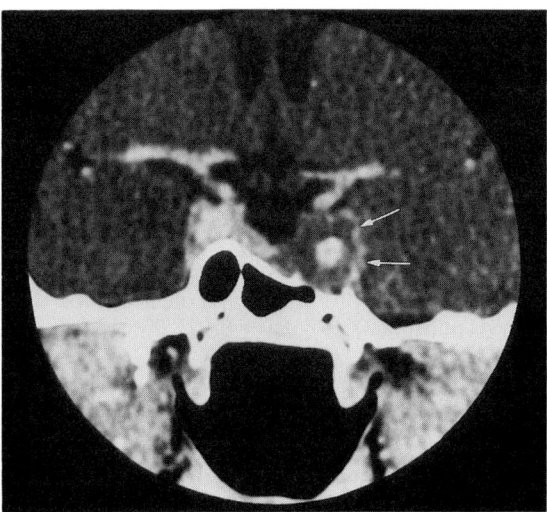

Figure 12. Residual intracavernous tumour after medical treatment of a macroprolactinoma. The left intracavernous internal carotid artery is surrounded by poorly enhanced tissue; note the bulging of the lateral wall of the cavernous sinus (arrows).

marked than usually. Dynamic CT is necessary here to demonstrate the encased internal carotid artery and often the lack of filling of the laterosellar veins, especially the vein of the carotid sulcus (Figure 13). Demonstration with dynamic CT of intracavernous tumoral extension is essential for planning adequate treatment since surgery is frequently unable to cure the intracavernous tumoral component.

Prolactin-secreting pituitary microadenomas

Prolactinomas are the most common pituitary adenomas. CT demonstration of intrasellar prolactinomas has been essential for the understanding of hyperprolactinaemias: this was a determining factor for modification of the

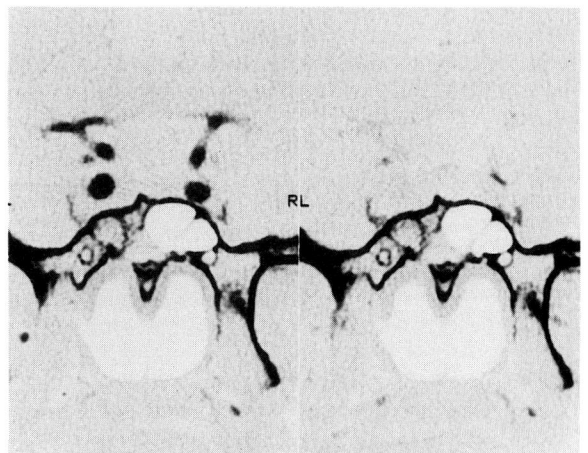

Figure 13. Acromegaly. Persistent abnormal GH level after surgery. On the left side, absence of the vein of the carotid sulcus in favour of cavernous sinus invasion.

therapeutic approach, demonstrating that tumour volume decreases with dopaminergic drug. For diagnosis of microadenomas, direct thin coronal sections and dynamic scanning have to be emphasized (Bonneville et al, 1982b). Nine signs should be discussed, and diagnosis of an intrasellar adenoma is increasingly reliable when a large number of these signs are found. Data from dynamic CT are essential.

1. Size of the pituitary

A pituitary gland with a height more than 8 mm is virtually always abnormal. When isolated, this sign is nevertheless insufficient to allow a definitive diagnosis of intrasellar adenoma. Besides cases of pituitary adenoma, a pituitary height greater than 8 mm can be seen in pregnancy and in hyperplasia due to dysfunction of a target organ. Furthermore, Swartz et al (1983) reported a mean height of 7.1 mm in 50 young women of childbearing age.

While we have not been able to confirm these data, we have seen a pituitary gland higher than 9 mm in the absence of any endocrine pathology or pregnancy in some cases where the gland width was less than 10 mm. Finally, one must always bear in mind that an intrasellar adenoma can be present in a gland the volume of which is not increased or with a maximal height not exceeding 2 mm. The height of the pituitary gland is normal in iatrogenic hyperprolactinaemias due to neuroleptics or due to renal dialysis.

2. Morphology of the superior pole

The superior pole of the pituitary is normally horizontal and frequently concave upwards when the gland is small. Swartz et al (1983) reported that the intrasellar content was convex upwards in 44% of women of childbearing age. However, an identical study carried out in France did not confirm this. We find that upward convexity always requires attention, even if its occurrence alone is not a criterion for a pituitary lesion. The concept of pituitary hyperplasia is not clearly defined and this term ought to be avoided: a convex pituitary gland must be considered radiologically either as a normal variant or as a manifestation of an isodense hidden adenoma. Asymmetrical bulging of the intrasellar contents is highly indicative of a microadenoma. On the other hand, a triangular or rounded median rise at the pituitary stalk passage is not pathological. The superior pole can also be visualized by reformation from axial sections. Asymmetry of the upper limit of intrasellar contents in right and left paramedian sagittal reformations can have some diagnostic value. The superior pole can remain entirely flat when the adenoma is small if the CT scan is done several months after the beginning of treatment with dopaminergic agents or where extension is exclusively inferior towards the sphenoid sinus.

3. Appearance of the sellar walls

Study of the appearance of the sella turcica is frequently disappointing and rarely of diagnostic value in intrasellar prolactinomas. When the adenoma is smaller than 5 mm in diameter, the sellar floor can be perfectly normal. Asymmetry, inclination, angulation, and differences in thickness of the floor can also be seen in the absence of microadenomas. In adenomas larger than 5 mm in diameter, localized thinning, especially when associated with a depression of the floor, is a supplementary diagnostic sign. Osseous thinning can also be generalized over the entire width of the floor in cases of intrasellar adenomas. Differential diagnosis between pathological thinning and a normally thin sellar floor is not always easy. Study of the sellar floor is interesting in adenomas treated with dopaminergic agents: a major osseous abnormality combined with an adenoma of very small size can suggest that the adenoma was far larger before treatment, and there is thus a risk of expansion upon withdrawal of dopaminergic agents (Bonneville et al, 1983b).

In axial sections, a pronounced posterior concavity of the anterior wall of the sella is highly characteristic of intrasellar adenoma. However, this appearance is also seen in empty sella. In holosellar adenomas, bulging of the anterior wall of the sella is frequently accompanied by a convexity of the medial limit of the cavernous sinus, pushing the internal carotid arteries outwards. In posteriorly located adenomas, asymmetrical erosion of the dorsum sellae is a useful supplementary sign; but physiological asymmetry of the dorsum sellae is not exceptional.

4. General non-contrast appearance of the gland

Native coronal CT before injection of contrast medium allows a rough identification of the gland for determination of height and morphology of the superior pole, and study of the osseous walls. The relationship between the sellar contents and the chiasm are readily visible in the suprasellar cistern. It can also suggest the presence of microadenoma if a rounded hypodense area is demonstrated within the gland. Thin tumoural calcifications, particularly in prolactin-secreting adenomas, may be identified. The frequency of such calcification visualized by CT scan is limited (approximately 2%) and is less than the 7% of histological series. A massive calcification of an intrasellar prolactinoma is highly uncommon (Rilliet et al, 1981).

5. Morphology and topography of the secondary pituitary capillary bed

Displacement of the pituitary capillary bed (Figure 14a,b) or its compression (Figure 15a,b) provide formal evidence for an intrasellar expansive process (Bonneville et al, 1983a). This can be the sole CT sign in prolactinomas presenting the same attenuation value as the healthy pituitary. In the cases where the capillary bed is not nodular but rather linear, parallel and in contact with the superior pole, localized defects in filling of the capillary bed take on particular significance (Figure 16a,b). These modifications in the capillary bed can be absent or minimal for midline or posteriorly located microadenomas. Finally, when the adenoma is larger than 8–10 mm in diameter, the secondary pituitary bed will generally not be seen due to its compression.

6. Attenuation value of the pituitary gland during dynamic CT

Contrast enhancement of the pituitary gland normally begins about 10 s after optimal opacification of the secondary pituitary capillary bed. In case of adenoma, enhancement of the parenchyma on the side of the lesion is delayed by comparison with the opposite side (see Figures 14–16). When CT scan is carried out after prolonged treatment with a dopamine agonist, the adenoma itself may no longer be directly visible due to the tumour-shrinkage action of the agent: asymmetrical enhancement of the pituitary gland during dynamic CT scan may be the sole sign of the presence of residual adenomatous cells (Bonneville et al, 1982a; Dietemann et al, 1983b; Barrow et al, 1984).

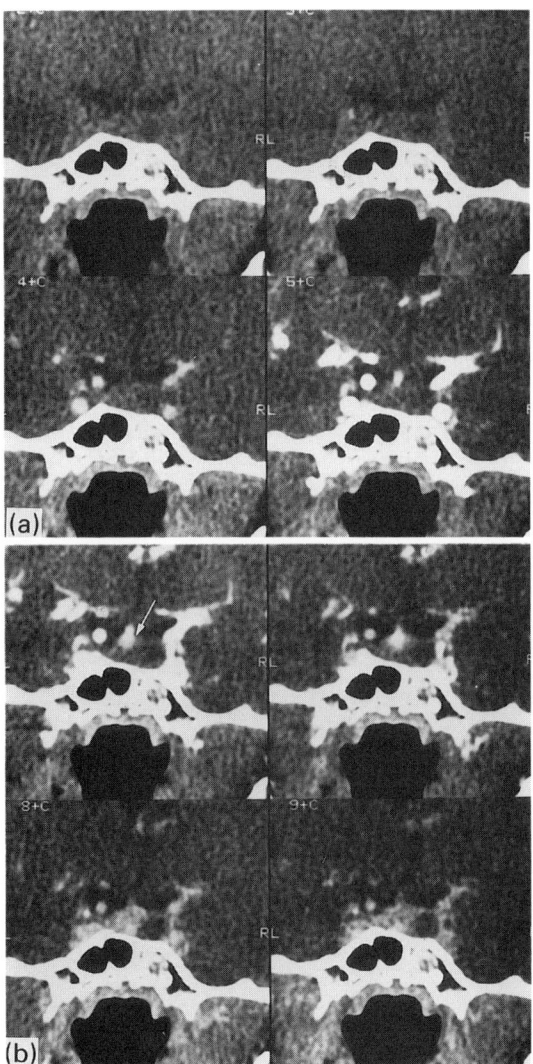

Figure 14. (a) (b) 9 mm prolactinoma. Dynamic coronal CT scan. Before contrast (upper left), low dense area within the pituitary. After bolus injection, displacement of the capillary bed (arrow) (upper right) and delayed enhancement of the pituitary adenoma. Note the displacement of the pituitary stalk (lower left).

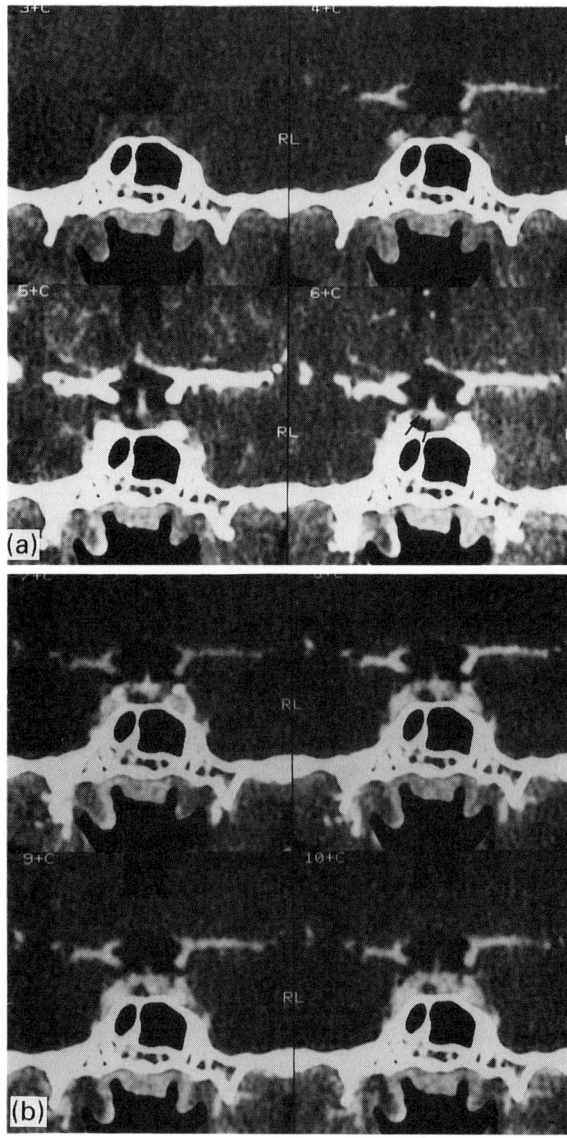

Figure 15. (a) (b) 4 mm prolactinoma. No displacement of the pituitary stalk, but localized compression of the capillary bed (arrows). The hypodense adenoma is well delineated at the end of the dynamic scan.

7. Attenuation value of the pituitary gland at some period after bolus injection

At the end of dynamic CT, intrasellar microadenomas virtually always appear as rounded or oval zones less dense than the normal pituitary. Infrequently, intrasellar adenomas present a rectilinear border, which can be the case after treatment with dopaminergic agents. An adenoma with a rectilinear border can be differentiated from a streak artefact going beyond the limits of the sella (Earnest et al, 1981). Hypodensity of the lesion by comparison with the healthy pituitary does not necessarily imply that the adenoma is necrotic except where density approximates 0 Hounsfield units (HU). Heterogeneity of the adenoma with greater density of the lower part of the tumour can be seen in the absence of any haemorrhagic process (Mohr

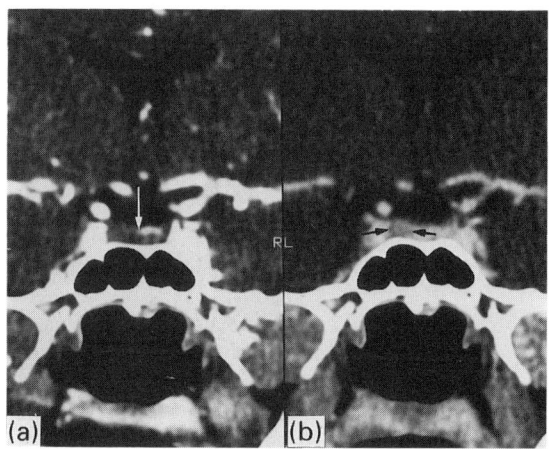

Figure 16. Prolactinoma. Dynamic coronal CT scan: (a) Localized defect in filling of the capillary bed (white arrow). (b) At the end of dynamic scanning a hypodense 3 mm microadenoma is demonstrated (black arrows).

and Hardy, 1982). Microadenomas denser than the normal pituitary are exceptional; we have seen only four cases in more than 3000 pituitary CT scans.

Demonstration of prolactinomas is far less reliable in axial sections even when thin. Only lesions greater than 4–5 mm in diameter are readily identifiable, and these should be differentiated from the normal posterior pituitary, a partial intrasellar expansion of the subarachnoid spaces and artefacts of reconstruction (streak artefacts resulting from inclusion of the petrous bones in the section) (Chambers et al, 1982). Frontal and sagittal reformations can also be useful, but they are not considered generally to be highly reliable for the detection of intrasellar prolactinomas.

Holosellar adenomas usually present a homogeneous enhancement with the density of the sellar content generally less than that of the normal pituitary. However, it is sometimes very similar, so that increase in volume of the gland, convexity of the superior pole and, especially, osseous deformation can constitute the sole diagnostic elements.

8. The posterior pituitary

The normal appearance of the posterior pituitary on thin axial sections has been considered in the section on 'Anatomy'. This characteristic pattern can rarely be deformed by pressure of an intrasellar adenoma.

9. Direction of the pituitary stalk

The pituitary stalk is frequently inclined from the normal vertical axis, even in cases of strictly intrasellar adenomas, due to its close relationship with the secondary pituitary capillary bed. Nevertheless, it must be borne in mind that the pituitary stalk can be inclined in the absence of any pituitary or hypothalamic disorder (Peyster and Hoover, 1984).

CT of growth hormone-secreting pituitary adenomas

Characteristic modifications of the skull base and vault are usually produced by growth hormone hypersecretion: thickening of the cranial vault, hyperostosis of the external occipital protuberance, extensive pneumatization of the paranasal sinuses and prognathism. Growth hormone-secreting adenomas vary in size from a few millimetres to several centimetres. Certain morphological features of the sella turcica are characteristic of this type of adenoma: enlarged square sellae, tapered tuberculum sellae, straightened and backward displaced dorsum sellae, increased density of the cortical bone of the sella turcica, intratumoural calcifications, and invasive characteristics and herniation of the tumour into the sphenoid sinus.

High-resolution CT usually demonstrates only a discrete low-density area corresponding to the adenoma. In rare cases the tumour may appear isodense. An upward bulging of the superior pole of the pituitary gland and a contralateral deviation of the pituitary stalk are noted in most of the cases.

A lateral invasion within the cavernous sinus should always be looked for. It is common to observe a partially empty sella while investigating an acromegalic patient. Such empty sella are secondary to partial spontaneous necrosis of a GH-secreting adenoma (Figure 17a–c). Dopamine agonists and somatostatin can also result in a shrinkage of the tumour.

CT of ACTH-secreting pituitary adenomas

Most cases of Cushing's disease are related to a very small ACTH-secreting pituitary adenoma. High resolution thin section dynamic CT scanning is today able to demonstrate microadenomas less than 3 mm in diameter (Figure 18a,b). Normal CT scan does not eliminate a pituitary microadenoma whose size can be less than 1 mm in Cushing's disease (Guthrie et al, 1981). In 30% of the patients with Cushing's disease,

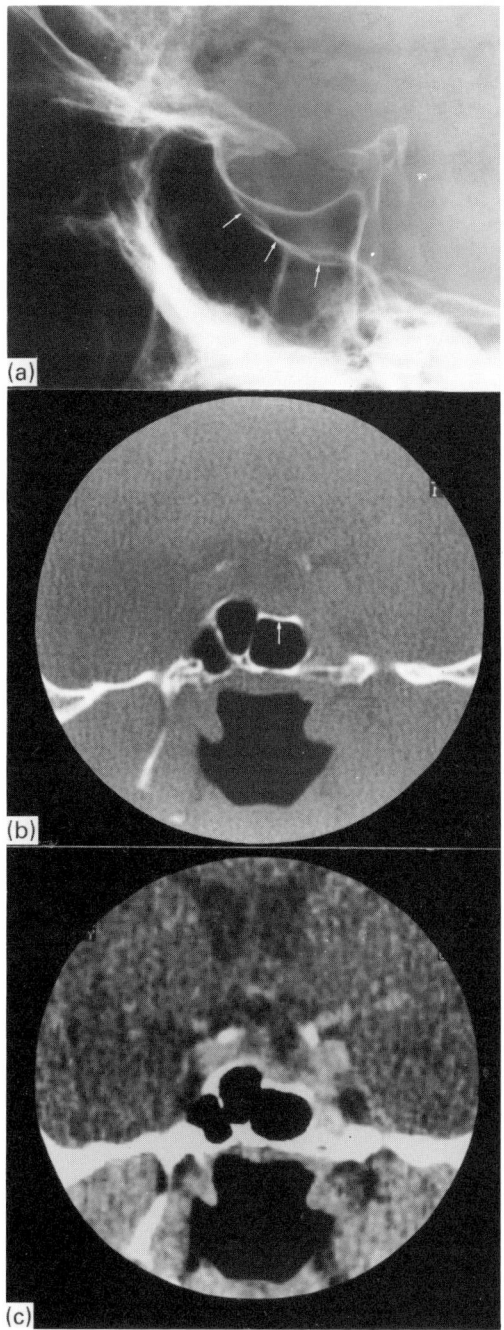

Figure 17. Acromegaly. Prolonged bromocriptine treatment. (a) Lateral magnified view of the sella turcica. Asymmetrical depression of the sellar floor (arrows). (b) Bone window. The sellar floor is depressed on the left, but is not eroded (arrow). (c) Coronal enhanced CT scan. Partially empty sella. No visible tumour. Probable shrinkage of a GH-secreting adenoma after medical treatment.

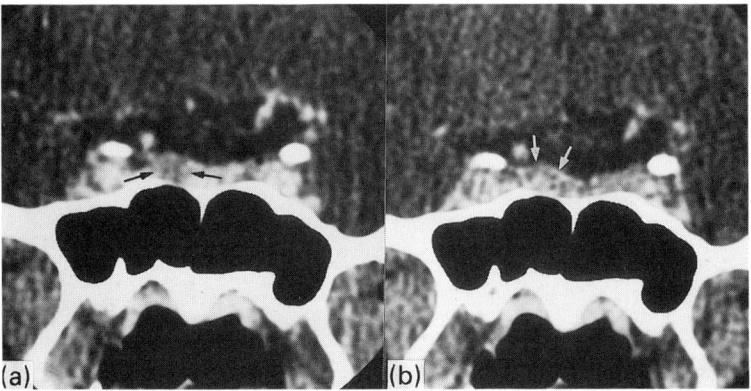

Figure 18. ACTH-secreting microadenoma. (a) The hypodense 3 mm adenoma is well demonstrated on the last cut of the dynamic CT scan (black arrows). (b) Conventional coronal CT, 60 s later. The hypodensity is no more visible. Note only the slight localized bulging of the superior aspect of the pituitary gland (white arrows).

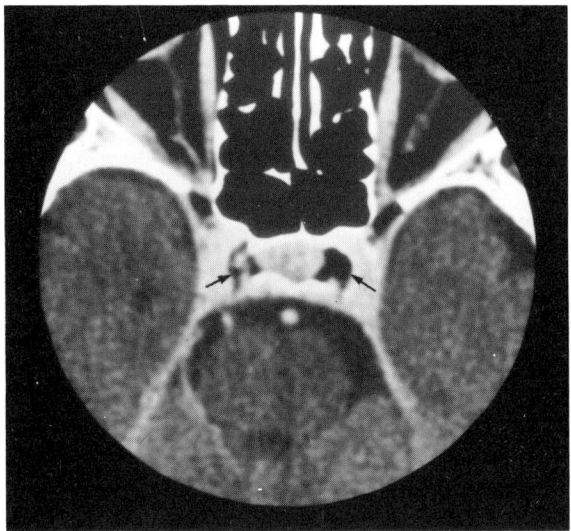

Figure 19. Cushing's disease. Axial enhanced CT scan. Large fat deposits within both cavernous sinus (arrows).

abnormal fat deposits can be noted within the cavernous sinus (Bachow et al, 1984) (Figure 19).

CT in other pituitary adenomas

Pituitary adenomas which secrete TSH, and those secreting follicle stimulating hormone–luteinizing hormone (FSH–LH), are rather rare. CT appearance of TSH-secreting adenomas is non-specific. Small adenomas determine a moderate mass effect and appear lower in density than the normal pituitary gland on enhanced CT scans. Macroadenomas look like non-secreting adenomas. FSH–LH-secreting adenomas have a tendency for rapid growth and generally present a prominent suprasellar extension by the time they are discovered. Moreover these adenomas may display an invasive tendency.

THE EMPTY SELLA SYNDROME

Empty sella turcica is characterized by an intrasellar herniation of the suprasellar subarachnoid spaces. Primary empty sella is related to a congenital dehiscence of the diaphragma sellae. Absence or large opening of diaphragma sellae may be noted in 20% of all individuals. The intrasellar herniation of the subarachnoid spaces is favoured by suprasellar promoting factors (raised intracranial pressure, postfixed chiasm) or by intrasellar promoting factors (menopause, multiparity, pituitary infarction related to diabetes mellitus, replacement therapy of primary end organ failure, or bromocriptine treatment) (Busch, 1951; Guibert-Tranier et al, 1980; Bonneville et al, 1986a; Tindall and Barrow, 1986). Secondary empty sella is usually related to surgical treatment or X-ray therapy. Rupture of an intrasellar cyst may also lead to an empty sella (Derome et al, 1980; Meyer et al, 1987). In children with idiopathic pituitary deficiency, due usually to hypothalamic defects, a small pituitary fossa associated with a gland of very low height and a partial empty sella is commonly observed (Bonneville et al, 1986a).

Empty sella is mainly encountered in middle-aged women. Clinical symptoms are rather rare, headaches and obesity being the commonest symptoms. Visual alteration (visual field defects, papilloedema), endocrine symptoms (pituitary deficiency, hyperprolactinaemia, diabetes insipidus), rhinorrhoea, or trigeminal neuralgia rarely reveal an empty sella. Hyperprolactinaemia associated with empty sella may be related to a stretched pituitary stalk or to a coincidental microprolactinoma (Bonneville and Dietemann, 1981; Burstzyn et al, 1983; Bonneville et al, 1986a; Nagao et al, 1987).

Diagnosis of empty sella is evoked in most cases on a lateral skull radiograph: sella is enlarged with a double floor. Frontal skull radiography reveals a regular, symmetric depression of the sellar floor without bony erosion in cases with a small sphenoid sinus. Empty sella is confirmed by axial and coronal enhanced CT scan. Cerebrospinal fluid (CSF) densities occupy a significant volume and the remaining pituitary may be difficult to

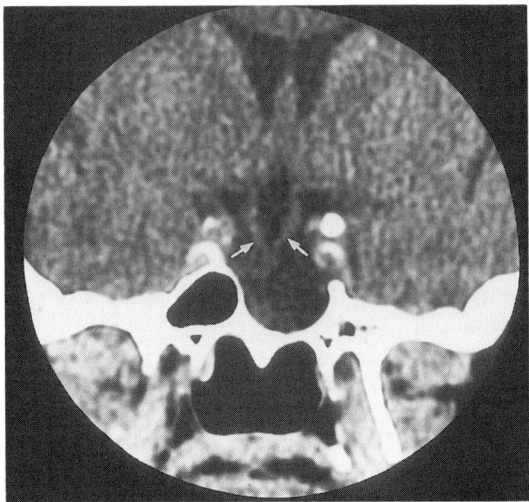

Figure 20. Totally empty sella. The whole pituitary fossa appears occupied by water density. No visible pituitary tissue. Asymmetrical depression of the sellar floor. Downward displacement of the optic chiasm (arrows) provoking visual disturbances.

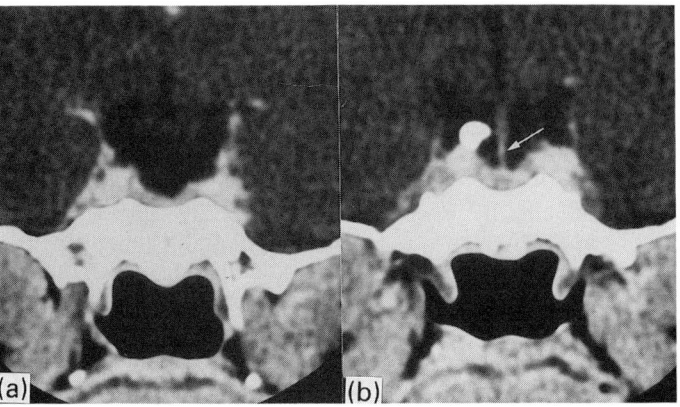

Figure 21. Partially empty sella. Coronal enhanced CT scans. (a) At the midsellar level. Remaining pituitary gland presents an upward concavity. Median symmetrical depression of the sellar floor above a non-pneumatized sphenoid sinus. (b) At the posterior part of the sellar, the pituitary stalk appears vertical in the midline and elongated (arrow).

identify (Figure 20). Coronal sections identify a stretched vertical median pituitary stalk (Figure 21a,b). On failure to identify the pituitary stalk prudence should dictate the use of CT cisternography or MRI to rule out an intrasellar or suprasellar cystic lesion (Haughton et al, 1980; Young et al, 1981; Meyer et al, 1987).

CRANIOPHARYNGIOMAS

Craniopharyngiomas arise from epithelial remnants of Rathke's pouch which are mainly located along the stalk and within the pituitary gland. Most craniopharyngiomas occur in patients under 25 years of age, but 20% are observed after the age of 40. Clinical symptoms are related to pituitary deficiency, hypothalamic dysfunction, visual disturbances and raised intracranial pressure.

Craniopharyngiomas can be both solid and cystic. The size of cranio- pharyngiomas ranges from 1 to 15 cm. From a surgical point of view it is important to know the precise topography of the tumour in relation to the pituitary stalk and the optic chiasm, which are usually located posterior to the craniopharyngioma. In one third of the cases the tumour is situated posterior to the optic chiasm (Baskin and Wilson, 1986; Tindall and Barrow, 1986).

Of craniopharyngiomas, 80% contain calcification and may be identified on plain films. Nodular and/or curvilinear calcifications are usually associ- ated with morphological changes within the sellar area. Enlargement of the sella, median symmetrical depression of the sellar floor, erosion of the dorsum sellae, and verticalization of the chiasmatic sulcus are the main

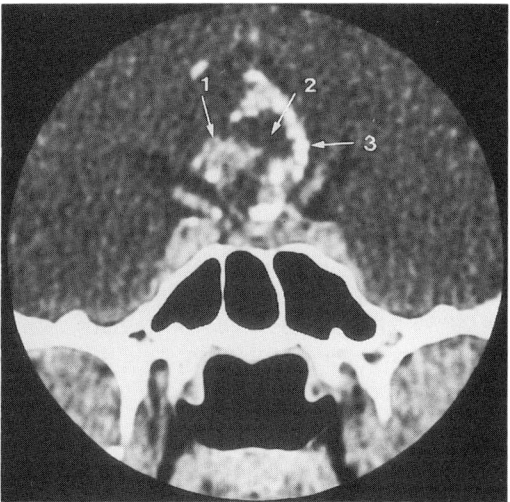

Figure 22. Suprasellar craniopharyngioma. Coronal contrast CT scan: 1, solid component; 2, cystic component; 3, calcified component.

morphological alterations observed on lateral and frontal radiographs (Bonneville and Dietemann, 1981).

Sensitivity of high-resolution CT is near 100%: only very small cystic tumours may be missed. The CT appearance is related to the presence of a solid, cystic or calcified component (Figure 22):

1. *The cystic portion* appears usually of low density with densities ranging from 0 to 20 HU. However isodense or hyperdense cysts are not exceptional. High attenuation values within cystic portions are related to a high cystic protein concentration (Braun et al, 1982; Dietemann and Bonneville, 1985a; Dietemann et al, 1985; Bonneville et al, 1986a; Diebler and Dulac, 1987; Young et al, 1987).
2. *The calcified portion* appears of high density. Calcifications may be nodular or linear with cyst walls (Gardeur et al, 1979).
3. *The solid portion* appears isodense or with low attenuation values. Enhancement is usually noted in the solid component (Fitz et al, 1978).

Intrasellar craniopharyngiomas may lead to an upward displacement of the pituitary gland (pseudoectopic pituitary gland) (Decker, 1985; Hori, 1985; Colohan et al, 1987).

Evaluation of tumour extension towards the foramen of Monro, the subfrontal area or the posterior fossa is possible with axial, coronal, and reformatted sagittal CT scans. However, MRI offers better delineation of the tumour and relation of the tumour to the optic chiasm is easily obtained on sagittal T1-weighted MRI (Freeman et al, 1987).

MENINGIOMAS

Meningiomas arise from meningoendothelial cells located in the arachnoid villi. Meningiomas of the suprasellar region arise usually in the presellar area (planum sphenoidale, chiasmatic sulcus), from the tuberculum sellae, the medial sphenoid wing, and exceptionally from the optic nerve sheath or the diaphragma sellae. Parasellar meningiomas occur mainly in adult women. When discovered, these tumours are usually large and cause stretching and compression of the optic pathways. Pituitary dysfunction or raised intracranial pressure is rather rare. The extensive use of CT allows incidental discovery of numerous small presellar meningiomas.

Frontal and lateral skull plain films reveal bony changes in 70% of the cases. Hyperostosis and blistering of the planum sphenoidale and/or chiasmatic sulcus, and calcifications are the usual findings in presellar meningiomas (Bonneville and Dietemann, 1981).

CT scan may establish diagnosis of presellar meningioma. The tumour appears either isodense or hyperdense. Marked homogeneous enhancement is usually noted after contrast infusion (Figure 23a,b). Calcifications are rather rarely observed. Low density areas reflect cystic or necrotic portions. Marked white matter oedema involving the frontal lobes is noted

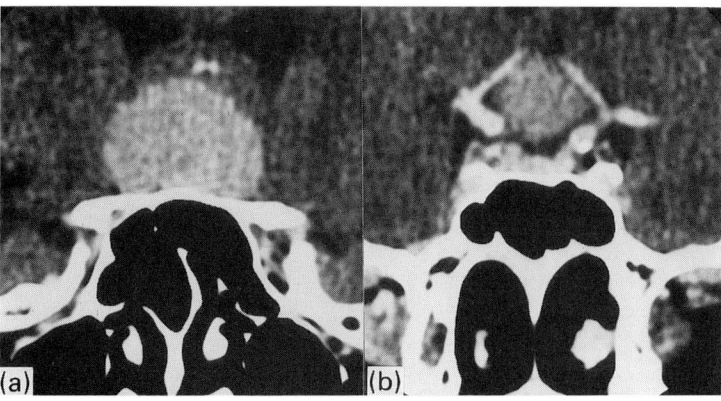

Figure 23. Meningioma of the planum sphenoidale. Coronal enhanced CT scans. (a) At the presellar level. Huge homogeneous enhanced tumour arising from the planum sphenoidale. Slight upward convexity of the planum ('blistering'). (b) At the midsellar level. The pituitary gland below the tumour appears normal.

in most of large presellar meningiomas. Coronal and sagittal reformatted scans are useful to demonstrate hyperostosis and blistering in the area of origin of the tumour (Bonneville et al, 1986a; Tindall and Barrow, 1986). Gadolinium-enhanced MRI using frontal, sagittal, and axial scans allows an accurate evaluation of presellar meningiomas.

OPTIC CHIASM AND HYPOTHALAMIC GLIOMAS

Gliomas of optic pathways usually occur before the age of 20. Von Recklinghausen's neurofibromatosis is present in 70% of single and in 100% of multicentric optic nerve gliomas, but only in 8% of optic chiasm gliomas (Tindall and Barrow, 1986). Visual failure appears progressively. Large tumours may involve the hypothalamus and the anterior third ventricle and result in endocrinopathies (panhypopituitarism, precocious puberty, diabetes insipidus) and in raised intracranial pressure.

Plain films often appear normal. Enlargement and excavation of the chiasmatic sulcus, erosion of the anterior clinoid processes, erosion of the dorsum sellae, and enlargement of the optic canals may be observed (Bonneville and Dietemann, 1981; Savoiardo et al, 1981).

Optic nerves and chiasma can be delineated on enhanced axial and coronal CT scans. In patients with a small suprasellar cistern, intrathecal contrast is needed. In optic chiasma glioma, coronal CT reveals a globulous chiasm. A chiasm more than 6 mm in thickness is suggestive of a tumour (Figure 24a,b). Optic chiasm glioma usually appears isodense with a more or less marked enhancement (Bonneville et al, 1986a; Flechter et al, 1986; Gillett and Symon, 1987), but MRI now offers precise delineation of the optic chiasm and optic tracts.

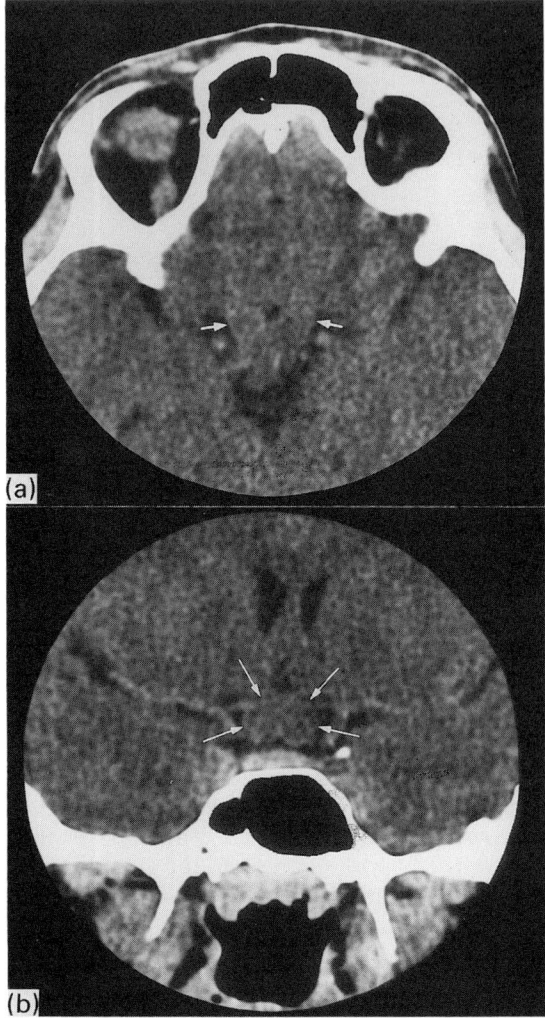

Figure 24. Optic nerves and chiasm glioma—native CT scan. (a) Axial section: enlargement of the optic chiasm and both intracranial optic nerves (arrows). (b) Coronal section: globulous optic chiasm (arrows). The pituitary gland is normal, separated from the chiasm by a thin layer of cerebrospinal fluid.

RARE PITUITARY AND PARASELLAR DISORDERS

Rare pituitary and parasellar lesions may appear spontaneously with low or high attenuation values, or enhance after contrast injection (Naidich et al, 1976; Daniels et al, 1981; Dietemann et al, 1985).

Vascular lesions

Intracavernous carotid artery aneurysms may extend into the pituitary fossa and compress the pituitary gland, causing hypopituitarism and/or hyper-prolactinaemia. Large suprasellar aneurysms may compress the pituitary stalk. Eggshell calcifications usually outline large aneurysms. Postcontrast CT scans delineate the non-thrombosed portion of the vascular malformation (MacPherson and Anderson, 1981; Kline et al, 1982; Bonneville et al, 1986a).

Malignant neoplastic lesions

Metastases to the pituitary are particularly frequent from breast and bronchial carcinomas. Posterior pituitary is more frequently involved than the anterior pituitary (Kovacs, 1973; Zager and Hedley-Whyte, 1987). However, clinical signs and radiological modifications related to pituitary metastases are rather unusual. Enhanced CT scans may reveal an enlarged pituitary gland. *Metastases to the pituitary stalk or the hypothalamus* appear on postcontrast CT as rounded, hyperdense suprasellar tumours.

   Primary pituitary carcinomas are rare and usually endocrine inactive. Extracranial metastases are possible (Tindall and Barrow, 1986). *Primary pituitary sarcomas* are usually reported after radiotherapy for pituitary adenoma (Martin et al, 1980). Rapid evolution, significant destruction of sellar walls and large parasellar extension may be observed in primary pituitary carcinomas and sarcomas.

Benign neoplastic lesions

Lesions with low attenuation values

Large pituitary *Rathke's cleft cysts* may become symptomatic. CT reveals an isodense or hypodense intrasellar mass and ring-enhancement may be noted (Figure 25) (Dietemann et al, 1983a; Kucharczyk et al, 1987). Supra- and intrasellar *arachnoid cysts* have CSF-like attenuation values (Bonneville et al, 1986a; Gentry et al, 1986; Diebler and Dulac, 1987; Meyer et al, 1987). *Parasitic cysts* (cysticercosis, hydatic cyst) are unusual findings. CSF densities are noted within the mass. *Dermoid* and *epidermoid cysts* usually appear hypodense on CT with, respectively, fatty and CSF densities. Rarely, epidermoid cysts appear spontaneously hyperdense (Schubiger et al, 1983).

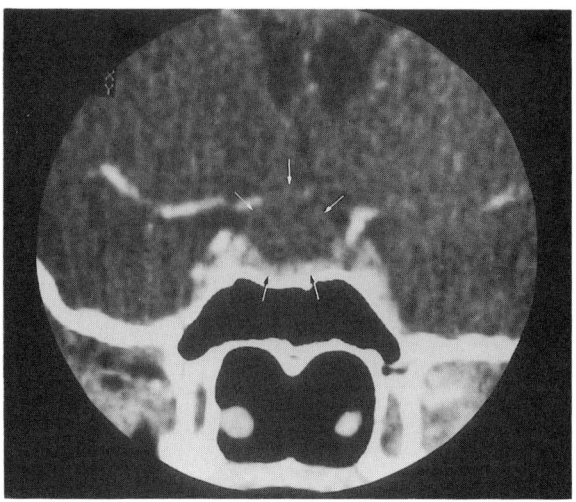

Figure 25. Rathke's cleft cyst. Coronal enhanced CT scan. The isodense rounded intrasellar tumour with suprasellar extent (white arrows) compresses the pituitary gland which is well identified below the cyst (black and white arrows).

Enhancing lesions

Inflammatory lesions are usually enhanced on postcontrast CT scans. Lepto-meningitis resulting from sarcoidosis or tuberculous meningitis are demon-strated by a massive enhancement in the suprasellar cisterns. Intrasellar tuberculoma may also be observed (Esposito et al, 1987). Histiocytosis X is usually located within the hypothalamus but may also be located in the pituitary gland (Nishio et al, 1987). Lymphocytic hypophysitis is a rare inflammatory pathology involving the pituitary during or after pregnancy (Bonneville et al, 1986a; Vanneste and Kamphorst, 1987). Pituitary abscess appears as a low attenuation lesion with ring-enhancement (Enzmann and Sieling, 1983).

Granular cell tumours (choristomas) and pituicytomas (pilocytic astro-cytomas) arise from the posterior lobe of the pituitary stalk and present as enhancing masses (Rossi et al, 1987).

Miscellaneous enhancing lesions may develop within the pituitary: haemangioblastoma, leiomyoma, melanoma, schwannoma, choriocarcinoma, haemangiopericytoma, germinoma, or myxoma (Bonneville et al, 1986a; Nagatami et al, 1987).

Calcified lesions

Pituitary 'calculus' is an amorphous intrasellar calcification lying within the anterior lobe of the pituitary gland. Patients are usually old and free of clinical and biological endocrine disorders (Bonneville et al, 1986a).

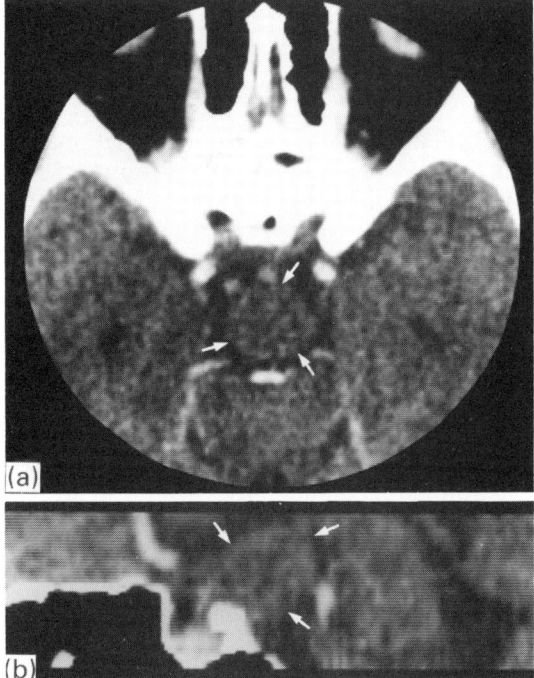

Figure 26. Hypothalamic hamartoma. (a) Axial and (b) Sagittal reformatted enhanced CT scans. Isodense suprasellar mass (arrows) located behind the optic chiasm and extending into the interpeduncular cistern.

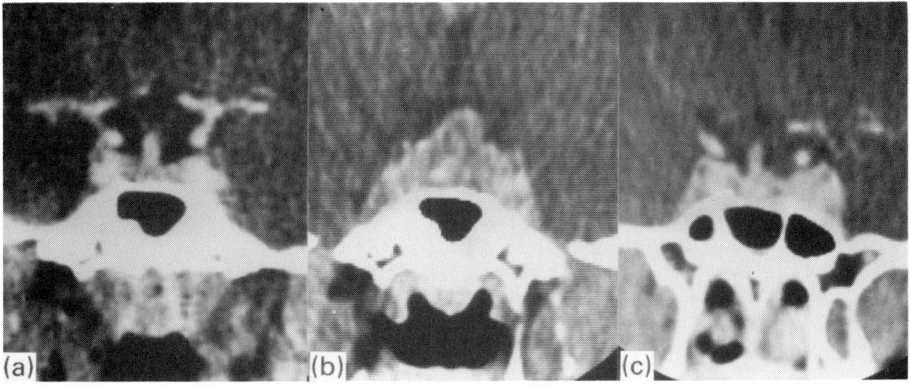

Figure 27. Intra- and suprasellar germinoma. Diabetes insipidus and progressive pituitary deficiency for 1 year. (a) Coronal enhanced CT scan. Discrete enlargement and marked enhancement of the pituitary stalk. (b) One year later. Marked enlargement of the pituitary stalk and sellar content. (c) After radiotherapy. The height and density of the pituitary gland appear normal. The pituitary stalk is also quite normal.

Endocrine disorders

Prolonged end organ failure may induce secondary hyperplasia or adenoma of the pituitary gland (Danzinger et al, 1979; Floyd et al, 1984; Fuji et al, 1987).

Precocious puberty leads sometimes to diagnosis of hypothalamic hamartoma. CT reveals an isodense non-enhancing suprasellar tumour located behind the pituitary stalk (Figure 26a,b) (Grosvalet et al, 1981; Kyuma et al, 1985; Bonneville et al, 1986a; Rieth et al, 1987).

Diabetes insipidus may be related to a suprasellar tumour, germinoma being the commonest one responsible (Figure 27a–c) (Manelfe and Louvet, 1976; Dietemann et al, 1983a; Dietemann et al, 1985).

Idiopathic pituitary dwarfism may be associated with a small partial empty sella. On coronal CT scans the height of the pituitary gland appears reduced (Bonneville and Dietemann, 1981; Bonneville et al, 1986a). MRI may reveal absence of the posterior lobe within the pituitary fossa associated with transection of the pituitary stalk. Ectopic posterior lobe may develop within the hypothalamus. Idiopathic pituitary dwarfism with an abnormal pituitary stalk may be related to an injury to the stalk probably at delivery (Fujisawa et al, 1987).

SUMMARY

High resolution CT with dynamic scanning, demonstrating the pituitary tuft, the pituitary enhancement and the related vascular structures, is of major benefit for the diagnosis of pituitary lesions. Perfection of examination techniques is essential for accurate application of the modality to detect subtle diagnostic signs. A good knowledge of normal anatomy and variants of the sella turcica and pituitary gland permits one to avoid most of the misdiagnoses. Since the CT findings are often non-specific to tissues, clinical endocrinological correlation is essential. The technique also allows consistent assessment of the extent of the disease to permit better treatment planning and effective follow-up of patients after therapy.

REFERENCES

Bachow TB, Hesselink JR, Aaron JO, Davis KR & Taveras JM (1984) Fat deposition in the cavernous sinus in Cushing's disease. *Radiology* **153:** 135–136.
Barrow DL, Tindall GT, Kovacs K, Thorner MO, Horvath E & Hoffman JC (1984) Clinical and pathological effects of bromocriptine on prolactin-secreting and other pituitary tumors. *Journal of Neurosurgery* **60:** 1–7.
Baskin DS & Wilson CB (1986) Surgical management of craniopharyngiomas. A review of 74 cases. *Journal of Neurosurgery* **65:** 22–27.
Besser GM (1976) The pituitary fossa: normal or abnormal. *British Journal of Radiology* **49:** 652–653.
Bonneville JF & Dietemann JL (1981) *Radiology of the sella turcica.* Berlin, Heidelberg, New York, Tokyo: Springer-Verlag.
Bonneville JF, Poulignot D, Cattin F, Couturier M, Mollet E & Dietemann JL (1982a) Computed tomographic demonstration of the effect of bromocriptine on pituitary

microadenoma size. *Radiology* **143**: 451–455.

Bonneville JF, Poulignot D, Coche G, Portha C, Cattin F & Bacha M (1982b) Radiological techniques in the diagnosis of microprolactinoma. In Molinatti GM (ed.) *A clinical problem: microprolactinoma. Diagnosis and treatment*, p 57. Amsterdam, Oxford, Princeton: Excerpta Medica.

Bonneville JF, Poulignot D, Cattin F, Couturier M, Mollet E & Dietemann JL (1982c) Apport des méthodes nouvelles dans l'exploration morphologique des tumeurs hypophysaires. *Annales d'Endocrinologie* (Paris), **43**: 303–308.

Bonneville JF, Cattin F, Moussa-Bacha K & Portha C (1983a) Dynamic computed tomography of the pituitary gland: the 'tuft sign'. *Radiology* **149**: 145–148.

Bonneville JF, Cattin F, Poulignot D, Dietemann JL & Couturier M (1983b) Value of high-resolution CT in the follow-up of prolactinomas treated with bromocriptine. In Tolis G (ed.) *Human Prolactin*. New York: Raven Press.

Bonneville JF, Dietemann JL, Cattin F & Portha C (1983c) Radiologie de la selle turcique: les grands principes de l'interprétation. *Feuillets de Radiologie* **23**: 103–118.

Bonneville JF, Cattin F, Portha C, Cuenin E, Clere P & Bartholomot B (1985) Computed tomographic demonstration of the posterior pituitary. *American Journal of Neuroradiology* **6**: 889–892.

Bonneville JF, Cattin F & Dietemann JL (1986a) *Computed tomography of the pituitary gland*. Berlin, Heidelberg, New York, Tokyo: Springer-Verlag.

Bonneville JF, Cattin F & Dietemann JL (1986b) The convex pituitary gland. *24th meeting of the American Society of Neuroradiology*, San Diego, 22 January 1986.

Braun IF, Pinto RS & Epstein F (1982) Dense cystic craniopharyngiomas. *American Journal of Neuroradiology* **3**: 139–141.

Bruneton JN, Drouillard JR, Sabatier JC, Elie GP & Tavernier JF (1979) Normal variants of the sella turcica. *Radiology* **131**: 99–104.

Bursztyn EM, Lavyne MH & Aisen M (1983) Empty sella syndrome with intrasellar herniation of the optic chiasm. *American Journal of Neuroradiology* **4**: 167–168.

Busch W (1951) Die Morphologie der Sella Turcica und ihre Beziehungen zur Hypophyse. *Virchows Archiv. Archives of Pathological Anatomy* **320**: 437–458.

Chambers EF, Turski PA, La Masters D & Newton TH (1982) Regions of low density in the contrast-enhanced pituitary gland: normal and pathologic processes. *Radiology* **144**: 109–113.

Colohan ART, Grady MS, Bonnin JM, Thorner MO, Kovacs K & Jane JA (1987) Ectopic pituitary gland simulating a suprasellar tumor. *Neurosurgery* **20**: 43–48.

Daniels DL, Williams AL, Thornton RS, Meyer GA, Cusick JF & Haughton VM (1981) Differential diagnosis of intrasellar tumors by CT. *Radiology* **141**: 697–701.

Danzinger J, Wallace S, Handel S & Samaan NB (1979) The sella turcica in primary end organ failure. *Radiology* **131**: 111–115.

Decker RE (1985) The ectopic pituitary gland in cases of craniopharyngioma. Report of two cases. *Journal of Neurosurgery* **62**: 291–292.

Derome PJ, Jedynak CP & Peillon F (1980) *Pituitary Adenomas*. Paris: Asclepios.

Diebler C & Dulac O (1987) Pediatric neurology and neuroradiology. Berlin, Heidelberg, New York, Tokyo: Springer-Verlag.

Dietemann JL & Bonneville JF (1985) Radiological Diagnosis of Pituitary Diseases. In Imura H (ed.) *The pituitary gland*, pp 341–361. New York: Raven Press.

Dietemann JL, Bonneville JF, Buchheit F, Cattin F, Heldt N & Wackenheim A (1983a) CT findings in symptomatic Rathke's cleft cysts of the pituitary gland. Report of three cases. *Neuroradiology* **24**: 263–267.

Dietemann JL, Portha C, Cattin F, Mollet E & Bonneville JF (1983b) CT follow-up of microprolactinomas during bromocriptine-induced pregnancy. *Neuroradiology* **25**: 133–138.

Dietemann JL, Bonneville JF, Hirsch E et al (1985) De la nécessité d'examens scanographiques itératifs en pathologie hypothalamo-hypophysaire. *Journal of Neuroradiology* **12**: 113–122.

Earnest FIV, McCullough EC & Frank DA (1981) Fact or artifact: an analysis of artifact in high-resolution CT scanning of the sella. *Radiology* **140**: 109–113.

Enzmann DR & Sieling RJ (1983) CT of pituitary abscess. *American Journal of Neuroradiology* **4**: 79–80.

Esposito V, Fraioli B, Ferrante L & Palma L (1987) Intrasellar tuberculoma: case report. *Neurosurgery* **21:** 721–723.

Fitz CR, Wortzmann G, Harwood-Nash DC, Holgate RC, Barry JF & Boldt DW (1978) CT in craniopharyngiomas. *Radiology* **127:** 687–691.

Flechter WA, Imes K & Hoyt WF (1986) Chiasmal gliomas: appearance and long-term changes demonstrated by computerized tomography. *Journal of Neurosurgery* **65:** 154–159.

Floyd JL, Dorwart RH, Nelson MJ, Mueller GL & Devroede M (1984) Pituitary hyperplasia secondary to thyroid failure: CT appearance. *American Journal of Neuroradiology* **5:** 469–471.

Freeman MP, Kessler RM, Allen JH & Price AC (1987) Craniopharyngioma: CT and MR imaging in nine cases. *Journal of Computer Assisted Tomography* **11:** 810–814.

Fujii T, Misumi S, Onoda K, Fukuda H & Buki Y (1987) Pituitary enlargement with target organ deficiency: hypothyroidism and hypogonadism. *Surgical Neurology* **28:** 390–394.

Fujisawa I, Kikuchi K, Nishimura K et al (1987) Transection of the pituitary stalk: development of an ectopic posterior lobe assessed with MR imaging. *Radiology* **165:** 487–489.

Gardeur D, Nachanakian A, Van Effenterre R, Zamora G & Metzger J (1979) Analyse tomodensitométrique des crâniopharyngiomes. *Journal de Radiologie* **60:** 51–57.

Gentry LR, Smoker WRK, Turski PA, Menezes AH, Ramirez L & Cornell H (1986) Suprasellar arachnoid cyst: CT recognition. *American Journal of Neuroradiology* **7:** 79–86.

Gillett GR & Symon L (1987) Hypothalamic glioma. *Surgical Neurology* **28:** 291–300.

Gold EB (1981) Epidemiology of pituitary adenomas. *Epidemiologic Reviews* **3:** 163–183.

Grosvalet A, Ernest C, Diebler C & Sauvegrain J (1981) CT in precocious puberty of central origin. *Annales de Radiologie* **24:** 32–38.

Guibert-Tranier F, Elie G, Guibert JL, Piton J & Caille JM (1980) Selles turciques vides. Diagnostic TDM. *Journal of Neuroradiology* **7:** 105–109.

Guthrie FW Jr, Ciric I, Hayashida S, Kerr WD Jr & Murphy ED (1981) Pituitary Cushing's syndrome and Nelson's syndrome: diagnostic criteria, surgical therapy and results. *Surgical Neurology* **16:** 316–323.

Haughton VM, Rosebaum AE, Williams AL & Drayer B (1980) Recognizing the empty sella by CT: the infundibulum sign. *American Journal of Neuroradiology* **1:** 527–529.

Hemminghytt S, Kalkhoff RK, Daniels DL et al (1983) Computed tomographic study of hormone-secreting microadenomas. *Radiology* **146:** 65–69.

Hori A (1985) Suprasellar peri-infundibular ectopic adenohypophysis in fetal and adult brains. *Journal of Neurosurgery* **63:** 113–115.

Kline LB, Acker JD & Post JD (1982) CT evaluation of the cavernous sinus. *Ophthalmology* **89:** 374–385.

Kovacs K (1973) Metastatic cancer of the pituitary gland. *Oncology* **27:** 533–542.

Kucharczyk W, Peck WW, Kelley WM, Norman D & Newton TH (1987) Rathke cleft cysts: CT, MR imaging, and pathologic features. *Radiology* **165:** 491–495.

Kyuma Y, Kato E, Sekido K & Kuwabara T (1985) Hypothalamic hamartoma successfully treated by operation. *Journal of Neurosurgery* **62:** 288–290.

Macpherson P & Anderson DE (1981) Radiological differentiation of intrasellar aneurysm from pituitary tumours. *Neuroradiology* **2:** 177–183.

Manelfe C & Louvet JP (1976) CT in diabetes insipidus. *Journal of Computer Assisted Tomography* **3:** 309–316.

Martin WH, Cail WS, Morris JL & Constable WC (1980) Fibrosarcoma after high energy radiation therapy for pituitary adenoma. *American Journal of Roentgenology* **135:** 1087–1090.

Mass S, Norman D & Newton TH (1978) Coronal computed tomography: indications and accuracy. *American Journal of Roentgenology* **131:** 875–879.

Meyer FC, Carpenter SM & Laws ER Jr (1987) Intrasellar arachnoid cysts. *Surgical Neurology* **28:** 105–110.

Mohr G & Hardy J (1982) Hemorrhage, necrosis, and apoplexy in pituitary adenomas. *Surgical Neurology* **18:** 181–189.

Nagao S, Kinugasa K & Nishimoto A (1987) Obliteration of the primary empty sella by transsphenoidal extradural balloon inflation: technical note. *Surgical Neurology* **27:** 455–458.

Nagatami M, Mori S, Takimoto N et al (1987) Primary myxoma in the pituitary fossa: case report. *Neurosurgery* **20:** 329–331.

Naidich TP, Pinto RS, Kushner MJ et al (1976) Evaluation of sellar and parasellar masses by computed tomography. *Radiology* **120:** 91–99.

Nishio S, Mizuno J, Barrow DL, Takei Y & Tindall GT (1987) Isolated histiocytosis X of the pituitary gland: case report. *Neurosurgery* **21:** 718–721.

Peyster RG & Hoover ED (1984) CT of the abnormal pituitary stalk. *American Journal of Neuroradiology* **5:** 49–52.

Popa G & Fielding U (1930) A portal circulation from the pituitary to the hypothalamic region. *Journal of Anatomy* **65:** 88–91.

Rhoton AL, Harris FS & Renn WH (1977) Microsurgical anatomy of the sellar region and cavernous sinus. *Clinical Neurosurgery* **24:** 54–85.

Rhoton AL Jr, Hardy DG & Chambers SM (1979) Microsurgical anatomy and dissection of the sphenoid bone, cavernous sinus and sellar region. *Surgical Neurology* **12:** 63–104.

Richmond IL & Wilson CB (1978) Pituitary adenomas in childhood and adolescence. *Journal of Neurosurgery* **49:** 163–168.

Rieth KG, Comite F, Dwyer AJ et al (1987) CT of cerebral abnormalities in precocious puberty. *American Journal of Neuroradiology* **8:** 283–290.

Rilliet B, Mohr G, Robert F & Hardy J (1981) Calcifications in pituitary adenomas. *Surgical Neurology* **15:** 249–255.

Roppolo HMN & Latchaw RE (1984) Normal pituitary gland: 2. Macroscopic anatomy CT correlation. *American Journal of Neuroradiology* **4:** 937–944.

Rossi ML, Bevan JS, Esiri MM, Hughes JT & Adams CB (1987) Pituicytoma (pilocytic astrocytoma). Case report. *Journal of Neurosurgery* **67:** 768–772.

Savoiardo M, Harwood-Nash DC, Tadmor R, Scotti G & Musgrane MA (1981) Gliomas of the intracranial anterior optic pathways in children. *Radiology* **138:** 601–610.

Schubiger O, Valavanis A & Gessaga E (1983) Dense supra-sellar epidermoid cyst. A case report. *Neuroradiology* **24:** 269–271.

Swanson JA, Sherman BM, Van Gilder JC & Chapler FK (1979) Coexistent empty sella and prolactin-secreting microadenoma. *American Journal of Obstetrics and Gynecology* **53:** 258.

Swartz JD, Russel KB, Basile BA, O'Donnell PC & Popky GL (1983) High-resolution CT appearance of the intrasellar contents in women of childbearing age. *Radiology* **147:** 115–117.

Syvertsen A, Haughton VM, Williams AL & Cusick JI (1979) The computed tomographic appearance of the normal pituitary gland and pituitary microadenomas. *Radiology* **133:** 385–391.

Tindall GT & Barrow DL (1986) *Disorders of the pituitary*. St Louis, Toronto, Princeton: Mosby.

Turski PA, Newton TH & Horten BH (1981) Sellar contour: anatomic-polytomographic correlation. *American Journal of Roentgenology* **137:** 213–216.

Vanneste JAL & Kamphorst W (1987) Lymphocytic hypophysis. *Surgical Neurology* **28:** 145–149.

Wislocki GB (1938) The vascular supply of the hypophysis cerebri of the rhesus monkey and man. *Research Publications—Association for Research in Nervous and Mental Disease* **17:** 48–68.

Wolpert SM, Post KD, Biller BJ & Molitch ME (1979) The value of computed tomography in evaluating patients with prolactinomas. *Radiology* **131:** 117–119.

Wortzman G & Rewcastle NB (1982) Tomographic abnormalities simulating pituitary microadenomas. *American Journal of Neuroradiology* **3:** 505–512.

Xuereb GB, Prichard MML & Daniel PM (1954) The hypophysial portal system of vessels in man. *Quarterly Journal of Experimental Physiology* **39:** 219–230.

Young WF, Ospina LF, Wesolowski D & Touma A (1981) The primary empty sella syndromes diagnosis with metrizamide cisternography. *Journal of the American Medical Association* **246:** 2611–2612.

Young SC, Zimmermann RA, Nowell MA et al (1987) Giant cystic craniopharyngiomas. *Neuroradiology* **29:** 468–473.

Zager EL & Hedley-Whyte ET (1987) Metastasis within the pituitary adenoma presenting with bilateral abducens palsies: case report and review of the literature. *Neurosurgery* **21:** 383–386.

3

Hypothalamic–pituitary region: magnetic resonance imaging

JULIAN C. CHEN
WALTER KUCHARCZYK

Magnetic resonance imaging (MRI) is an excellent means of assessing the hypothalamic–pituitary axis. Many reports have demonstrated the utility of MRI in delineating the intricate anatomy of this region and in detecting various neoplastic and infiltrative disorders. MRI, still early in its development, already compares favourably with computed tomography (CT). As more research and clinical experience accumulates, MRI shows promise of becoming the imaging modality of choice for pituitary and hypothalamic lesions. This chapter focuses on the MRI findings of various disorders from the clinical perspective.

THE PITUITARY GLAND

Disorders of the pituitary gland may conveniently be categorized functionally as disorders of the anterior lobe (the adenohypophysis) or the posterior lobe (the neurohypophysis). It is also useful to consider the various disease states as disorders of hyper- or hyposecretion of each of the two lobes. Many hypopituitary disorders are related to pathologies affecting the hypothalamus.

Hypersecretory states of the anterior lobe

Pituitary adenomas

Pituitary adenomas are benign neoplasms arising from the anterior lobe. They may be secretory or non-secretory. Clinically and biochemically the secretory tumours may be further subclassified according to the hormone produced—prolactin-, growth hormone- and ACTH (adrenocorticotrophic hormone)-secreting adenomas are the commonest. Thyroid stimulating hormone (TSH) and, rarely, gonadotropin-producing types are also recognized. 'Mixed tumours' also occur and are most often a prolactin–growth hormone combination.

In general, secretory adenomas present at an earlier stage of their

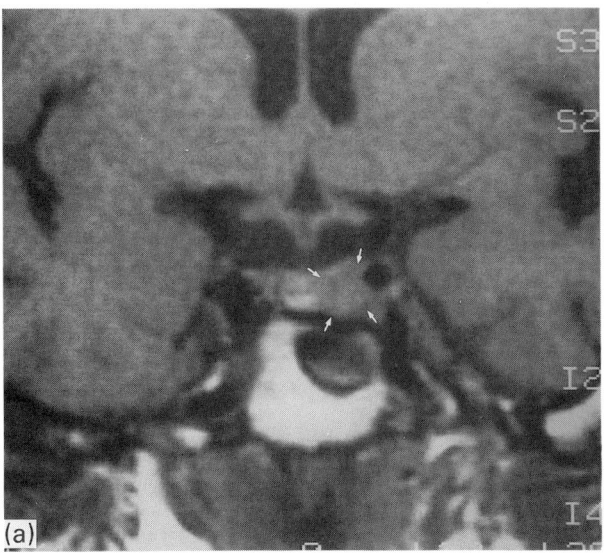

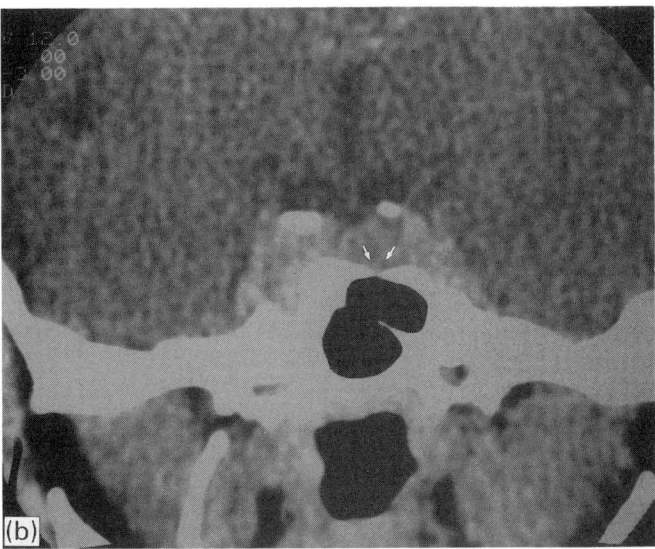

Figure 1. *Pituitary microadenoma.* This 45-year-old woman presented with Cushing's disease. The T1-weighted coronal image (a) shows a low signal nodule in the left pituitary (arrows) typical of pituitary adenomas. Coronal sella CT performed earlier (b) was interpreted as negative, but in retrospect the tumour location is appreciated by the local erosion of the floor of the sella (arrows).

evolution because of their clinically manifest hormonal effects and hence are generally smaller at the time of discovery than non-secretory adenomas. Non-secretory adenomas present at a larger size and usually only when the parasellar structures are disturbed. As no reliable MRI criteria exist to distinguish between non-functioning and the various types of secretory adenomas, the traditional radiological classification of adenomas based on size is still preferred. By convention, microadenomas are less than 1 cm in diameter and macroadenomas are those greater than 1 cm in diameter.

Microadenomas are common. Although the incidence is not known exactly they are often detected incidentally at autopsy and on unrelated MRI studies. Presumably, these incidental adenomas represent non-secretory or low-grade secretory tumours. Their small size and/or lack of significant hormonal activity are the probable reasons for the lack of clinical manifestations. In some autopsy studies, the incidence of 'sub-clinical' adenomas is as high as 45% (Kulkrani et al, 1988).

Microadenomas are best seen on T1-weighted MR images. The most common appearance of a microadenoma on MRI is a focal low signal intensity lesion in the lateral aspect of the gland. On the T2-weighted images the signal intensity is variable. Often there is contralateral displacement of the pituitary stalk or a focal protrusion of the superior margin of the gland upwards. Using these criteria the reported detection rate of microadenomas on MRI has ranged from 55 to 100% depending on the centre, the MR imager, the pulse sequence and the method of patient selection. These figures are comparable to those reported for CT (Figure 1) (Kulcharczyk et al, 1986; Pojunas et al, 1986; Marcovitz et al, 1987; Kulkrani et al, 1988).

As might be expected, the sensitivity of detection decreases for small lesions. For lesions smaller than 3 mm in diameter detection is unreliable, principally due to the limits of spatial resolution of current scanners. Thus small secretory tumours, particularly those that cause Cushing's disease continue to present a diagnostic problem. Further refinements of MR technology and the use of MR contrast agents may improve the detection rate of such lesions. One early report on the use of gadolinium-DPTA (an MR contrast agent) for the detection of ACTH-secretory adenomas documented such an improvement, although the series was small (Dwyer et al, 1987). The authors advocated the use of delayed scanning (longer than 45 min following contrast injection) as a means of further improving the detection rate.

Adenomas grow and expand in a fairly predictable manner. Usually by the time they reach 1 cm or greater in diameter, they have enlarged the sella turcica and extended beyond its confines. Upward expansion above the sella is the commonest direction of extrasellar spread and may result in compression of the optic chiasm, supraclinoid carotid artery or hypothalamus. Often there is a characteristic narrowing or 'waisting' around the equator of the tumour as it grows through the diaphragma sella. On occasions, an adenoma may obtain sufficient size to cause obstructive hydrocephalus by invagination and compression of the third ventricle.

With downward growth, erosion of the sella turcica occurs. Although high-resolution coronal CT is better suited for assessment of bony involvement, the actual lower tumour margin is better appreciated on MRI (Figure 2). Downward extension *per se* does not result in any significant clinical problems in most cases but on rare occasions it may cause CSF rhinorrhea due to complete erosion of the roof of the sphenoid sinus.

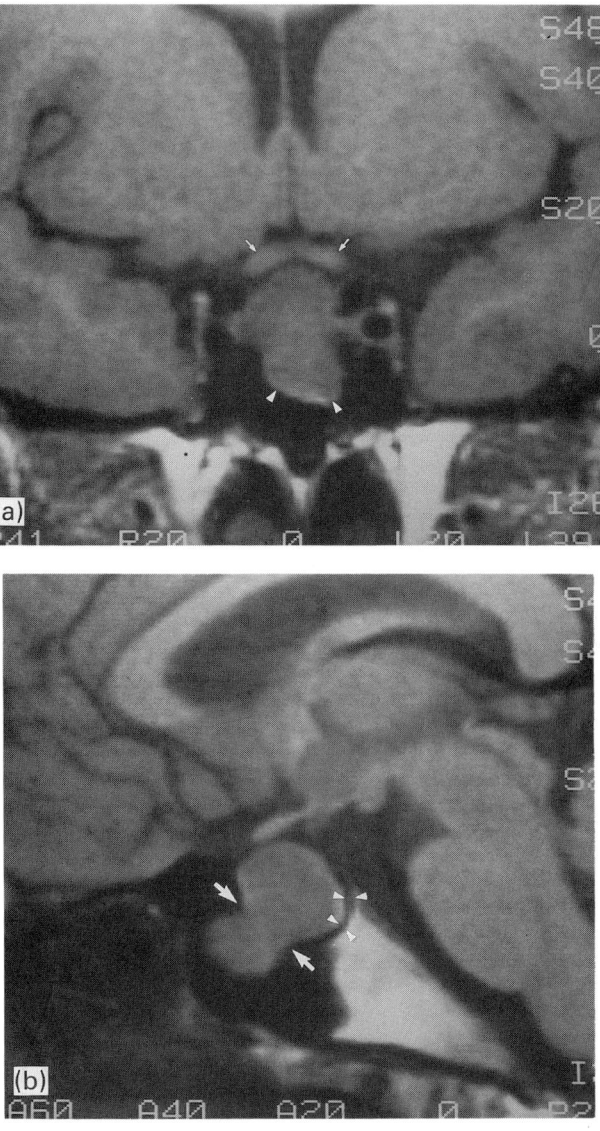

Figure 2. *Large pituitary adenoma.* The T1-weighted coronal image (a) shows the optic chiasm (arrows) which is displaced superiorly. Inferior margin of the adenoma (arrowheads) is within the sphenoid sinus. The sagittal image (b) shows a grossly expanded sellar with an attenuated dorsum sellae (arrowheads). A waist-like narrowing (arrows) demarcates the point where the tumour erodes through the sellar floor into the sphenoid sinus.

Lateral extension is problematic because of the difficulty in determining cavernous sinus involvement. It is difficult to assess accurately early cavernous sinus extension because of the difficulty in delineating the medial dural walls of the cavernous sinus. With gross extension, the tumour may completely fill the cavernous sinus and cause lateral deflection of the lateral cavernous sinus dura. Interestingly, the carotid artery lumen is usually preserved even if completely surrounded by adenoma. Constriction of the arterial lumen should arouse suspicion of another lesion, in particular of meningioma (Scotti et al, 1988).

Although they are histologically benign, invasive pituitary adenomas are an aggressive subset of adenomas which demonstrate a predilection to invade the bony and dural margins of the pituitary gland irrespective of their size or secretory activity. Adenomas with these invasive characteristics are associated with a poor prognosis because total surgical resection is impossible. The only distinguishing imaging feature between these aggressive lesions and their more benign counterparts is the dural and bony extension of tumour spread in the former group.

Pituitary hyperplasia

Pituitary hyperplasia may occur as a primary event, or with failure of a peripheral endocrine organ such as primary hypothyroidism (Floyd et al, 1984). The MR findings are symmetrical enlargement of the pituitary gland without evidence of a well-defined focal lesion within the parenchyma of the gland.

Hyperprolactinaemia due to suprasellar lesions

Pituitary prolactin secretion is under inhibitory control of the hypothalamus. Therefore, interference with any part of the hypothalamohypophyseal-portal venous system may result in disinhibition of prolactin secretion and thereby cause hyperprolactinaemia. This is most often seen with tumours in the suprasellar cistern, in particular craniopharyngioma, but may also occur with hypothalamic tumours or with physical disruption of the pituitary infundibulum (Lundberg et al, 1981) (Figures 3 and 4). The clinical findings may be difficult to distinguish from a pituitary adenoma. Therefore, the role of MRI in patients with unexplained hyperprolactinaemia is to localize the lesion to the gland or to the suprasellar cistern.

Hypersecretory states due to hypothalamic lesions

The hypothalamus is the major regulatory centre of pituitary function. However, except for one case of a large craniopharyngioma invaginating the hypothalamus causing hyperprolactinaemia, we have never encountered a lesion in the hypothalamus responsible for a hypersecretory state using MRI, nor are we aware of any such reports in the literature. If such lesions exist, they are either exceedingly rare or they are not visible by MRI (or CT for that matter).

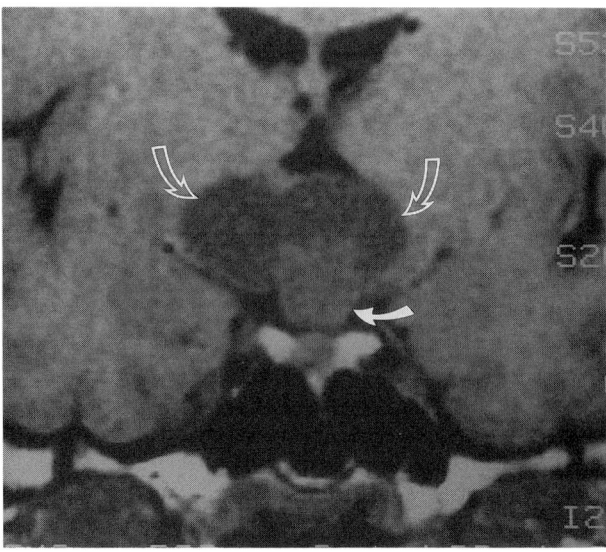

Figure 3. *Craniopharyngioma*. T1-weighted coronal image. This patient presented with hyper-prolactinaemia. A large suprasellar mass with cystic (open arrows) and solid (solid arrow) components is seen. The floor of the third ventricle is pushed superiorly by the tumour. In most cases craniopharyngioma cyst is bright on T1-weighted images. This case is unusual in this regard.

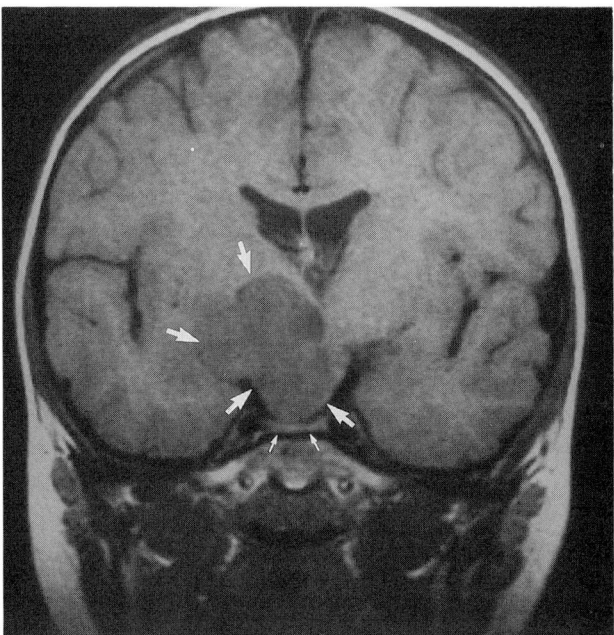

Figure 4. *Hypothalamic glioma*. T1-weighted coronal image. A lobulated mass (large arrows) is seen arising from the hypothalamic area, slightly displacing the lateral ventricle and obliterating the third ventricle. Compressed pituitary gland can be seen below the tumour (small arrows). Hypothalamic dysfunction was demonstrated clinically.

Hyposecretory states of the anterior lobe

Virtually any destructive or compressive lesion originating in the hypo-thalamus, pituitary stalk, optic chiasm, parasellar vessels, or the pituitary gland can lead to endocrine failure of the pituitary gland. Usually these lesions cause global loss of hormonal secretion rather than selective loss of any one type of hormone. Many times hypopituitarism is dominated by other clinical findings such as visual loss, headache or opthalmoplegia and the hormonal deficiency only discovered on laboratory testing. The various lesions that can cause hypopituitarism are herein discussed although very often the degree of pituitary dysfunction is minimal.

Congenital/developmental

Absence of the pituitary gland or various degrees of pituitary hypoplasia may occur in isolation, or in association with other midline congenital anomalies such as sphenoid encephaloceles. Depending on the degree of the anomaly, MRI may show complete absence or hypoplasia of gland, a small sella turcica, and other midline anomalies if they exist.

Pituitary-deficient dwarfs have been found to have a unique combination of findings on T1-weighted MR images: a small sella turcica, a small pituitary gland and absence of the distal pituitary stalk. The proximal pituitary stalk is thickened and contains a small, high intensity nodule, the nodule represent-ing an ectopic posterior pituitary lobe (Figure 5). Abnormalities of the hypothalamus have not been observed on MRI. It is thought that a perinatal ischaemic or traumatic insult to the distal stalk and pituitary gland results in

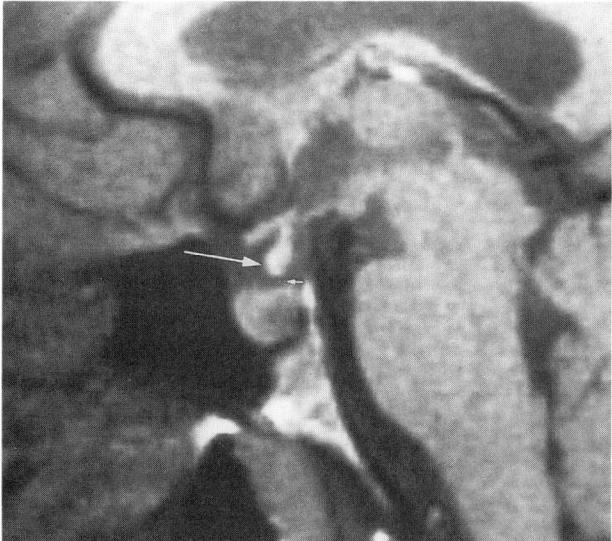

Figure 5. *Pituitary dwarfism.* T1-weighted sagittal image. A high signal area (large arrow) is seen in the pituitary stalk which is thought to represent an ectopic posterior lobe. Pituitary stalk is absent (small arrow). This 27-year-old man was 4 feet 11 inches tall. He presented with global reduction in anterior pituitary lobe function without diabetes insipidus.

arrest of development. The gland remains hypoplastic and the neurohypophysis ceases in its descent, remaining at the tip of the truncated infundibulum. The neurohypophysis is functionally intact, albeit in an aberrant position, and therefore there is no clinical deficit in posterior lobe function. However, the anterior lobe becomes atrophic resulting in deficiencies of anterior lobe hormones (Kelly et al, 1988).

Trauma

Transection of the pituitary stalk results from an acceleration–rotation type injury, most commonly occurring in motor vehicle accidents. Disruption of the delicate reticular network of vessels around the stalk may lead to ischaemic damage of the pituitary gland. However, the severity of associated head injuries is such that patients rarely survive long enough to manifest hypopituitarism.

Neoplasms

Meningioma. Meningiomas arise from the dural reflections in and around the suprasellar region particularly on the tuberculum sellae. They have a wide-based dural attachment. Their signal characteristics are similar to grey matter. In addition, their slow growth and minimal tissue reaction make detection difficult. Because of the frequent incidence of calcification and marked X-ray contrast enhancement, CT is the diagnostic method of choice. MRI contrast agents have been shown to enhance the intensity of meningiomas on MRI similar to that seen on CT. The use of MR contrast agents will undoubtedly improve the accuracy of MR imaging for the detection of this type of tumour.

Craniopharyngioma. Craniopharyngiomas and related Rathke's Pouch-derived tumours can occur anywhere along the remnant of the craniopharyngeal tract. Of craniopharyngiomas, about 25% are found in an intrasellar location, about 50% in the suprasellar cistern and the remaining 25% bridge both locations. They are most commonly seen in children but can also occur throughout adulthood. Most often they consist of cystic and solid parts (see Figure 3). The cyst often contains degraded blood products, cholesterol crystals or proteinatious materials. The solid phase of the tumour may be fleshy or mineralized. The MRI appearance closely reflects these physical components of the tumour. On the T1-weighted images the solid phase is an intermediate grey intensity, calcified portions dark, and the cystic portion from very bright to dark (Pusey et al, 1987).

Rathke's cleft cysts are common as incidental findings at autopsy but they seldom cause hormonal disturbances because they are too small to affect the gland. Occasionally they may enlarge sufficiently to produce a neurological or endocrine disturbance through compression. Most often they arise anterior to the pituitary stalk or in the anterior half of the sella turcica. The cyst contents usually appear identical to CSF on both the T1- and T2-weighted images. However the cyst may also contain abundant desquamated cellular material or mucinous fluid and thus they may be indistinguishable from craniopharyngiomas (Kucharczyk et al, 1987).

Other tumours. The area around the sella turcica is host to many different types of neoplasms including but not limited to optic glioma, germinoma, teratoma, chordoma, nasopharyngeal carcinoma, and metastases. These are all relatively uncommon. They may all cause different types of pituitary disturbance but usually other clinical deficits are more prominent and they will not be discussed further.

Ischaemia and vascular disease

Sheehan's syndrome used to be one of the commoner causes of hypo-pituitarism in women. The currently accepted explanation is that hypo-perfusion of the gland in the peri- and post-partum period is followed by reperfusion resulting in haemorrhage into the gland (Figure 6). It is thought that the enlarged pituitary gland present in pregnancy is more susceptible to such ischaemic insults. Clinically there is sudden loss of pituitary function, headache and often visual loss, a symptom complex at times termed 'pituitary apoplexy'. Pituitary apoplexy may also occur in patients with a previously unrecognized adenoma.

Aneurysms of the distal internal carotid artery or its branches can

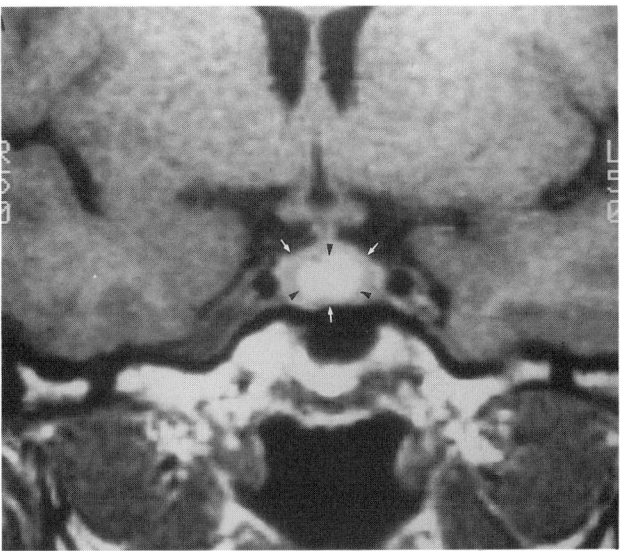

Figure 6. *Pituitary haemorrhage.* T1-weighted coronal image. This patient had a prolactinoma. The images obtained one day after delivery show a high signal intensity lesion (black arrow-heads) corresponding to an acute haematoma centrally in the grossly expanded pituitary gland (white arrows). She did not have any specific endocrine problem on follow-up medical investigations, probably due to the small size of haemorrhage. Larger haemorrhagic lesions can cause pituitary apoplexy leading to hypopituitarism.

occasionally cause compression of the hypothalamus or pituitary gland (Figure 7). This may also occur with a large basilar tip aneurysm. On MRI, the lesion appears as a globular sac, dark if the lumen is patent and bright if the lumen is thrombosed. Vasculitis and cerebral vascular occlusive disorders can also rarely be causes of hypopituitarism.

Inflammation

Granulomatous processes sporadically cause hypopituitarism through hypothalamic and pituitary involvement. In sarcoidosis (Figure 8) and tuberculosis, the lesion appears as a focus of increased signal intensity on T2-weighted images in the hypothalamus, pituitary gland or brain parenchyma. Usually, hypothalamic disturbances predominate over those referable to the pituitary gland.

Metabolic disorders

Haemochromatosis may affect the pituitary gland. The blood–brain barrier offers protection of the brain from excess plasma iron. However, the median eminence and the pituitary lack an effective blood–brain barrier and hence are vulnerable to iron toxicity. If sufficient iron is deposited, the affected regions appear dark on the T2-weighted images (Drayer et al, 1986).

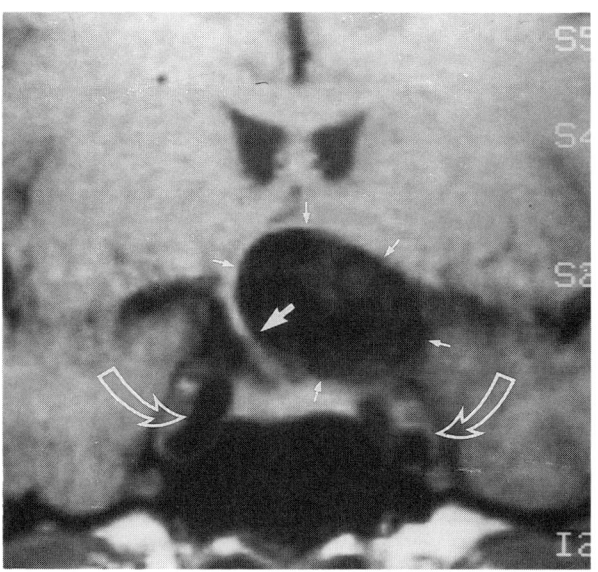

Figure 7. *Giant aneurysm.* T1-weighted coronal image. Gross displacement of the pituitary stalk (large solid arrow), hypothalamus, and chiasm is caused by a large low signal mass (small arrows) corresponding to a giant aneurysm arising from the termination of the left internal carotid artery. Patent left and right carotid arteries are seen in the cavernous sinuses bilaterally (open arrows).

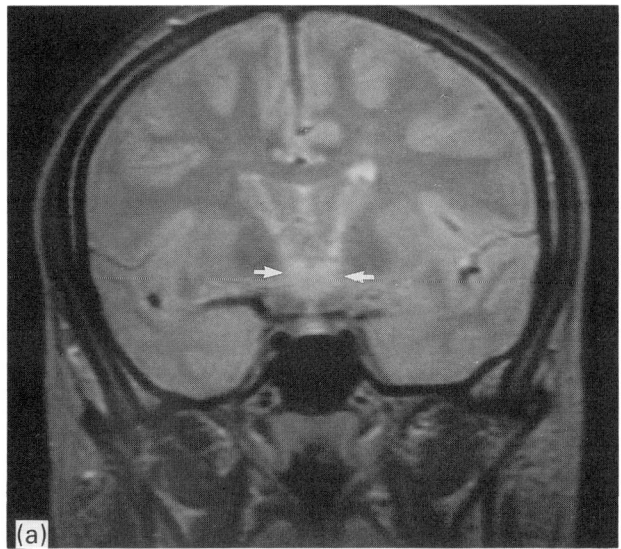

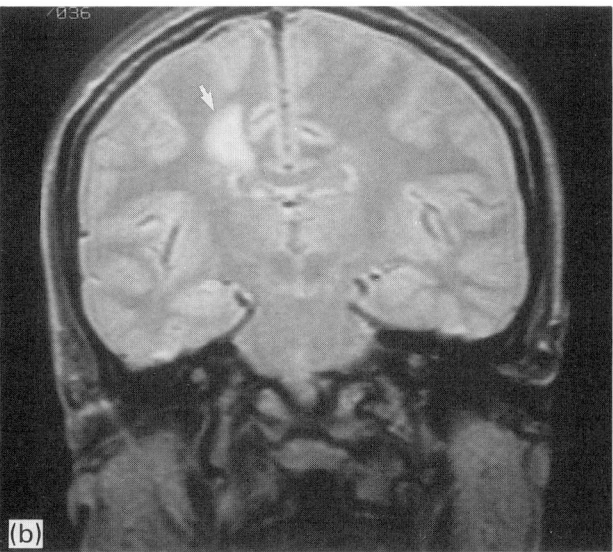

Figure 8. *Diabetes insipidus secondary to sarcoidosis.* Proton-Density Coronal Images A and B. (a) Increased signal from the hypothalamic area (two arrows) and (b) paraventricular cortical white matter (single arrow) are seen in this young black woman with a history of sarcoidosis. Both the clinical and MR findings resolved with steroid therapy.

Radiation

Pituitary failure can occur in patients receiving therapeutic irradiation for lymphoma, leukaemia, pituitary adenoma, optic tract glioma and other intracranial tumours. The dose at which this occurs is uncertain. The affected area is of high signal intensity on the T2-weighted image and generally has sharp borders corresponding to the margins of the radiation field. It is not certain whether it is primarily hypothalamic failure or pituitary failure responsible for the hormone deficiency. It may be both as both tissues are usually in the same radiation field.

Posterior pituitary lobe dysfunction

The posterior lobe of the pituitary gland can readily be seen as a structure distinct from the rest of the pituitary gland. It is a high signal intensity area occupying the posterior quarter of the sella turcica. The nature of the material responsible for the high signal is unexplained. Vasopressin, the protein carrier (neurophysin), and lipid droplets have all been proposed as the possible sources (Kelly et al, 1988). In patients with diabetes insipidus, this high signal intensity is consistently absent. This absence occurs whatever the cause of the diabetes insipidus whether it be idiopathic, or secondary to the destructive lesions of the hypothalamus, stalk or posterior lobe.

Central (idiopathic) diabetes insipidus is thought to be due to hypothalamic failure of vasopressin secretion. However a hypothalamic lesion has not been identified. The only abnormality noted on MRI is absence of high intensity in the posterior lobe (Figure 9).

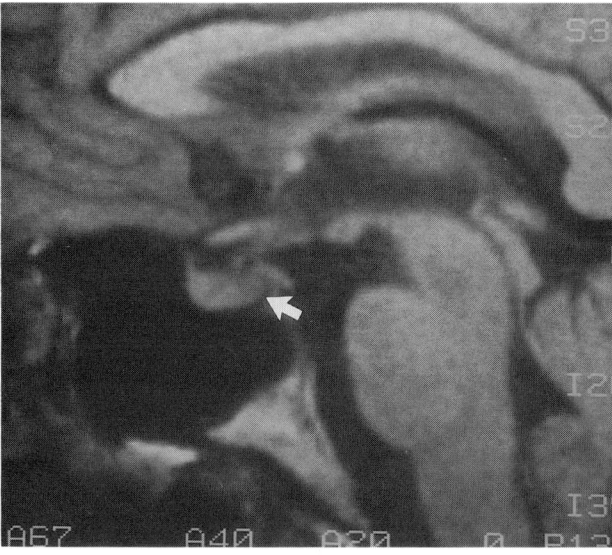

Figure 9. *Idiopathic diabetes insipidus.* T1-weighted sagittal image. There is an absence of the normal hyperintense signal from the posterior lobe (arrow). This 40-year-old man had idiopathic diabetes insipidus.

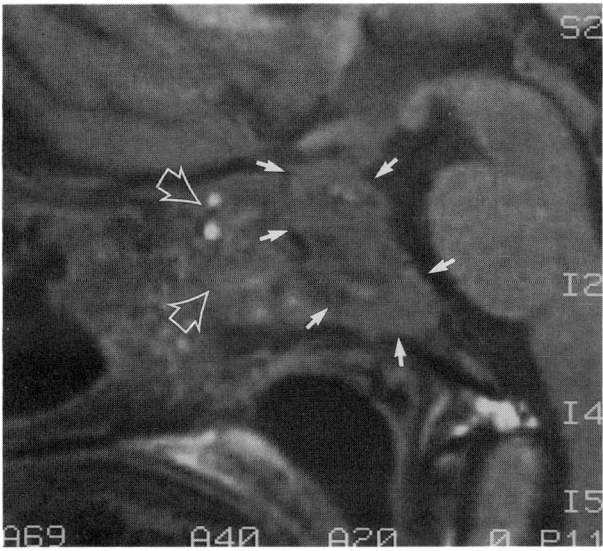

Figure 10. *Diabetes insipidus secondary to metastatic neoplasm.* T1-weighted sagittal image. Breast carcinoma metastasis causing extensive destruction of the sella turcica and sphenoid sinus, and its extension into the nasopharynx are seen (arrows). Postbiopsy changes are noted anteriorly to the tumour (open arrows). This 33-year-old woman presented with diabetes insipidus and amenorrhoea 1 year after radiation treatment.

The secondary causes of diabetes insipidus vary with age groups. In children, histiocytosis-X, hamartomas of the tuber cinereum, suprasellar germinomas and craniopharyngiomas are common. Histiocytosis-X causes thickening of the stalk with an increase in signal on the T2-weighted images. Hamartomas appear as enlargement of the tuber cinereum, usually mildly hyperintense on the T2-weighted images. The various tumours causing diabetes insipidus are visible as nodules or masses in the stalk or in the suprasellar cistern. In adults, the tumours causing diabetes insipidus are most often metastases (Max et al, 1981) (Figure 10), although primary gliomas of the stalk or posterior lobe do occur rarely. Granulomatous processes such as sarcoidosis and tuberculosis can also cause diabetes insipidus (see Figure 8).

THE HYPOTHALAMUS

Many disorders causing hypothalamic dysfunction have been discussed in earlier sections within this chapter with the exception of the hypothalamic glioma. This tumour is most often seen in children and presents usually as a disorder of hypothalamic regulatory function or occasionally as visual loss particularly if there is a large exophytic component compressing the optic chiasm (see Figure 4). The direct multiplanar capability of MRI is helpful in correctly localizing the lesion to the hypothalamus. Occasionally, if the tumour is large it may be inseparable from the optic chiasm. There are no unique distinguishing features in terms of signal intensity. The tumour usually appears dark compared to brain parenchyma on the T1-weighted and bright on the T2-weighted images.

THE 'EMPTY SELLA TURCICA'

The empty sella turcica is a very common finding and in the vast majority of cases can be considered to be a normal variant. On MRI the sella appears as a symmetrically expanded space containing cerebrospinal fluid (Figure 11). The gland is seen as a thin rim of tissue lining the floor of the sellar. The infundibulum traverses the 'empty sella', connecting the hypothalamus to the pituitary gland in the normal manner. The major use of MRI is in excluding a mass lesion as a cause of the expanded sella turcica.

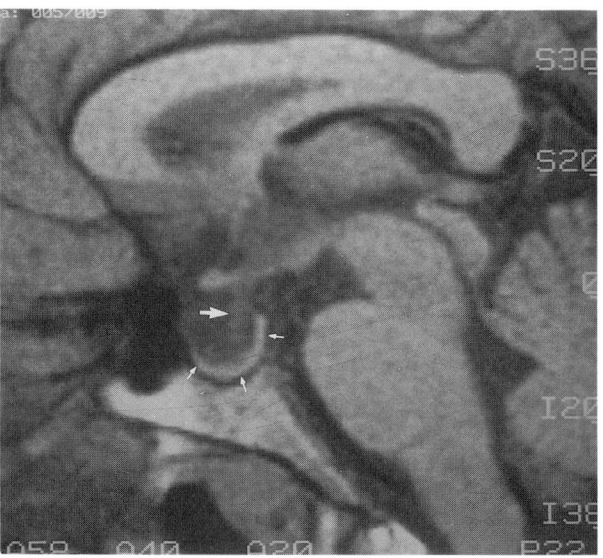

Figure 11. *Empty sella turcica.* T1-weighted sagittal image. Enlargement of the sella turcica and a rim of pituitary tissue (small arrows) are seen. The pituitary stalk is seen in its normal position (larger arrow). This patient had a history of hypertension and recurrent headache; probably unrelated to the MRI findings.

SUMMARY

Endocrine disorders of the hypothalamus and pituitary gland are often caused by lesions which can be accurately detected and delineated by MRI, often with specific findings. MRI has emerged as the imaging modality of choice for pathology of the hypothalamus and other suprasellar structures, and for extrasellar extension of pituitary tumours. The advantage is mainly based on the high contrast resolution, vascular visualization without the need for intravascular contrast and direct multiplanar imaging capability inherent with the technique. CT, however, enjoys much wider availability and better spatial resolution at present. CT is still the method used to detect pituitary microadenomas in most centres, although high field-strength MR scanners and gadolinium enhancement permit thinner sections with improved sensitivity in certain institutes. Further advances in MRI technology are expected to broaden its usefulness in endocrinology.

REFERENCES

Drayer B, Burger P, Darwin R et al (1986) Magnetic resonance imaging of brain iron. *American Journal of Neuroradiology* **7:** 373–380.
Dwyer AJ, Frank JA, Doppman JL et al (1987) Pituitary adenomas in patients with Cushing's disease: initial experience with Gd-DPTA-enhanced MR imaging. *Radiology* **163:** 421–426.
Floyd JL, Dorwart RH, Nelson MJ et al (1984) Pituitary hyperplasia secondary to thyroid failure: CT appearance. *American Journal of Neuroradiology* **5:** 469–471.
Kelly WM, Kucharczyk W, Kucharczyk J et al (1988) Posterior pituitary ectopia: an MR feature of pituitary dwarfism. *American Journal of Neuroradiology* **9:** 453–460.
Kucharczyk W, Davis DO, Kelly WM et al (1986) Pituitary adenomas: high resolution MRI at 1.5-T. *Radiology* **161:** 761–765.
Kucharczyk W, Peck WW, Kelly WM, Norman D & Newton TH (1987) Rathke cleft cysts: CT, MR and pathological features. *Radiology* **165:** 491–495.
Kulkrani MV, Lee KF, McArdle CB, Yeakley JW & Haar FL (1988) 1.5-T MR imaging of pituitary microadenomas: technical consideration and CT correlation. *American Journal of Neuroradiology* **9:** 5–11.
Lundberg PO, Osterman PO & Wide L (1981) Serum prolactin in patients with hypothalamus and pituitary disorders. *Journal of Neurosurgery* **55:** 194–199.
Marcovitz MV, Wee R, Chan J & Hardy J (1987). The diagnostic accuracy of preoperative CT scanning in the evaluation of pituitary ACTH-secreting microadenomas. *American Journal of Neuroradiology* **8:** 641–644.
Max MB, Deck MDF & Rottenberg DA (1981) Pituitary metastasis: incidence in cancer patients and clinical differentiation from pituitary adenoma. *Neurology* **31:** 998–1002.
Pojunas KW, Daniels DL, Williams AL & Haughton VM (1986) MR imaging of prolactin-secreting microadenomas. *American Journal of Neuroradiology* **7:** 209–213.
Pusey E, Kortman KE, Flannigan BD et al (1987) MR of craniopharyngiomas: tumor delineation and characterization. *American Journal of Neuroradiology* **8:** 439.
Scotti G, Yu C-Y, Dillon WP et al (1988) MR imaging of cavernous sinus involvement by pituitary adenomas. *American Journal of Neuroradiology* **9:** 657–664.

4

Multimodality imaging of the thyroid gland

MARTIN P. SANDLER
JAMES A. PATTON
BARRY M. McCOOK

Thyroid disorders affect a wide spectrum of the human population from the neonate to the elderly. Numerous imaging modalities including nuclear medicine, ultrasonography, X-ray fluorescent scanning, computed tomography (CT) and, more recently, magnetic resonance imaging (MRI) have been used for diagnosis in affected patients. This chapter evaluates and correlates the non-invasive imaging procedures currently available to diagnose thyroid disorders.

IMAGING PRINCIPLES

The imaging principles of nuclear medicine, X-ray fluorescent scanning, ultrasonography, and CT are well established. Nuclear medicine techniques enable the assessment of thyroid size, location, and function at the time the study is performed through the use of chemical as well as imaging procedures. They utilize the physiological processes of the glands and radiolabelling of chemicals taken up by the glands. X-ray fluorescent scanning utilizes an external source of radiation to map the stable iodine that has been trapped and stored by the thyroid, in order to assess its past functional status. Ultrasonography utilizes reflected sound waves to identify and evaluate gland size, location, the presence of nodules, and to differentiate between cystic and solid lesions. CT makes use of the attenuation of transmitted X-ray to provide high resolution images of neck anatomy.

MRI makes use of magnetic fields and radiofrequency (RF) waves applied in specific pulse sequences to selected slices in the body. Image contrast is determined by tissue characterization. The advantage of MRI, but also one of its complexities, is the multitude of different types of images that can be produced by varying the RF pulse length and the sequence in which the pulses are applied. High resolution images of neck anatomy can be obtained using sequences that emphasize proton density. To demonstrate pathological lesions, either T1- or T2-weighted images are usually necessary.

The spin–lattice relaxation time (TI) of a tissue depends upon the relationship of the hydrogen atoms to their molecular lattice. Measurements are short where water (rich in hydrogen) is closely bound to proteins, such as in muscle or in fat. In general, malignant tissue has a longer T1 than its normal native tissue, as does oedematous and infected tissue. The T1 parameter is the major constituent of inversion recovery images and produces images of high contrast. The appearance of inversion recovery images may be altered by varying the pulse sequence, a phenomenon that must be understood in order to interpret the images obtained. In addition, signal intensity decreases with increasing T1, a factor that may cause confusion in image interpretation. Calculated T1 images may be obtained using MRI techniques. However calibration of an MR imager must be continually performed to assure precise determination of T1 values in thyroid nodules. In addition, the absolute value of T1 is dependent upon the strength of the magnetic field utilized. Thus, comparison of values between instruments with different magnetic field strengths and resonant frequencies is complex.

Spin–spin relaxation times (T2) are often more sensitive to differences in tissue make-up and therefore T2-weighted images are important in MRI. T2-weighted images are acquired using a spin–echo technique with signal intensity increasing with increasing T2 values. T2 values also are determined by the environment in which the hydrogen protons exist. T2-weighted images tend to be of high spatial resolution and to have high contrast between areas of differing T2 values. Similar attention to the pulse sequence employed in the production of T2 images must be paid, as is necessary when viewing T1-weighted images.

MRI may be applied in any plane and images are routinely produced from axial, coronal, and sagittal planes. An advantage of MRI over CT in sagittal and coronal imaging is that images are constructed directly from data acquired in the chosen image plane and not reconstructed from that acquired in another plane.

CLINICAL APPLICATION

Radionuclides used for thyroid imaging

Technetium-99m (^{99m}Tc) pertechnetate is the most readily available radionuclide employed for thyroid imaging. Pertechnetate ions (TcO_4^-) are trapped by the thyroid in the same manner as iodine through an active transport mechanism, but they are not organified (Andros et al, 1965; Sodee, 1966; Atkins and Richards, 1968; dos Remedios et al, 1971; Burke et al, 1972). Iodine-123 (^{123}I) is both trapped and organified by the thyroid gland, allowing overall assessment of thyroid function. Iodine-123 is produced in a cyclotron, making it scarce and expensive. It also has a relatively short half-life of 13.6 h, making therefore long-term storage a problem: advance notice is usually necessary prior to imaging with this radionuclide. Iodine-131 (^{131}I) was frequently used in thyroid imaging in the past, but due to the high thyroid and total-body radiation dose from its beta emission (Table 1) it is now rarely used outside the study of metastatic thyroid cancer.

Table 1. Radionuclides for thyroid imaging. From Sandler et al (1986).

Radionuclide	Half-life	Photon energy (keV)	Usual dose	Radiation dose to adults (rads) Thyroid	Whole-body
[131]I	8.1 days	364	50 µCi (oral)	75	0.22
[125]I	60 days	28–35	50 µCi (oral)	52	0.17
[123]I	13 h	159	200–400 µCi (oral)	3–6	0.01
[99m]Tc	6 h	140	5–15 mCi (i.v.)	1	0.06

The choice of radionuclide for routine imaging of the thyroid gland is therefore between ^{99m}Tc and [123]I. A disadvantage of imaging with pertechnetate is that it is only trapped and not organified in the follicles. In addition, early imaging following intravenous administration is associated with high background activity. Imaging with ^{99m}Tc, however, frequently provides enough information to serve as an acceptable alternative to [123]I. In those instances where it is thought essential to assess both organification and trapping, ^{123}I scanning can be performed subsequently.

Normal thyroid gland

The normal thyroid gland and anatomic variants can be visualized by numerous imaging modalities including scintigraphy, ultrasound, CT and MRI.

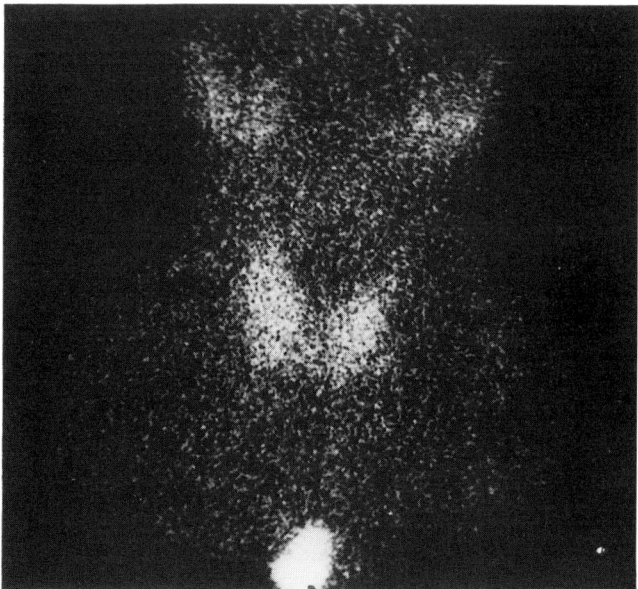

Figure 1. Normal ^{99m}Tc thyroid scan. Note symmetry and uniform activity with salivary gland activity. Background activity is secondary to blood-pool effect. Inferior activity is due to hot marker.

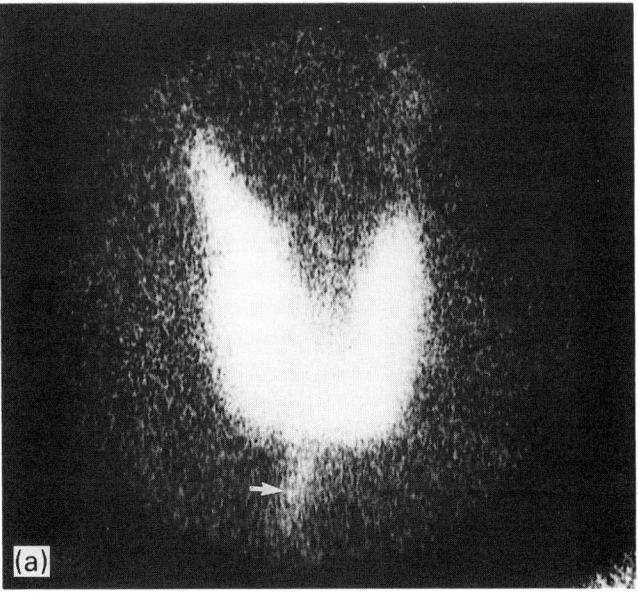

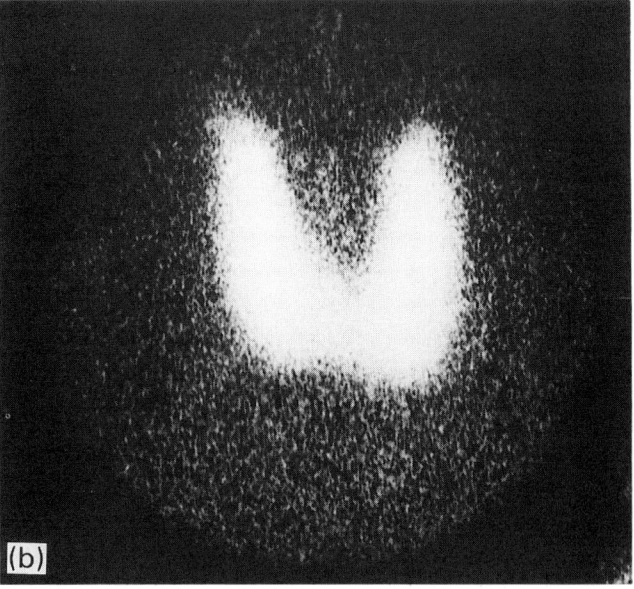

Figure 2. Midline oesophageal activity (white arrow, a) that disappeared when the patient swallowed water (b). From Sandler et al (1986), with permission.

Thyroid scintigraphy

The thyroid gland appears as two ellipsoid columns slightly angled toward each other and connected by a narrow isthmus. The gland exhibits uniform activity, with slight increase in activity occasionally noted in the central part of the lobes, secondary to their ellipsoid configuration. Areas of radioactivity that may be visualized outside the thyroid gland with pertechnetate imaging include the salivary glands, buccal mucosa, oesophagus, and blood-pool background (Figure 1).

Anatomical variations in normal thyroid imaging include the following:

1. Asymmetry in size of lobes.
2. Congenital absence of a lobe or isthmus.
3. Angulation of the lobes toward each other forming either a U- or V-shaped configuration.
4. Presence of a pyramidal lobe (remnant of the distal part of the thyroglossal duct) present in 10% of patients.
5. Extrathyroidal activity in the region of the oropharynx or hyporopharynx. Such activity is usually located medial and inferior to the thyroid gland and disappears with changes in location and/or intensity after swallowing a small amount of water (Figure 2a, b).

Ultrasound

The sonographic appearance of the normal thyroid gland is one of homo-

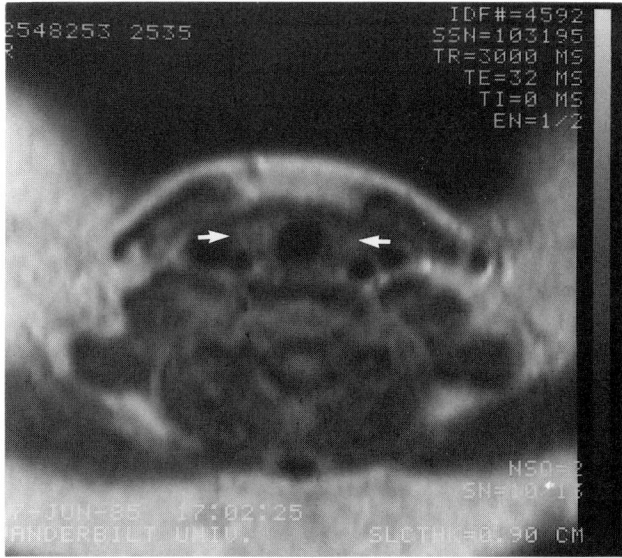

Figure 3. Transverse section through a normal thyroid gland using a spin–echo 3000/32 pulse sequence. White arrows show right and left lobes of the thyroid. From Sandler and Patton (1987), with permission.

geneous echogenicity, which is greater than that of the proximal strap muscles in the neck. The homogeneous echogenic pattern within the thyroid gland emanates from the numerous follicles that comprise the thyroid.

Magnetic resonance imaging

MRI is capable of providing excellent anatomical detail of the thyroid gland using proton density imaging (Figure 3).

Multinodular goitre

The pathophysiology of multinodular goitre is thought to be the consequence of cycling periods of hyperstimulation, followed by involution of the stimulated areas in most instances. In some patients the hyperplastic tissue fails to return to normal. Hormonal synthesis is maintained even though some of the stimulated thyroid follicles may be unable to mobilize colloid, the net effect of which is an imbalance between synthesis and mobilization, resulting in both an increase in size and occasional rupture of the follicle. The rupture and release of colloid from the follicles may result in areas of fibrosis within the thyroid gland. If these fibrotic areas are scattered irregularly throughout the gland, a typical multinodular colloid goitre may develop. The importance of identifying a multinodular goitre relates to the lower incidence of malignancy in these patients (1–6%) compared with a higher incidence in patients with a single 'cold' nodule (15–25%).

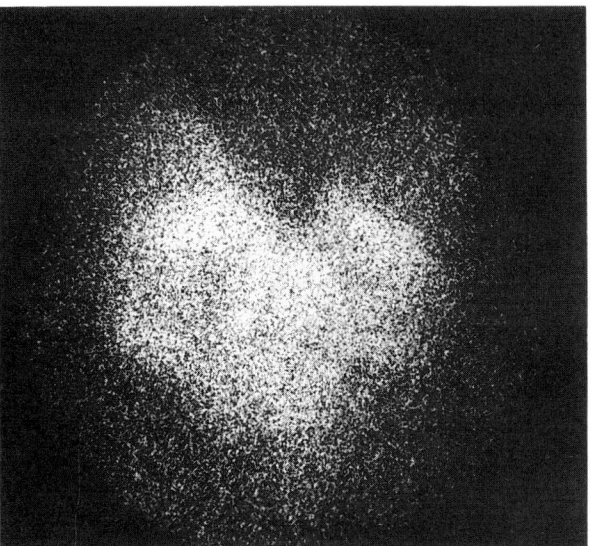

Figure 4. Multinodular goitre. Multiple functioning 'cold' areas occupy both lobes of the asymmetrically enlarged thyroid gland.

The scintigraphic appearance of a multinodular goitre is that of multiple non-functioning cold areas interdispersed between focal areas of increased activity in an asymmetrically enlarged thyroid gland (Figure 4). Ultrasound is also an excellent imaging modality for identifying multinodular goitre. High-resolution, real-time sonography allows the visualization of adenomas of 2–3 mm, increasing the detection of multinodular goitre when only a solitary thyroid nodule was detected by clinical palpation (Simeone et al, 1982). Since current available data on the incidence in malignancy in a multinodular goitre is related to clinically palpable goitres, the significance of small non-palpable nodules detected by real-time sonography remains uncertain. Multinodular goitres are easily identifiable by MRI on the basis of their anatomic appearance (Figure 5a-f).

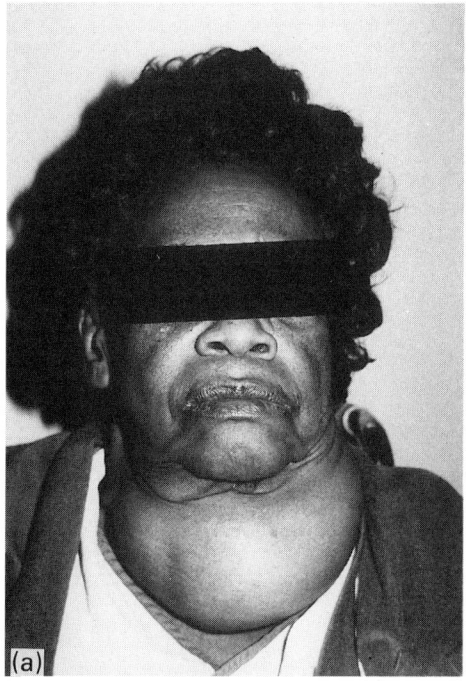

Figure 5. (a) Patient with large multinodular goitre presenting with neck discomfort without symptoms of superior mediastinal obstruction. (b) Chest radiograph reveals a large mediastinal mass. Also present is a right middle lobe consolidation and a small right pleural effusion. (c) [131]I thyroid scintigram shows a large diffuse multinodular goitre with retrosternal extension (white arrows). (d) Sagittal MRI 500/32 pulse sequence shows large goitre with anterior and posterior mediastinal extension. (e) Sagittal MRI 2000/160 pulse sequence (T2-weighting) shows diffuse increase in signal intensity in most areas of multinodular goitre, probably related to colloid and haemorrhage. (f) Transverse MRI 500/32 pulse sequence shows extension of goitre from anterior through middle to posterior mediastinum. (a)–(e) From Sandler and Patton (1987), with permission.

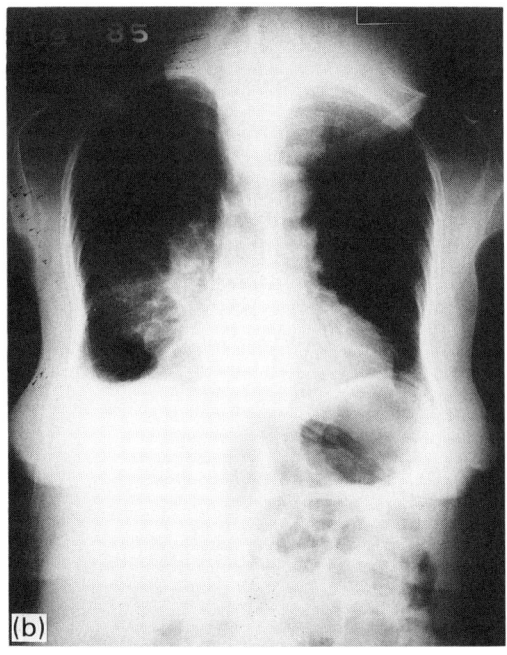

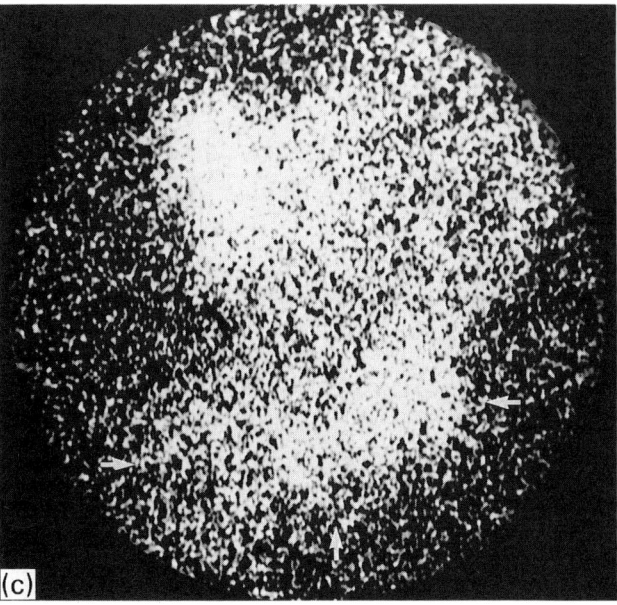

Figure 5 (*continued*)

Non-functioning thyroid nodules

The investigation of a solitary thyroid nodule should be performed in a logical sequence. It is important to identify those patients with functioning thyroid nodules and further differentiate this group into hypertrophic versus autonomous nodules which have the potential to become toxic. The recent move to make thyroid biopsy the only investigative procedure in patients with solitary thyroid nodules may prevent the diagnosis of a functioning autonomous thyroid nodule (Van Herle et al, 1982).

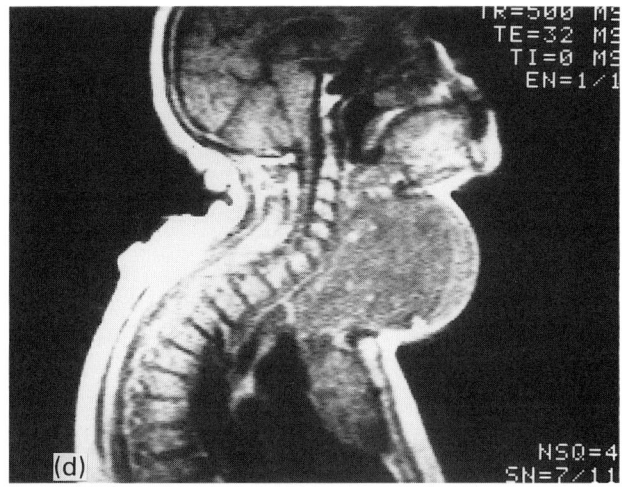

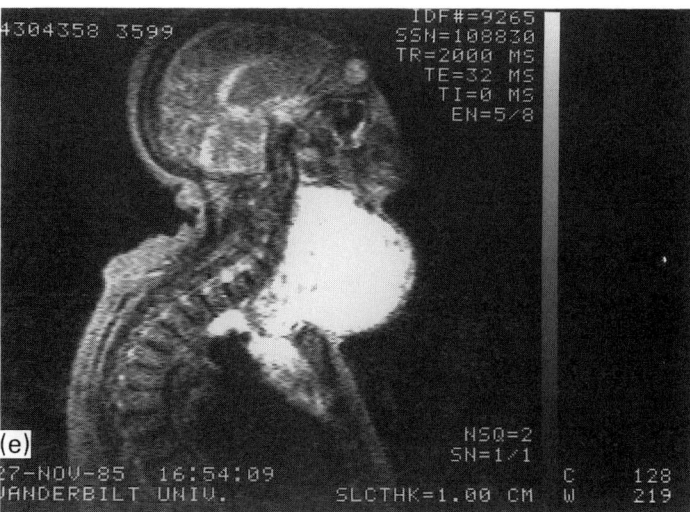

Figure 5 (*continued*)

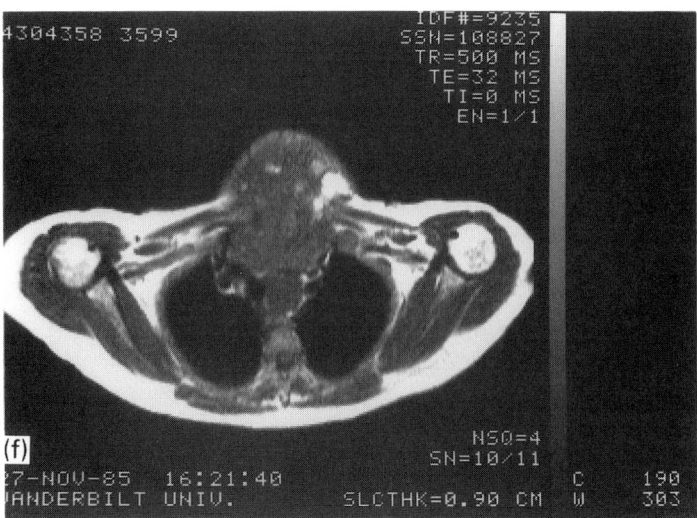

Figure 5 (*continued*)

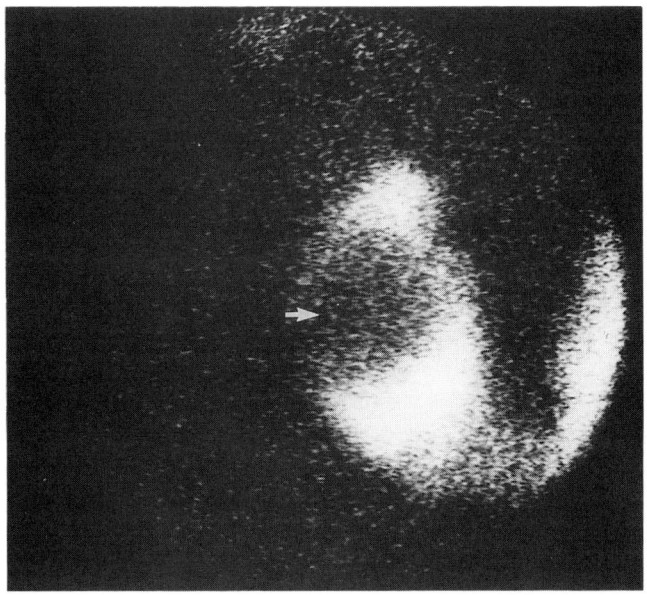

Figure 6. Solitary non-functional 'cold' nodule situated in the mid portion of the right lobe (white arrow).

Scintigraphy

Non-functioning ('cold') nodules, are regions that do not concentrate radio-isotopes as much as the rest of the thyroid gland (Figure 6). Although thyroid malignancies do not effectively concentrate radiosotopes, only ~ 20% or less of 'cold' nodules are caused by cancerous lesions (Psarra et al, 1974). The remaining 80% of 'cold' nodules, degenerative nodules, nodular haemorrhage, cysts, inflammatory nodules (including Hashimoto's thyroiditis or de Quervain's thyroiditis), infiltrative disorders (including amyloid or haemochromatosis), are non-thyroid neoplasms (Table 2). A

Table 2. Aetiology of the solitary palpable nodule. From Sandler et al (1986).

	Malignant	
Benign	Primary	Secondary
Adenoma	Carcinoma	Kidney
	Papillary adenocarcinoma	Pancreas
Adenomatous hyperplasia	Follicular carcinoma	Oesophagus
in a goitre	Clear cell carcinoma	Rectum
	Oxyphil carcinoma	Melanoma
Adenomatous nodule	Medullary carcinoma	Lung
	Undifferentiated carcinoma	Lymphoma
Cyst	Small cell carcinoma	
	Giant cell carcinoma	
Colloid nodules	Epidermoid carcinoma	
Chronic thyroiditis	Other malignant tumours	
	Lymphoma	
Subacute thyroiditis	Sarcoma	
	Malignant teratoma	
Miscellaneous:		
Amyloid		
Haemochromatosis		

functioning thyroid stimulating hormone (TSH)-dependent adenoma may appear as a cold nodule in patients with Graves' disease where impaired radionuclide uptake by the nodule is secondary to low TSH levels. This entity is known as the Marine–Lenhart syndrome. Confirmation of the diagnosis can be made by TSH stimulation.

The detection of extrathyroidal activity on a routine thyroid scan in a patient with palpable lymph nodes and a solitary thyroid nodule, although rare, most likely indicates metastatic thyroid cancer.

Ultrasound

Ultrasound has been used in thyroid imaging in an attempt to differentiate benign from malignant thyroid nodules. Two signs have been proposed by the ultrasonographer as markers of benignancy: pure cystic lesions and the halo sign (Propper et al, 1980; Sykes, 1981) (Figure 7). On the other hand, hypoechogenicity of the nodule compared to the surrounding tissue has been presented as a sign indicative of malignancy (Simeone et al, 1982).

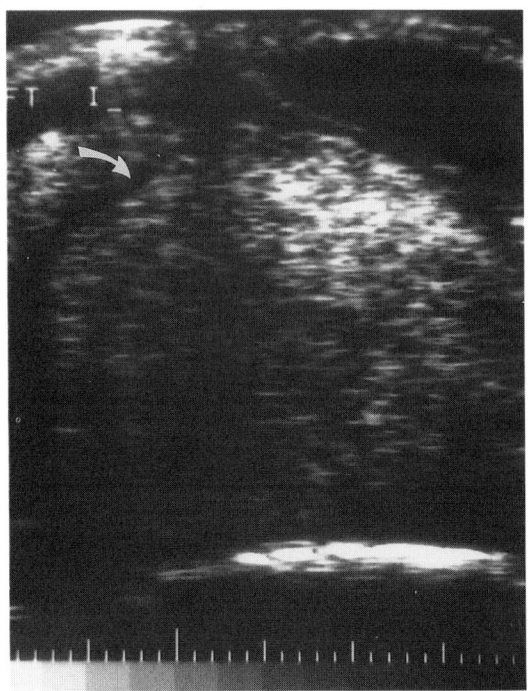

Figure 7. Solitary echogenic solid nodule with surrounding sonolucent 'halo' (arrow). Scintigraphy identified a non-functioning thyroid nodule.

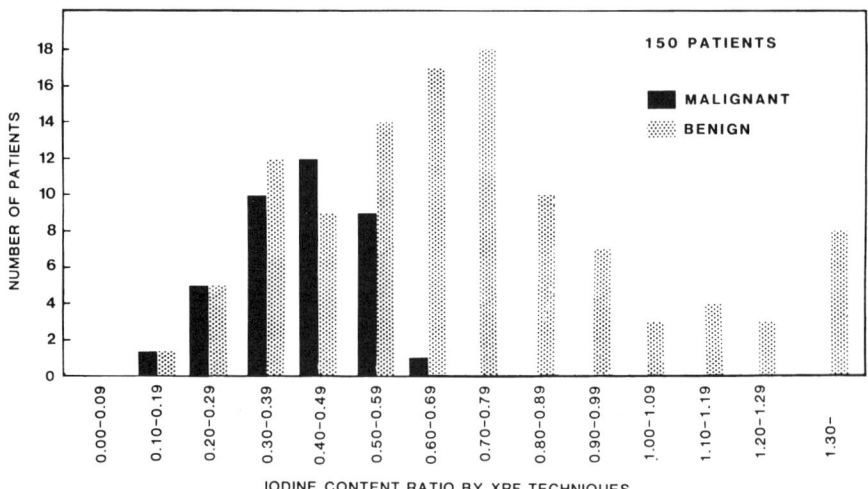

Figure 8. Bar graph of iodine content ratio determined before surgery from 150 patients with solitary 'cold' thyroid nodules in which histological diagnoses were obtained from surgical specimens. From Patton et al (1985), with permission.

None of these signs, however, has proven to be specific for either malignant or benign lesions.

Serial sonograms have also been used to follow changes in the size of solid nodules in patients taking suppressive therapy, allowing precise evaluation of the growth pattern of these nodules. In general, a reduction of 50% of nodule size over a 3- to 6-month period on chronic thyroid suppression is required as an indicator of benignancy.

X-ray fluorescent scanning

Quantitative X-ray fluorescent (XRF) scanning is an established technique for the investigation of thyroid disorders and has proven to be especially

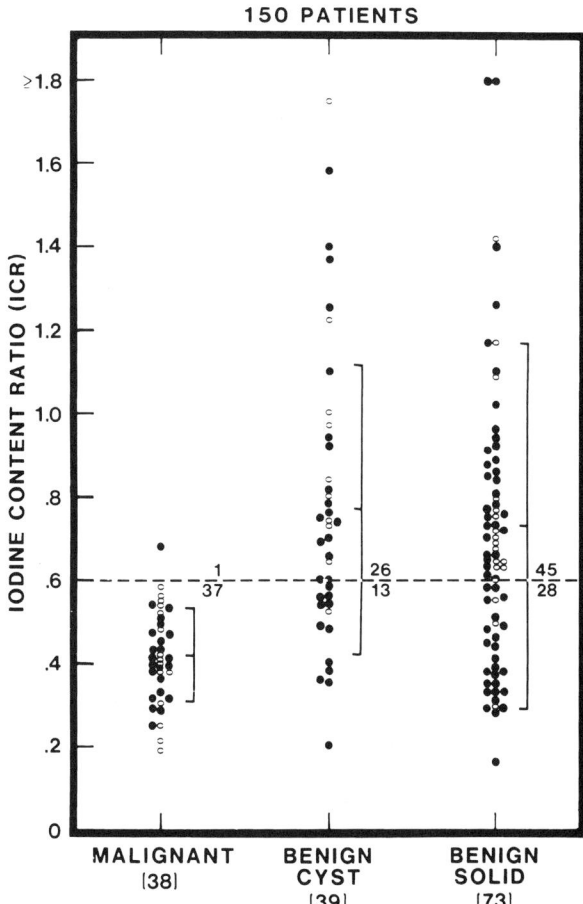

Figure 9. Iodine content ratios determined before surgery from 150 patients with solitary 'cold' nodules. Groupings are based on histological study of surgical specimens. Open circles correspond to the 42 patients in the original retrospective study. From Patton et al (1985), with permission.

useful in the evaluation of solitary cold thyroid nodules (Patton et al, 1976, 1980, 1985). With this technique, the in vivo iodine content of a solitary thyroid nodule and that of a corresponding region of normal thyroid tissue in the contralateral lobe are measured. The iodine content ratio (ICR) of the thyroid nodule versus normal tissue is calculated and used as a predictor of benignancy. In a study of 150 patients with histological diagnosis, it has been shown that an iodine content ratio above 0.6 is excellent as an indicator of

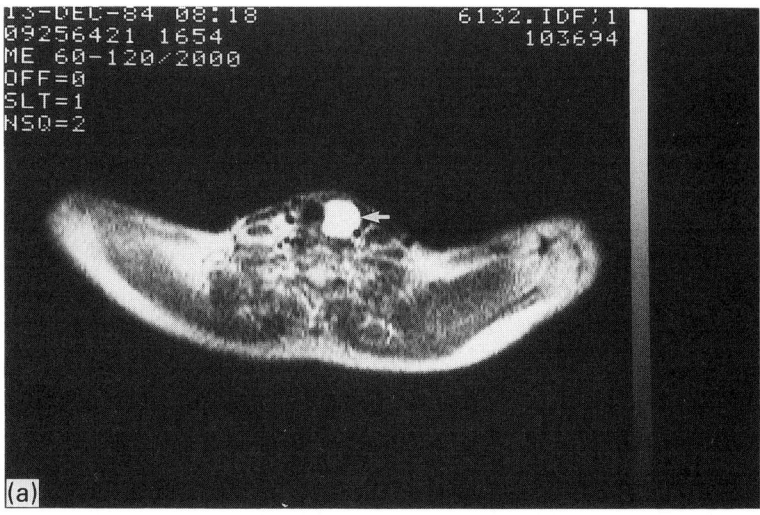

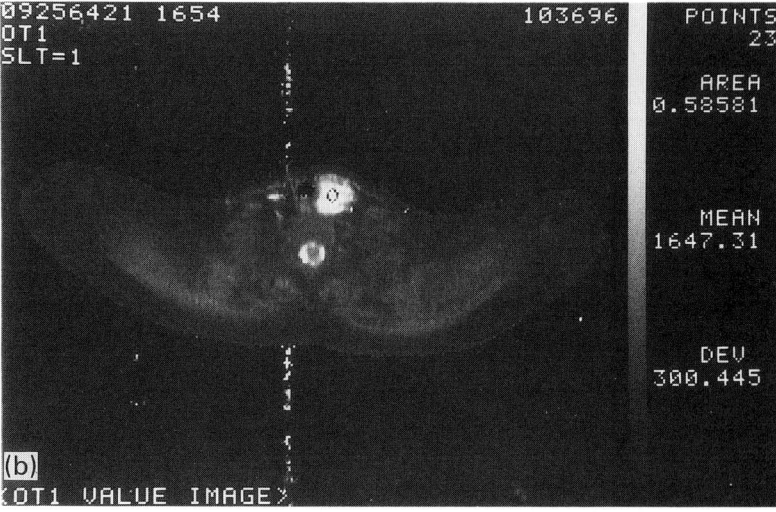

Figure 10. Transverse MRI section through a benign functioning hypertrophic adenoma. (a) Spin-echo 2000/120 pulse sequence (white arrow). (b) Calculated observed T1 value 1647 ms. From Sandler and Patton (1987), with permission.

benignancy with a sensitivity of 63% and a specificity of 99% (Figures 8 and 9).

XRF scanning of solitary cold thyroid nodules is only valid when investigating single nodules. Separation between the various pathological types of thyroid malignancy is not possible using XRF scanning. This technique, in conjunction with careful clinical judgement, can be used to identify those patients who are at low risk for malignancy and can probably undergo conservative clinical management. Because there is no administration of a radio-isotope, this technique becomes the method of choice in the evaluation of thyroid nodules in both paediatric and pregnant patients.

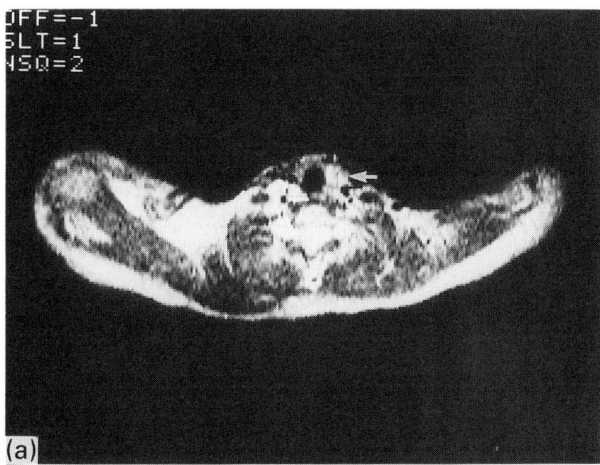

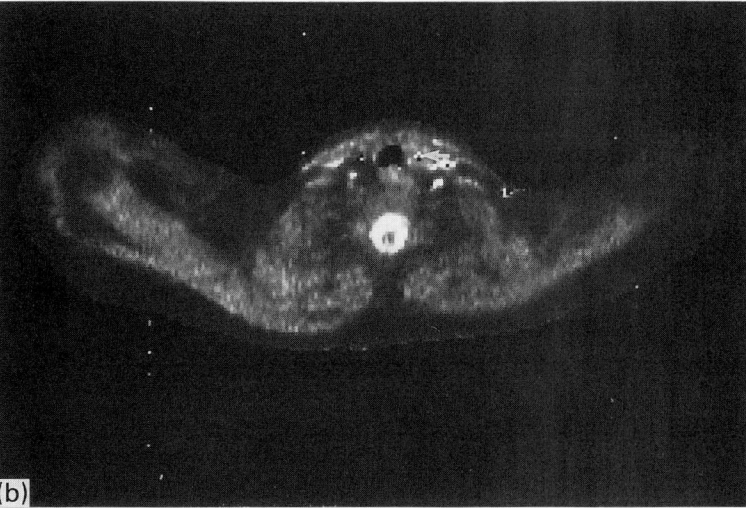

Figure 11. Transverse MRI section through a well-differentiated follicular carcinoma. (a) Spin–echo 2000/120 pulse sequence (T2-weighting) (white arrow). (b) Calculated observed T1 value 567 ms. From Sandler and Patton (1987), with permission.

Magnetic resonance imaging

In vitro magnetic resonance studies on thyroid biopsy specimens performed by de Certaines and coworkers revealed abnormal T1 and T2 values in both benign and malignant lesions with no clear differentiation possible (de Certaines et al, 1982). Nodules showing increased radionuclide uptake showed a marked degree of variability in T1 values with nine out of ten having significantly increased T2 values compared with normal extranodular tissue. Solitary benign cold nodules ($n = 9$) all showed increased T1 and T2 values. T1 and T2 values showed considerable variation in four patients with thyroid carcinoma. An increase in T1 was observed in two patients and a decrease in one. T1 was not measured in the fourth patient. T2 values were increased in two cases and decreased in two. There was no significant difference in the relaxation times between nodular and extranodular tissue in patients with multinodular goitre.

The in vivo differentiation between benign and malignant thyroid lesions does not appear to be possible on the basis of T1 and T2 measurements alone (Figures 10–13). Benign and malignant thyroid tissue may, in part, be distinguished using MRI by the degree of disruption of thyroid anatomy, and the invasion of normal thyroid tissue and surrounding structures. Colloid cysts exhibit greater prolonged T1 values characteristic of simple fluids. Haemorrhage into a cyst should lower the T1 value. Adenomas exhibit a wide range of T1 values, although generally prolonged, encompassing those of thyroid carcinomas. The ability of magnetic resonance spectroscopy to differentiate benign versus malignant thyroid nodules in vivo awaits further investigation.

Functioning thyroid nodules

A nodule that concentrates the administered radiosotope to a greater degree than the surrounding tissue appears either hot or warm relative to the thyroid gland. A hot thyroid nodule in most cases is benign, because maligant tissue rarely demonstrates normal scintigraphic activity (Jackson and Thomson, 1967; Goldsmith, 1978; Sisson et al, 1978). The incidence of hot nodules in patients with discrete thyroid nodules varies from 6.6 to 25% (Jackson and Thomson, 1967; Goldsmith, 1978; Sisson et al, 1978). Functioning thyroid nodules in the euthyroid patient may be classified as either hypertrophic nodules or autonomous adenoma.

Hypertrophic nodules are TSH-dependent and are thought to develop as a result of either inflammatory or degenerative insult to the gland. Those areas of the thyroid that survive the insult respond to elevated levels of TSH and become hypertrophied to compensate for defective hormone synthesis in the gland. The net effect is the appearance of a hot or warm nodule. Autonomous adenomas are nodules that arise independently of TSH stimulation.

Hypertrophic vs. autonomous functioning thyroid nodules

The T3 suppression test allows the differentiation of autonomous vs. hyper-

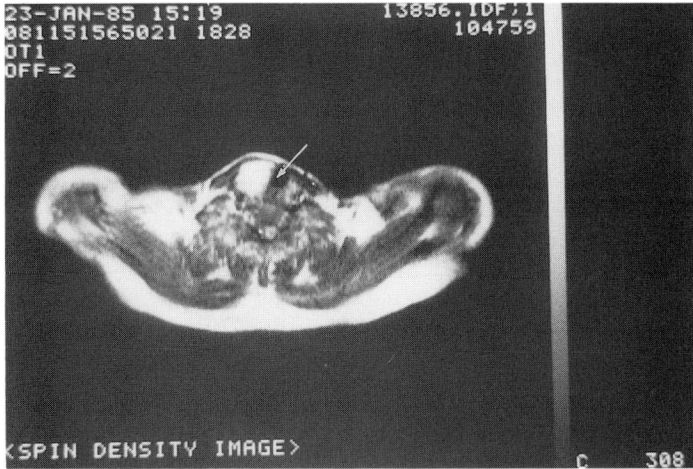

Figure 12. Transverse MRI section through a metastatic melanoma to the right lobe of the thyroid in a patient with a previous left hemilobectomy. Note right-sided tracheal compression (white arrow). Calculated OT1 value 400 ms. From Smith et al (1986), with permission.

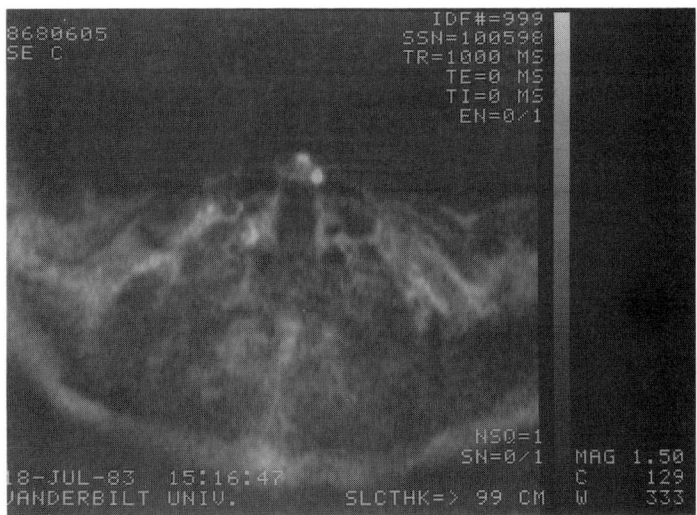

Figure 13. A thyroglossal ductal cyst on transverse section using a spin–echo 1000/120 (T2-weighting). This lesion was also identified on ultrasound but could not be seen on nuclear medicine studies. At surgery, this patient was noted to have a papillary carcinoma. The lesion is seen as two discrete areas of high signal intensity in the midline and in the left lobe of the thyroid. From Smith et al (1986), with permission.

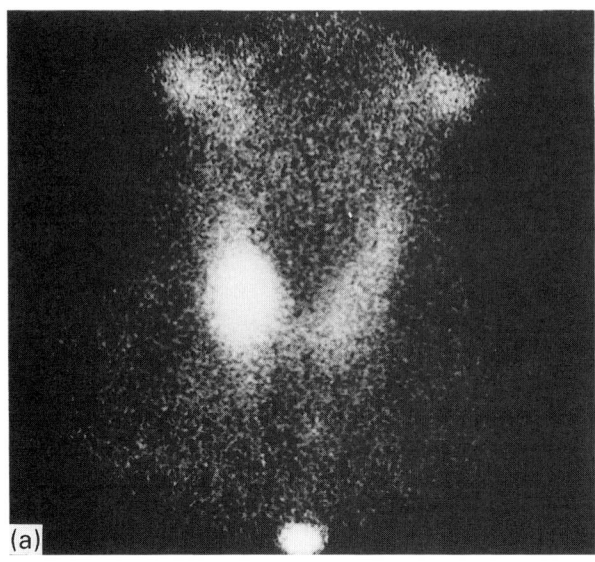

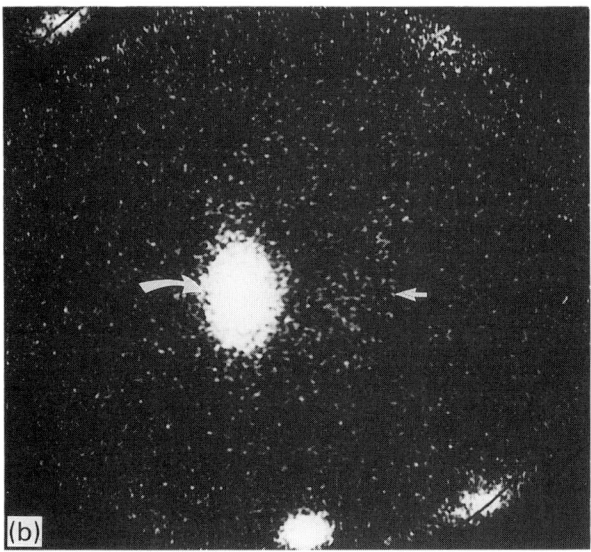

Figure 14. Effect of cytomel suppression on an autonomous thyroid nodule. (a) Initial scan. (b) Postcytomel suppression using 7-day course reveals activity in autonomous nodule (curved arrow) with suppression of remaining gland (straight arrow). From Sandler et al (1986), with permission.

trophic nodules. In this test, patients are administered 75–100 µg/day of tri-iodothyronine (T3) daily for a period of 7–10 days. This is followed by a ^{99m}Tc scan. As autonomous nodules function independently of TSH, they will continue to appear 'hot', demonstrating no significant change in overall appearance from earlier studies (Figure 14). Hypertrophic nodules, on the other hand, will no longer show evidence of increased trapping since the hypothalamic–pituitary–thyroid axis has been 'turned off' by the exoge-nously administered T3. The separation of these two entities is important, as the management of patients with a hypertrophic nodule should be thyroid suppression (thyroxine 150–200 µg/day), whereas patients with an auto-nomous nodule need only be observed.

Disparate thyroid imaging

Disparate thyroid imaging is a dissociation between trapping and organi-fication, measured respectively with ^{99m}Tc and ^{123}I (Figure 15). It occurs in 2–3% of individuals with thyroid disorders and is not specific for malignant disease, having been described in patients with adenomatous goitre and follicular adenoma (Strauss et al, 1970; Atkins et al, 1973; Shambaugh et al, 1974). A common subcellular defect has been postulated to account for the non-specificity of this finding.

In view of the low incidence of disparity between trapping and organi-fication, initial thyroid imaging in patients with solitary thyroid nodule using ^{123}I should be reserved for those who have an increased risk of thyroid malignancy, i.e. individuals with a previous history of head and neck irradi-ation during childhood, prepubertal patients, adult males, and patients with a positive family history of thyroid malignancy. Similarly, if a hot or warm nodule is demonstrated by ^{99m}Tc imaging, it should be reimaged with ^{123}I to ascertain the true functioning status of the nodule.

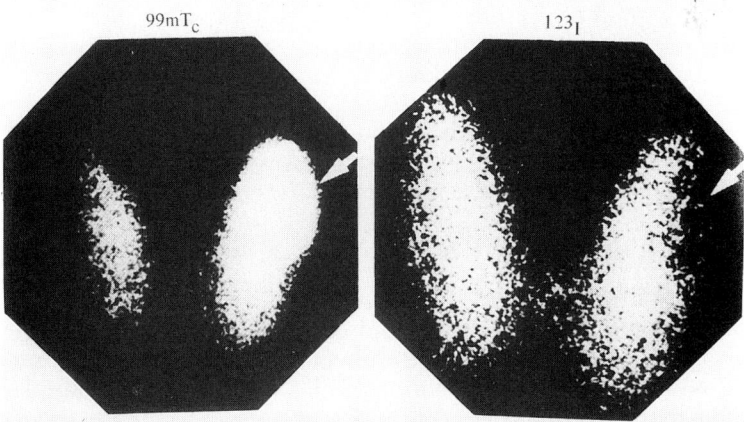

Figure 15. Discrepancy between ^{99m}Tc and ^{123}I scans. Scan with ^{99m}Tc shows a hot nodule in the left upper thyroid (arrow). The nodule appeared cold at repeat scan with ^{123}I (right arrow). From Pinsky and Yun Ryo (1981), with permission.

Malignancy and functioning thyroid nodules

Focal hot nodules on iodine thyroid scintigrams are associated with an exceedingly low incidence of malignancy (Freitas et al, 1985). Most reported hot carcinomas represent the coexistence of small malignancies adjacent to a benign hot lesion (Mulnar et al, 1958; Becker et al, 1963; Dische, 1964; McLaughlin et al, 1970; Meier and Hamburger, 1971; Fujimoto et al, 1972; Hamburger, 1975; Wolfstein, 1978; Abdel-Razzak and Christie, 1979; Blitzer and Son, 1979; Khan et al, 1981). A cold area within a hot nodule is suggestive of carcinoma within a hyperfunctioning adenoma, and this finding has the same significance as a cold nodule within an otherwise normal gland.

There are only two well-documented cases of 'hot carcinoma' reported in the literature (Ghose et al, 1971; Sandler et al, 1988). The case described by Ghose et al (1971) showed a high radio-iodine content in the carcinoma by autoradiography, whereas that described by Sandler et al (1988) showed a low in vitro iodine content measured by X-ray fluorescence.

When a palpable nodule corresponds in position to a uniformly 'hot' area on iodine scintigraphy, malignancy is unlikely but not completely excluded. Thus, hyperfunctioning thyroid nodules that have clinically suspicious features or occur in patients with risk factors for thyroid carcinoma should not be presumed benign by scintigraphic criteria.

Needle biopsy of the thyroid

Random reports of fine needle aspiration of the thyroid gland have appeared in literature since the turn of the century. This procedure is relatively benign and simple and may yield important diagnostic information about the thyroid nodule. However it is important to approach the routine processing and interpretation of thyroid lesions in a standardized, systematic fashion. Early biopsy experience may be gained by examining resected surgical specimens with the aspiration technique. Additionally, during the early clinical experience, most solitary nodules should be removed and the histology compared to the cytology.

The evaluation of aspirated cells requires specialized expertise, which often limits this procedure to major medical centres. The most important aspect of needle biopsies for a physician to be aware of is that '*a non-diagnostic biopsy is of no value in the prediction of benignancy of the solitary thyroid nodule*'.

Retrosternal goitre

Although substernal aberrant thyroid goitre accounts for only 10% of all mediastinal masses, it remains one of the major diagnostic considerations in the assessment of mediastinal abnormalities (Daniel et al, 1960). The pre-operative diagnosis of a thyroidal mediastinal mass frequently requires the use of sophisticated imaging techniques including, either alone or in combination: thyroid scintigraphy, CT and MRI (Bashist et al, 1983; Cohen et al, 1983).

Scintigraphy

Radionuclide imaging has been the standard method for evaluating whether or not a mediastinal mass represents functioning thyroid tissue (see Figure 5c). False-negative thyroid scans in mediastinal goitre may occur when there is too little uptake of radio-active iodine by the goitre either due to low iodine concentrating capacity of the tissue or recent exposure of the patient

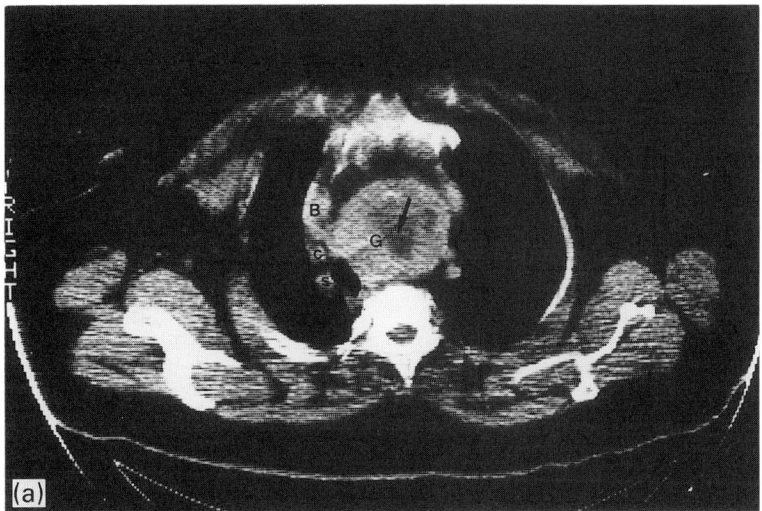

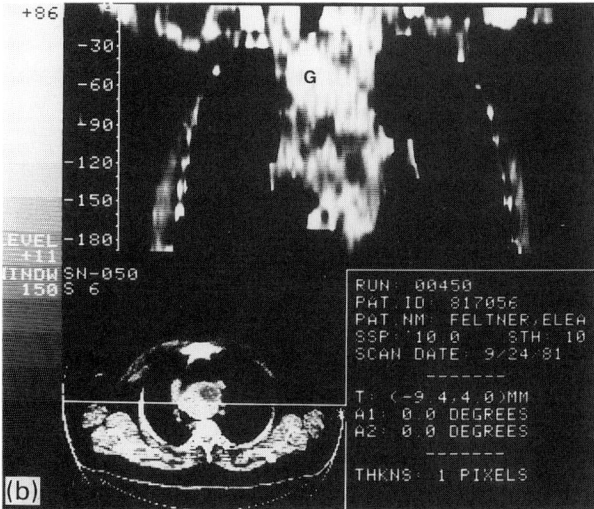

Figure 16. (a) A complete intrathoracic goitre (G) with areas of low attenuation due to cyst formation (arrow). The brachiocephalic veins (B), carotoid artery (c), and subclavian artery (s) surround the mass on both sides. (b) A multiplanar coronal reconstruction of the lesion in (a) showing the location of the goitre (g). From Shaff et al (1986), with permission.

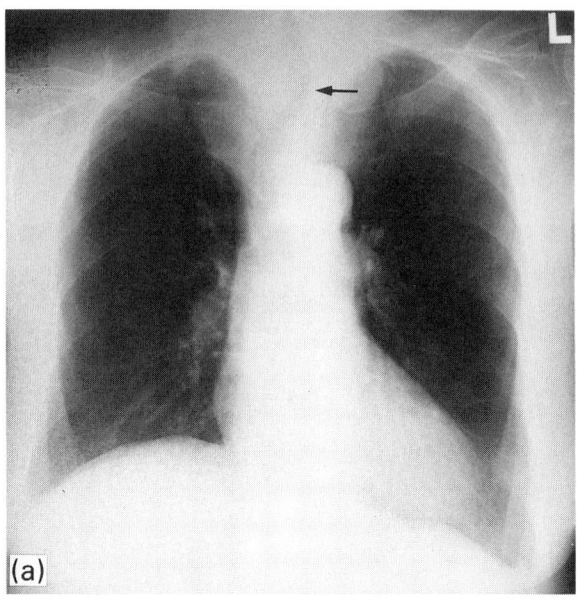

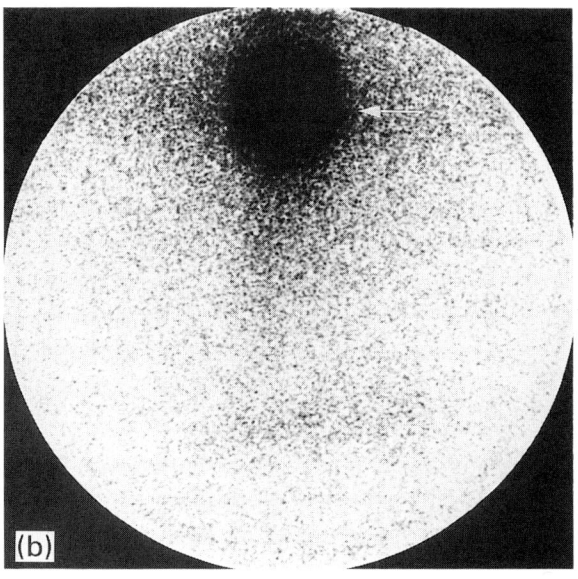

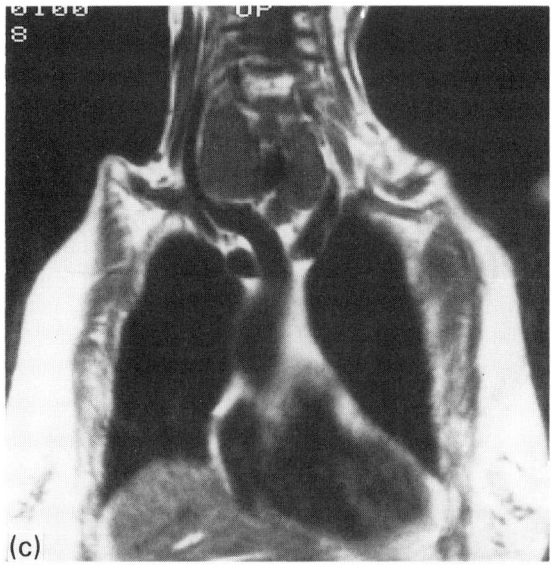

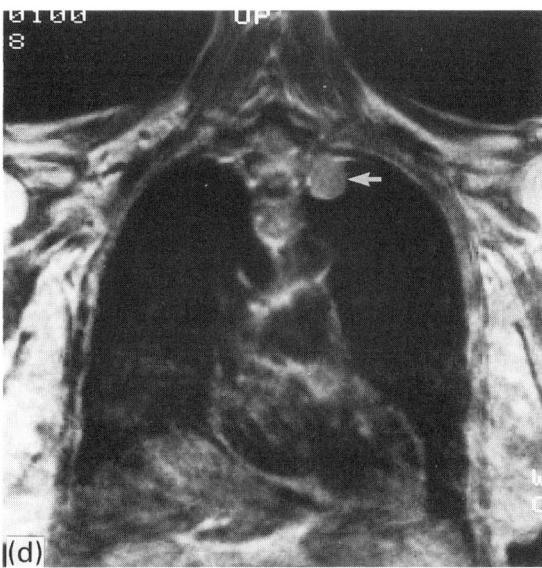

Figure 17. (a) Chest X-ray reveals a mediastinal mass with tracheal deviation (arrow) in a patient with a past history of total thyroidectomy. (b) Iodine-131 thyroid scintigram shows a large functioning thyroid goitre (arrow). (c) Coronal MRI 500/32 pulse sequence shows large goitre compressing right internal jugular vein. (d) Coronal MRI 500/32 pulse sequence identifies extension of goitre into the posterior mediastinum (arrow).

to exogenous iodine. False-positive scans for mediastinal thyroid tissue may occur: one has been reported in a patient with papillary adenocarcinoma of the lung (Fernandez-Ulloa et al, 1976).

Computed tomography

CT findings of intrathoracic goitre have noted the continuity with the cervical gland (Figure 16), focal calcifications, high non-contrast attenuation values of the goitre, and postintravenous contrast enhancement (Brasch et al, 1978). These features, although suggestive, are not specific for the diagnosis of intrathoracic goitre. It is more likely that the early enhancement of intrathoracic masses following intravenous contrast represents the vascularity of the mass rather than significant trapping and organification of iodine by the thyroid gland (Sekiya et al, 1979).

Magnetic resonance imaging

MRI is an excellent modality to image the mediastinum, producing high resolution tomographic or three-dimensional images without the use of ionizing radiation (Figure 17a–d). MRI of the mediastinum also differentiates vascular structures from solid hilar or mediastinal masses without the use of contrast agents (Sandler et al, 1984). Volume calculations of thyroid mediastinal masses are possible with MRI, permitting quantitative assessment of the response of the mass to TSH suppression.

Hyperthyroidism

Hyperthyroidism, a chemical syndrome that results from supraphysiological levels of thyroid hormones, may occur as a consequence of numerous diseases (Table 3). Clinical history and physical examination, combined with thyroid scintigraphy, thyroid uptake (Table 4) and thyroid antibodies, allows identification and differentiation of the various disease processes.

Graves' disease

Patients with Graves' disease exhibit prolonged T1 values; the physiologic basis of which remains unexplained (Figure 18). MRI of patients with Graves' disease, however, is of limited value when compared to the numerous modalities currently available to diagnose this disorder and differentiate it from other causes of hyperthyroidism.

Toxic nodular goitres

Toxic nodular goitres may be either multinodular or secondary to a solitary hyperfunctioning adenoma. Patients with toxic multinodular goitre are usually older than those with diffuse toxic goitre and, on an average, are between the fourth and fifth decades. Patients with a solitary toxic nodule, on the other hand, often are younger and vary in age from adolescents to

Table 3. Classification of hyperthyroidism. From Sandler et al (1986), with permission.

A. *Thyroid gland* (± 95%)
    Diffuse toxic goitre (Graves' disease)
    Toxic nodular goitre
        Multinodular (Plummer's disease)
    Thyroiditis (subacute)
B. *Exogenous thyroid hormone-iodine* (± 4%)
    Iatrogenic
    Factitious
    Iodine-induced (Jod-Basedow)
C. *Rarely encountered causes* (± 1%)
    Hypothalamic–pituitary neoplasms
    Struma ovarii
    Excessive HCG production by trophoblastic tissue
    Metastatic thyroid carcinoma

Table 4. ^{131}I Thyroid uptake in thyrotoxicosis. From Sandler et al (1986).

Increased	Normal	Decreased
Graves' disease (diffuse goitre)	Trophoblastic disease	Thyroiditis (subacute chronic)
Plummer's disease (multinodular goitre)		Iatrogenic/factitious
Trophoblastic disease (HCG)		Jod-Basedow (iodine-induced)
		Functioning thyroid metastases

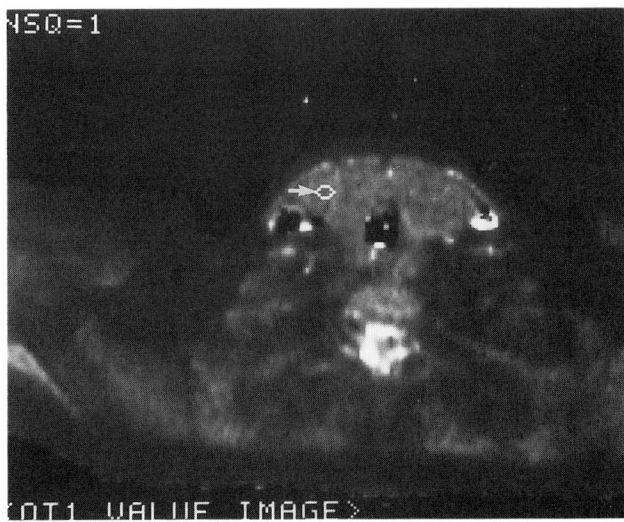

Figure 18. Transverse MRI section through a symmetrically enlarged gland in a patient with Graves' disease. Calculated T1 value 477 ms (arrow). From Sandler and Patton (1987), with permission.

adults. A solitary toxic nodule is slightly more common in males, whereas the sex incidence is roughly equal in those patients with toxic multinodular goitre. The aetiology of toxic nodular goitres is uncertain but may represent solitary or multiple functioning autonomous adenomas within the thyroid gland. Physical examination of patients with either a solitary toxic nodule or toxic multinodular goitre generally is not a problem. However, the presence of a clinically palpable multinodular goitre in association with hyper-thyroidism is not specific for toxic multinodular goitre (Plummer's disease), since this combination may occur in patients with either subacute thyroiditis or iatrogenic hyperthyroidism (suppression of TSH with exogenous thyroid hormone in a patient with a euthyroid multinodular goitre). Scintigraphy of patients with a toxic multinodular goitre reveals areas of increased and decreased radionuclide activity within the gland. The areas of increased activity invariably are present in both lobes, corresponding to islands of autonomously hyperfunctioning tissue, whereas the areas of decreased activity represent those that have been suppressed by excessive thyroid activity. There is also a decrease in both background and salivary gland activity (Figure 19).

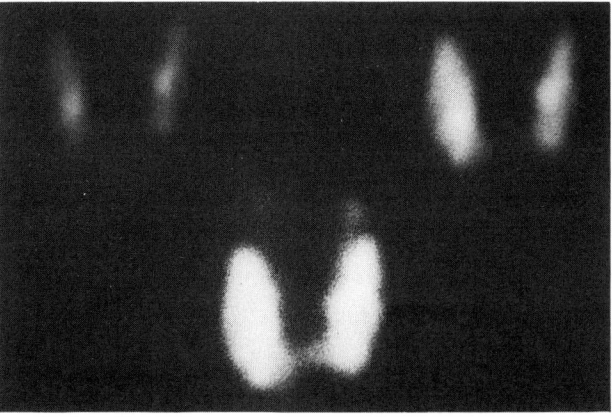

Figure 19. Toxic multinodular goitre [99mTc]. Multiple hyperfunctioning areas interspersed with non-functioning areas occupy both lobes. Decreased background and salivary gland activity secondary to increased trapping of the radionuclide by the hyperactive areas of the gland. From Sandler et al (1986), with permission.

The presence of cancer in toxic nodule goitres is extremely rare and varies from 0.1–0.9%. The 24-hour thyroid radio-iodine uptake in patients with toxic multinodular goitres may be elevated but often is within the normal range.

Detection of thyroid carcinoma and metastatic thyroid disease

In recent years, in view of the lack of specificity of other imaging modalities, the list of radionuclides used for diagnosing thyroid carcinoma has been significantly expanded.

Iodine-131

Radionuclide uptake by functioning thyroid neoplasms and their metastases is far less efficient than normal thyroid tissue. As a result, metastases are not usually demonstrated if normal thyroid tissue is present. Thus, the initial step prior to performing a total-body ^{131}I scan for metastatic disease is the assessment of thyroid gland remnants by routine scanning techniques. If significant residual thyroid tissue is present, it is first necessary to ablate the thyroid remnant with large doses of radioiodine.

The most important factor for a successful baseline or follow-up total-body ^{131}I scan is the induction of endogenous TSH levels that are high enough to stimulate ^{131}I uptake by the neoplastic tissue. Adequate TSH levels usually can be achieved (> 20 uU/ml) 2 weeks after the discontinuation of T3 or 4–6 weeks after the discontinuation of thyroxine (T4).

Whole-body scanning is performed 48–72 hours after the administration of 1–5 mCi of ^{131}I orally. Of the various types of thyroid neoplasms or their metastases, only follicular and mixed papillary follicular carcinomas are able to concentrate iodide (Haynie et al, 1963). Occasional reports of radio-iodine uptake in medullary carcinoma have appeared in the literature. Further evaluation of these cases have questioned the cell origin being of the follicular type in some patients and also has raised the possibility of the presence of two distinct tumours coexisting with both medullary and follicular cell types (Spencer et al, 1982). Metastatic lesions from medullary carcinoma to both bone and liver can frequently be detected by radionuclide bone and hepatic scintigraphy (Johnson et al, 1984).

Following the administration of millicurie doses or ^{131}I, radio-activity is demonstrable routinely in several physiological sites: salivary glands, gastric mucosa and contents, small and large bowel, urinary bladder, liver, and breast (especially during lactation). These areas of normal physiological uptake should not be confused with functioning metastatic disease.

Thallium-201

Successful tumour imaging with [^{201}Tl] chloride has been described in thyroid carcinoma, bronchial carcinoma, breast carcinoma, lymphoma, osteosarcoma, Ewing's sarcoma, soft-tissue sarcoma, liver-cell carcinoma and oesophageal cancer. Increased ^{201}Tl uptake in ^{99m}Tc or ^{123}I cold nodules is correlated with a high risk of malignancy. In this respect, [^{201}Tl] chloride so far is the most successful tumour-seeking agent in the evaluation of thyroid nodules (Tonami et al, 1978). However, the method is not specific enough to differentiate between malignant and benign disease of the thyroid.

In postoperative detection of thyroid carcinoma the specificity of ^{201}Tl scintigraphy is less of a problem (Tonami and Hisada, 1980). There are several reports of cases of thyroid carcinoma that did not concentrate ^{131}I, but were ^{201}Tl-positive (Muller-Brand et al, 1983; Nemec et al, 1984). Since ^{131}I therapy is not feasible in these patients, it is helpful to localize the metastases by means of ^{201}Tl scintigraphy to facilitate the appropriate therapy.

[⁹⁹ᵐTc] (V) Dimercaptosuccinic acid

⁹⁹ᵐTc phosphates and [²⁰¹Tl] chloride have been used with limited success to localize medullary carcinoma of the thyroid (MCT) (Spencer, 1984). Two additional radiopharmaceuticals have been introduced recently: [¹³¹I] meta-iodobenzylguanidine ([¹³¹I]MIBG), which is useful in the detection of phaeochromocytoma and other neoplasms of neuroectodermal origin (Shapiro et al, 1985), and [⁹⁹ᵐTc] (V) dimercaptosuccinic acid (DMSA), in which ⁹⁹ᵐTc core exhibits characteristics comparable to the orthophosphate ion (Ohta et al, 1984a). Ohta et al have postulated that since pentavalent DMSA resembles the phosphate ion that this is the mechanism by which [⁹⁹ᵐTc] (V) DMSA accumulates in tumours, particularly MCT where calcification is a well-recognized phenomenon. Uptake of [⁹⁹ᵐTc] (V) DMSA into tumours has also been observed in patients with soft tissue sarcoma, osteosarcoma and prostatic carcinoma (Ohta et al, 1984b, 1985; Jeghers et al, 1986). Both [¹³¹I]MIBG and [⁹⁹ᵐTc] (V) DMSA have been reported to be valuable in localizing medullary thyroid carcinoma.

A recent study, however, has failed to confirm the diagnostic ability of either [⁹⁹ᵐTc] (V) DMSA or [¹³¹I]MIBG to detect medullary thyroid carcinoma reliably (Hilditch et al, 1986). The limited uptake of [¹³¹I]MIBG by such tumours indicates that this radiopharmaceutical has questionable value in primary diagnosis or in the detection of recurrence, but its potential role in therapy in patients with significant uptake warrants further investigation.

SUMMARY

The continued development of high technology in the rapidly expanding field of computer-based imaging has had a significant impact on many areas of diagnostic imaging. The problem of rising medical costs emphasizes the importance of reaching a diagnosis by the most straightforward and cost-effective method while providing minimal patient discomfort. This responsibility to the patient and the medical care system rests with the physician. It is therefore essential that both imaging and referring physicians have a broad background of information regarding the potential limitations and relative merits of both old and new technologies available to patients with thyroid disorders. The appropriate utilization and relative roles of these imaging modalities have been discussed with respect to the individual clinical problem in this chapter.

Acknowledgement

The authors extend their appreciation to Ms Virginia Brocker for her patience and perseverance during the preparation of the manuscript.

REFERENCES

Abdel-Razzak M & Christie JH (1979) Thyroid carcinoma in an autonomously functioning nodule. *Journal of Nuclear Medicine* **20**: 1001–1002 (letter).

Andros G, Harper PV, Lathrop KA (1965) Pertechnetate-99m localization in many with applications to thyroid scanning and the study of thyroid physiology. *Journal of Clinical Endocrinology and Metabolism* **25**: 1067–1076.

Atkins HL & Richards P (1968) Assessment of thyroid function and anatomy with technetium-99m pertechnetate. *Journal of Nuclear Medicine* **9**: 7–15.

Atkins HL, Klopper JF, Lambrecht RM et al (1973) A comparison of technetium-99m and iodine-123 for thyroid imaging. *American Journal of Roentgenology, Radium Therapy and Nuclear Medicine* **117**: 195–201.

Bashist B, Ellis K & Gold RP (1983) Computed tomography of intrathoracic goiters. *American Journal of Roentgenology* **140**: 45–460.

Becker FO, Economou PG & Schwartz TB (1963) The occurrence of carcinoma in 'hot' thyroid nodules: report of two cases. *Annals of Internal Medicine* **58**: 877–882.

Blitzer A & Son ML (1979) Thyroid carcinoma in a patient with a coexisting functional adenoma. *Otolaryngology and Head and Neck Surgery* **87**: 768–774.

Brasch RC, Boyd DP & Gooding CA (1978) Computer tomographic scanning in children: comparison of radiation dose and resolving powers of commercial CT scanners. *American Journal of Roentgenology* **131**: 95–101.

Burke GA, Halko A, Silverstein GE et al (1972) Comparative thyroid uptake studies with I-131 and 99m-Tc04. *Journal of Clinical Endocrinology and Metabolism* **34**: 630–637.

de Certaines J, Herry JY, Lancien G et al (1982) Evaluation of human thyroid tumors by proton nuclear magnetic resonance. *Journal of Nuclear Medicine* **23**: 48–51.

Cohen AM, Crevistom S, LiPuma JP et al (1983) NMR evaluation of hilar and mediastinal lymphadenopathy. *Radiology* **148**: 739–742.

Daniel RA Jr, Diveley WL, Edwards WH et al (1960) Mediastinal tumors. *Annals of Surgery* **151**; 783–795.

Dische S (1964) The radioscope scan applied to the detection of carcinoma in thyroid swellings. *Cancer* **17**: 473–479.

Fernandez-Ulloa M, Maxon HR, Mehta S et al (1976) Iodine-131 uptake by primary lung adenocarcinoma: misinterpretation of I-131 scan. *Journal of the American Medical Association* **236**: 857–858.

Freitas JE, Gross MD, Ripley S et al (1985) Radionuclide diagnosis and therapy of thyroid cancer: current status report. *Seminars in Nuclear Medicine* **15**: 106–131.

Fujimoto Y, Oka A & Nagataki S (1972) Occurrence of papillary carcinoma in hyper-functioning thyroid nodule: report of a case. *Endocrinologia Japonica* **19**: 371–374.

Ghose MK, Genuth SM, Abellera RM et al (1971) Functioning primary thyroid carcinoma and metastases producing hyperthyroidism. *Journal of Clinical Endocrinology and Metabolism* **33**: 639–646.

Goldsmith SJ (1978) Thyroid in vivo test of function and imaging. In Rothfeld B (ed.) *Nuclear Medicine Endocrinology*, pp. 19–26. Philadelphia: JB Lippincott.

Hamburger JI (1975) Solitary autonomously functioning thyroid lesions. *American Journal of Medicine* **58**: 740–748.

Haynie TP, Nofal NM & Beierwaltes WH (1963) Treatment of thyroid carcinoma with [131]I. *Journal of the American Medical Association* **183**: 303–306.

Hilditch TE, Connell JMC, Elliott AT et al (1986) Poor results with technetium-99m(V) DMS and ^{131}I MIBG in the imaging of medullary thyroid carcinoma. *Journal of Nuclear Medicine* **27**: 1150–1153.

Jackson IMD & Thomson JA (1967) The relationship of carcinoma to the single thyroid nodule. *British Journal of Surgery* **54**: 1007–1009.

Jeghers O, Puttemans N, Urbain D et al (1986) Technetium-99m DMSA uptake by metastatic carcinoma of the prostate. *Journal of Nuclear Medicine* **27**: 1223–1225.

Johnson DG, Coleman RE, McCook TA et al (1984) Bone and liver images in medullary carcinoma of the thyroid gland: concise communication. *Journal of Nuclear Medicine* **25**: 419–422.

Khan, O, Ell PJ, Maclennan KA et al (1981) Thyroid carcinoma in a autonomously hyperfunctioning thyroid nodule. *Postgraduate Medical Journal* **57:** 172–175.

McLaughlin RP, Scholz DA, McConahey WM et al (1970) Metastatic thyroid carcinoma with hyperthyroidism: two cases with functioning metastatic follicular thyroid carcinoma. *Mayo Clinic Proceedings* **45:** 328–335.

Meier DA & Hamburger JI (1971) An autonomously functioning thyroid nodule, cancer, and prior radiation. *Archives of Surgery* **103:** 759–761.

Muller-Brand J, Fridrich R, Spicher E et al (1983) Thyroglobulin als tumormarker and thalliumszintigraphie zur verlaufskontrolle beim differenzierten schildrusen karzinom. *Schweizerische Medizinische Wochenschrift* **113:** 325–327.

Mulnar GD, Childs DS & Woolner LB (1958) Histologic evidence of malignancy in a thyroid gland bearing a 'hot' nodule. *Journal of Clinical Endocrinology and Metabolism* **18:** 1132–1134 (letter).

Nemec J, Zamrazil V, Pohunkova D et al (1984) The rational use of ^{201}Tl scintigraphy in the evaluation of differentiated thyroid cancer. *European Journal of Nuclear Medicine* **9:** 261–264.

Ohta H, Yamamoto K, Endo K et al (1984a) A new imaging agent for medullary carcinoma of the thyroid. *Journal of Nuclear Medicine* **25:** 323–325.

Ohta H, Endo K, Fujita T et al (1984b) Imaging of soft tissue tumors with Tc(V)-99m dimercaptosuccinic acid. A new tumor-seeking agent. *Clinical Nuclear Medicine* **9:** 568–573.

Ohta H, Ishii M, Yoshizumi M et al (1985) Is ECT imaging with Tc(V)-99m dimercaptosuccinic acid useful to detect lung metastases of osteosarcoma? *Clinical Nuclear Medicine* **10:** 13–15.

Patton JA, Hollifield JW, Brill AB et al (1976) Differentiation between malignant and benign solitary thyroid nodules by fluorescent scanning. *Journal of Nuclear Medicine* **17:** 17–21.

Patton JA, Sandler MP, Sacks GA et al (1982) Prediction of benignancy of solitary 'cold' thyroid nodules using x-ray fluorescent scanning. *Endocrine Society Abstract*, San Francisco, 64, 281.

Patton JA, Sandler MP & Partain CL (1985) Prediction of benignancy of the solitary 'cold' thyroid nodule by fluorescent scanning. *Journal of Nuclear Medicine* **26:** 461–464.

Pinsky S and Yun Ryo U (1981) *Nuclear Medicine Annual.* New York: Raven Press.

Propper RA, Skolnick ML, Winstein BJ et al (1980) The non-specificity of the thyroid halo sign. *Journal of Clinical Ultrasound* **8:** 129–132.

Psarra A, Papadopoulos SN, Livada D et al (1974) The single thyroid nodule. *British Journal of Surgery* **59:** 545–548.

dos Remedios LV, Weber PM & Jasko IA (1971) Thyroid scintiphotography in 1000 patients; rational use of 99m-Tc and I-131 compounds. *Journal of Nuclear Medicine* **12:** 673–677

Sandler MP & Patton JA (1987) Multimodality imaging of the thyroid and parathyroid glands. *Journal of Nuclear Medicine* **28:** 123.

Sandler MP, Patton JA, Sacks GA et al (1984) Evaluation of intrathoracic goitre with I-123 scintigraphy and nuclear magnetic resonance imaging. *Journal of Nuclear Medicine* **25:** 874–876.

Sandler MP, Patton JA, Sacks GA et al (1986) Scintigraphic thyroid imaging. In Sandler MP, Patton JA & Partain CL (eds) *Thyroid and Parathyroid Imaging*, p. 121. East Norwalk: Appleton-Century-Crofts.

Sandler MP, Fellmeth B, Salhany KE et al (1988) Thyroid carcinoma masqerading as a solitary benign hyperfunctioning nodule. *Clinical Nuclear Medicine* **13:** 410–415.

Sekiya T, Tade A, KawaKami et al (1979) Clinical application of computed tomography to thyroid disease. *Computerized Tomography* **3:** 185–193.

Shaff MI, Price AC, Sandler MP & Kulkarni MV (1986) Computed tomography in thyroid disease. In Sandler MP, Patton JA & Partain CL (eds) Thyroid and Parathyroid Imaging. East Norwalk: Appleton-Century-Crofts.

Shambaugh GE III, Quinn JL, Oyasu R & Freinkel N (1974) Disparate thyroid imaging: combined studies with sodium pertechnetate Tc-99m and radioactive iodine. *Journal of the American Medical Association* **228:** 866–869.

Shapiro B, Copp JE, Sisson JC et al (1985) Iodine-131 metaiodobenzylguanidine for the locating of suspected paeochromocytoma: experience in 400 cases. *Journal of Nuclear Medicine* **26:** 576–585.

Simeone JR, Daniels GH, Mueller RP et al (1982) High-resolution real-time sonography of the thyroid. *Radiology* **145:** 431–435.

Sisson JC, Bartold SP & Bartold SL (1978) The dilemma of a solitary thyroid nodule: resolution through decision analysis. *Seminars in Nuclear Medicine* **8:** 59–71.

Smith FW, Runge VM, Sandler MP, Patton JA & Partain CL (1986) Magnetic resonance imaging in thyroid disease. In Sandler MP, Patton JA & Partain CL (eds) *Thyroid and Parathyroid Imaging*, p. 346. East Norwalk: Appleton-Century-Crofts.

Sodee DB (1966) The study of thyroid physiology utilizing intravenous sodium pertechnetate. *Journal of Nuclear Medicine* **7:** 564–567.

Spencer RP (1984) Radiotracers in therapy and evaluation of primary or metastatic sites. *Journal of Nuclear Medicine* **25:** 514–517.

Spencer RP, Garg V, Ralsz LG et al (1982) Radioiodide uptake and turnover in a pseudo-medullary thyroid carcinoma. *Journal of Nuclear Medicine* **23:** 1006–1010.

Strauss HW, Hurley PJ & Wagner HN Jr (1970) Advantages of ^{99m}Tc pertechnetate for thyroid scanning in patients with decreased radioiodine uptake. *Radiology* **97:** 307–310.

Sykes D (1981) The solitary thyroid nodule. *British Journal of Surgery* **68:** 510–512.

Tonami N & Hisada K (1980) ^{201}Tl scintigraphy in postoperative detection of thyroid cancer: a comparative study with ^{131}I. *Radiology* **136:** 461–464.

Tonami N, Bunko H, Michigish T et al (1978) Clinical application of ^{201}Tl scintigraphy in patients with cold thyroid nodules. *Clinical Nuclear Medicine* **3:** 217–221.

Van Herle AJ, Rich P, Ljung BME et al (1982) The thyroid nodule. *Annals of Internal Medicine* **96:** 221–232.

Wolfstein RS (1978) Enigma of the 'hyperfunctioning' thyroid carcinoma resolved? *Journal of Nuclear Medicine* **19:** 441–442 (letter).

5

Gastrointestinal and pancreatic endocrine
tumours

JEFFREY T. HALL
SIDNEY WALLACE
C. HUMBERTO CARRASCO
CHUSILP CHARNSANGAVEJ
WILLIAM R. RICHLI
JAFFER AJANI
NAGUIB SAMAAN
GERALD D. DODD JR

In an attempt to create a unified concept, Pearse (1968) suggested that neuroendocrine cells are diffusely distributed in many organ systems and include cells of the anterior pituitary gland, the parafollicular thyroid cells, the chromaffin cells of the adrenal medulla and extra-adrenal paraganglia, the enterochromaffin and peptide-secreting cells of the gastrointestinal tract and pancreatic islet cells, and the Feyrter cells of the tracheobronchial tree. The acronym APUD was derived from their most prominent features, i.e. the fluorogenic amine content, *a*mine *p*recursor *u*ptake and the presence of amino acid *d*ecarboxylase (Larsson et al, 1975; Pearse, 1977; Launay et al, 1983). Although there is no common embryonic origin, functional and physiological similarities and complex neurohormonal interactions continue to support an integrated APUD concept.

Nearly 40 polypeptides which serve as endocrine, paracrine or neuro-transmitter agents have been found in the endocrine cells of the gut and in the pancreatic islet cells of Langerhans: the gastroenteropancreatic endocrine axis (Krejs, 1987). These include:

1. In the stomach—gastrin, adrenocorticotropin hormone-like polypeptide (ACTH), somatostatin, serotonin and vasoactive polypeptides (VIP).
2. In the duodenum and jejunum—cholecystokinin, gastric inhibitory polypeptides, gastrin, glucagon, motilin, somatostatin, secretin, substance P, serotonin, VIP and bombesin.
3. In the small and large bowels—glucagon, neurotensin, serotonin and bombesin.
4. In the pancreas—insulin, glucagon, somatostatin, serotonin, melano-cyte stimulating hormone (MSH), VIP, ACTH, growth hormone

releasing factor (GHRF) and pancreatic polypeptide (Larsson et al, 1975; Friesen, 1982; Rivier et al, 1982; Krejs, 1987).

The APUD cells and their corresponding neoplasms, APUDomas, are closely related in terms of their biosynthetic mechanisms, their histochemical and ultrastructural features. APUDomas may produce abnormal quantities of amines or peptide hormones that may be identical to the secretory products of their non-neoplastic counterparts. APUDomas may be benign or malignant; hyperplasia is included among them because of the functional resemblance. These neoplasms also occur as part of the multiple endocrine neoplasms (MEN) syndrome. Generally, APUDomas grow slowly and even after metastasizing they are associated with prolonged survival.

This chapter describes the radiological contributions to the diagnosis and management of primary neuroendocrine neoplasms of the gastrointestinal tract and their metastases as well as the clinical syndromes they manifest.

PRIMARY GASTROINTESTINAL ENDOCRINE TUMOURS

Carcinoid

Carcinoid tumours develop in the Kulchitsky's enterochromaffin cells in the crypts of Lieberkuhn and are characterized by the presence of neurosecretory granules (Oberndorder, 1907; Pearse et al, 1974). About 85% of the carcinoid tumours are found in the gastrointestinal tract, 10% in the lung mostly as bronchial carcinoids and the rest in various organs such as the larynx, thymus, kidney, ovary, prostate and skin (Godwin, 1975). In the gastrointestinal tract, the carcinoid tumours originate most frequently in the appendix, ileum and rectum but rarely in the pancreas. Carcinoid is by far the most common tumour of the appendix comprising 77% of all appendiceal tumours; the second most frequent (23%) of the small bowel tumours, and 47% of all malignant small bowel tumours. The incidence of gastrointestinal carcinoid has been reported from 0.2% to 1.1%, with a female : male ratio of 1.5 : 1.0 (Linnell and Mansson, 1966; Ostermiller and Joergenson, 1966; Godwin, 1975; Jager and Polk, 1977).

Carcinoid tumours are all potentially malignant and may secrete metabolically active substances including serotonin; kallikrein (bradykinin); substance P, neurokinin A, and neuropeptide K (tachykinins); and prostaglandins. These substances are responsible for the 'carcinoid syndrome'—cutaneous flushing, asthma (wheezing), diarrhoea, cyanosis, right-sided valvular heart disease (tricuspid regurgitation and/or stenosis and pulmonic stenosis) (Thorson et al, 1954), pellagra-like dermatitis and arthritis. The foregut and midgut carcinoids (bronchial and small bowel) are frequently associated with the carcinoid syndrome,.while those in the hindgut (colon and rectum) are seldom, if ever, associated. This syndrome occurs in 6.7% of all patients with carcinoid tumours and 10% of patients with small bowel carcinoids (which comprise 90% of all patients with carcinoid syndrome).

The carcinoid syndrome is almost always associated with liver metastases since the tumours in the liver secrete hormonal products directly into the systemic circulation with avoidance of hepatic detoxification. Of all patients with carcinoid liver metastases, 45% experience the syndrome. In cases of bronchial carcinoid and carcinoid arising from teratoma of the ovary, the syndrome may be present without evidence of metastatic disease. This is explained by the venous drainage from the lung and ovary which bypasses the liver where serotonin from gastrointestinal carcinoids is metabolized by monoamine oxidase (Ostermiller and Joergenson, 1966; Davis et al, 1973; Godwin, 1975; Brennan and MacDonald, 1985; Cruetzfeldt and Stockman, 1987).

In the classical 'carcinoid syndrome', the most practical laboratory test has been the determination of the urinary 5-hydroxyindoleacetic acid levels (5HIAA). Abnormal values do not necessarily indicate a gastrointestinal carcinoid; they may be associated with tumours in the bronchi, ovary and testes as well as oat-cell carcinoma of the lung. Moertel et al (1961) found the median survival from the first determination of elevated 5HIAA to be 23 months. It is not uncommon for patients with metastatic carcinoid tumour with no treatment to live many years (Moertel, 1973; Davis et al, 1973).

Radiologically, the tumours present a variety of appearances directly reflecting the method of spread as well as the extent of disease (Bluth, 1960; Hudson and Margulis, 1964; Boijsen et al, 1974; Bancks et al, 1975; Goldstein and Miller, 1975; Dodd, 1978, 1985). Since the tumours arise from the Kulchitsky's cells, they appear in their uncomplicated form as submucosal nodules. This is particularly true in the stomach and duodenum (Figure 1).

In our series of 75 patients with gastrointestinal carcinoids the majority originated in the terminal ileum or appendix (Goldstein and Miller, 1975). Three of 18 cases with positive small bowel series presented smooth, solitary, intraluminal defects in the distal ileum. The tumour may extend

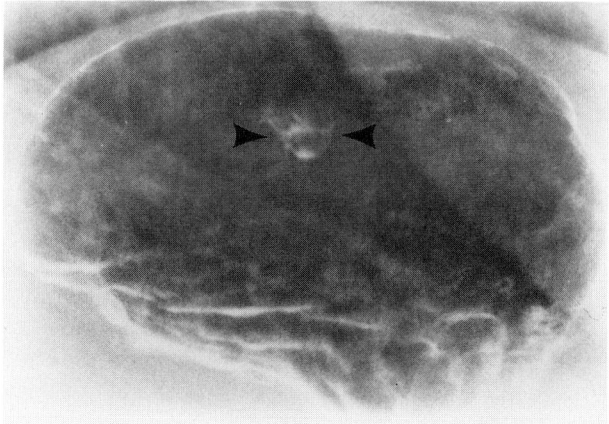

Figure 1. Carcinoid of the stomach. A sessile polyp (arrowheads) presenting as a submucosal nodule in the gastric fundus on barium study.

intraluminally with eventual obstruction, and may also serve as a lead point for intussusception. The differential diagnosis includes any benign tumour arising from the mucosa or submucosa, aberrant gastric mucosa and solitary metastases. Carcinoids may ulcerate particularly in the ileum and colon: the differential diagnosis for such a 'target lesion' includes lymphoma, melanoma and Kaposi's sarcoma. Multiple nodules occur in approximately one third of the patients and may result from metastases to other parts of the bowel, or from multiplicity of primary tumours.

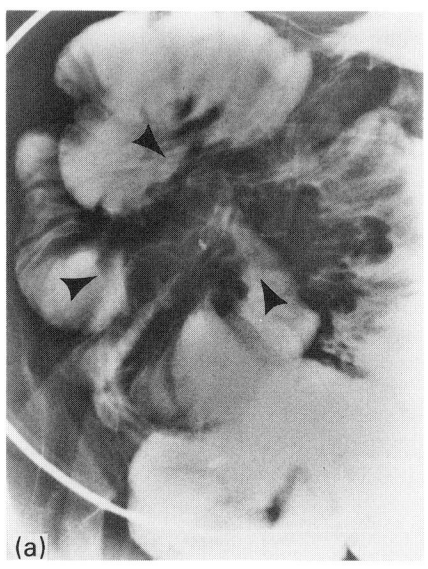

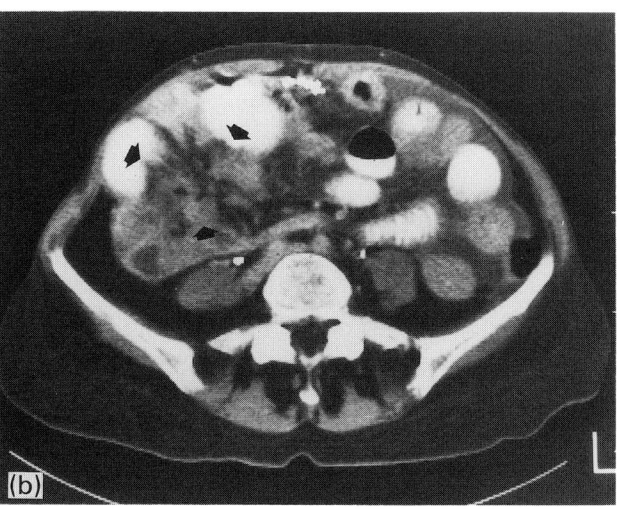

Figure 2. Desmoplastic reaction as the result of a small bowel carcinoid. (a) Small bowel barium examination; (b) Abdominal CT scan. Note the sharp angulation and traction effects on the loops of small bowel—arrowheads in (a) and arrows in (b).

As the carcinoid enlarges, the intraluminal component is often exceeded by submucosal extension and outward growth through the bowel wall, with characteristic hypertrophy of the involved muscle layers. Barium studies demonstrate thickening of the mucosal folds. The tumour may also be predominantly extraluminal with a minimal or absent intraluminal component: radiologically presenting a purely extrinsic mass with compression and stretching of the adjacent bowel.

If a carcinoid extends exoenterically, it eventually involves the mesentery and tends to incite a pharmacologically-mediated fibroblastic response. Manifestations of mesenteric desmoplastic reaction, sometimes isolated without evidence of a mass component, were the most frequent and striking radiological findings present in at least 13 of our 18 patients with small bowel carcinoids. There is rigidity and fixation of the bowel loops with retraction toward the root of the mesentery (Figure 2). Sharp angulation and kinking of the loops occur, accounting for the frequency of obstructive symptoms. Traction effects or tethering of the mucosal folds are also common. Extensive mesenteric fibrosis may encase the bowel and, in conjunction with hypertrophic muscular thickening, may cause diffuse luminal narrowing. Differential diagnosis of such a radiological appearance includes a number of diseases that have significant mesenteric involvement such as abdominal carcinomatosis, postoperative adhesions, radiation enteritis, granulomatous enteritis etc.

Visceral angiography may be helpful in the evaluation of a suspected carcinoid tumour when clinical and laboratory findings are suggestive but the barium studies are normal. If the barium examinations are abnormal, angiography can aid in differentiating carcinoid tumour from other neoplastic process (Figure 3) (Goldstein and Miller, 1975).

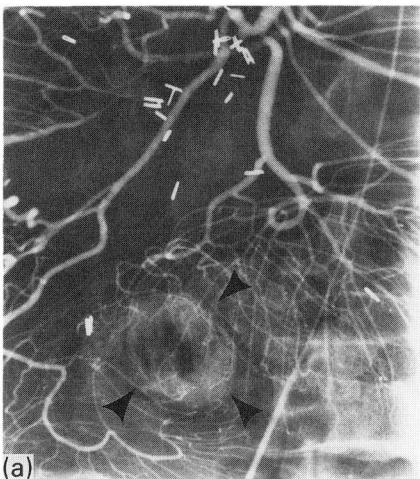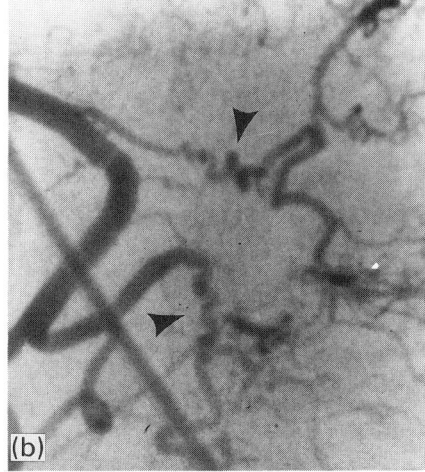

Figure 3. Small bowel carcinoid: angiography. (a) Superior mesenteric arteriography (SMA) reveals recurrent hypervascular carcinoid (arrowheads). (b) SMA with digital subtraction demonstrates the effects on the mesenteric arteries (arrowheads) of the desmoplastic reaction as the result of a carcinoid tumour.

Table 1. Neuroendocrine tumours of the pancreas.

Tumour	Cell	Syndrome	Age and sex ratio	Size at presentation	Location	Malignancy	Radiological strategy	Incidence
Insulinoma	B	Fasting, hypoglycaemia, sweating, trembling, palpitations, apprehension	40 yr M = F	40% < 1 cm 90% < 5 cm 95% discrete neoplasm 5% adenomatosis	Throughout pancreas	90% benign 10% regional metastases	1. Dynamic or arterial CT 2. Arteriography 3. PVS 4. Intraoperative US	75–80% of all FCT islet cell
Gastrinoma	G	Zollinger–Ellison: PUD–ABD pain, vomiting, melaena, weight loss	Middle-age M 65% 30% MEN I	Variable	60–70% Multifocal	60% Malignant 30% Adenoma 10% Hyperplasia	1. UGI (for DX) 2. CT dynamic 3. US 4. Arteriography 5. PVS	2nd most common
Glucagonoma		Diabetes, migratory necrolytic erythema, weight loss, thrombophlebitis	4th decade	> 3 cm	Tail/body	75% Malignant	1. CT dynamic 2. Angiography (± 100%)*	Rare
WDHA/Verner–Morrison		Secretory diarrhoea, hypokalaemia, renal insufficiency (watery diarrhoea, hypokalaemia, achlorhydria syndrome) cutaneous flushing	45 yr F 67%	Variable	Tail or proximal body	50% With metastases 30% Benign 15% Hyperplasia	1. UGI, SBFT (for DX) 2. CT dynamic 3. Angiography	Rare
Somatostinoma	D	Mild diabetes, steatorrhoea, weight loss gastric hyposecretion, diarrhoea	Unknown	> 3 cm	Body/tail	Frequent	1. CT 2. US 3. Angiography	Rare
Non-functioning tumours		None		6–20 cm		If malignant usually not aggressive	1. CT 2. Angiography 3. US	

* Prinz et al (1979).

M, male; F, female; CT, computed tomography; FCT, functioning computed tomography; PVS, portal vein sampling; US, ultrasound; PUD, peptic ulcer disease; ABD, abdomen; MEN I, multiple endocrine neoplasm I; UGI, upper gastrointestinal examination; DX, diagnosis; CT dynamic, dynamic computed tomography; SBFT, small bowel followthrough examination.

PANCREATIC ENDOCRINE TUMOURS (Table 1)

The islets of Langerhans comprise approximately 2% of the bulk of the pancreas with the greatest concentration of these cells in the tail of the pancreas, less numerous in the body and even less in the head. The islets are composed of four different cell lines: the alpha cells which secrete glucagon; the beta cells which produce insulin; the delta cells, somatostatin; and the PP cells, pancreatic polypeptides. The PP cells are also scattered among the acinar cells. In addition, a variety of other pharmacologically active substances are produced by the islet cell (Schein et al, 1973; Larsson et al, 1975; Friesen, 1982; Rivier et al, 1982).

Pancreatic endocrine tumours, even when very small, may produce complex clinical syndromes with symptoms based upon the hormones secreted. Those neoplasms which do not secrete any metabolically active substances or which do so below the current levels of detection are termed non-functioning islet cell tumours (Kent et al, 1981). These lesions tend to become clinically apparent by their local mass effect, metastases or by invasion of surrounding structures. The localization of these lesions usually require radiological and/or surgical intervention (Wolf et al, 1977; DiBisceglie et al, 1984).

The non-hereditary sporadic islet cell tumours tend to occur in the fourth and fifth decades of life, without sex preference. Most of these tumours arise within the pancreas, though they may originate within the duodenum, stomach, splenic hilum and mesentery when part of the MEN syndromes (Ballard et al, 1964; Wilson SD, 1978; O'Berg et al, 1982; Dodd, 1985; Dodds et al, 1985; Doppman, 1985).

MEN I or Wermer's syndrome consists of lesions of the parathyroid, islet cells and pituitary gland. Parathyroid hyperplasia and gastrin-producing islet cell hyperplasia are the major clinical presentations. In a review of 85 patients with MEN I, the glandular involvement was as follows: parathyroid 88%, pancreatic islet cells 81%, anterior pituitary 65%, adrenal cortex 38% and thyroid 19%. Nearly all patients with MEN I syndrome eventually develop an abnormality, hyperplasia or neoplasm, of the pancreas. This pancreatic abnormality frequently manifests itself 5–10 years after the patient starts experiencing symptoms of hyperparathyroidism (Ballard et al, 1964). The main pancreatic hormone is gastrin, although secretion of the various other pancreatic hormones (VIP, pancreatic polypeptides) has been described in patients with this syndrome (Hutcheon et al, 1979; Friesen et al, 1983).

The MEN II syndrome consists of parathyroid hyperplasia, medullary thyroid carcinoma and phaeochromocytoma. MEN IIb, otherwise known as MEN III or Sipple's syndrome, is a variant of MEN II combining medullary carcinoma of the thyroid, phaeochromocytoma and tumours of neuronal tissue (Hill et al, 1973).

Gut hormone-producing tumours are rare, with an incidence of one per 200 000 population per year. Gastrinomas are found in one person per two million per year, VIPomas in one per 10 million, and glucagonomas in one per 20 million (Buchanan KD, Irish Registry, 1986, quoted in Brennan MF and MacDonald JS, 1985; Krejs, 1987).

Insulinoma

Insulinoma is the commonest of the pancreatic islet cell tumours. The average age at the time of diagnosis is 40 years. Most insulinomas present at an early stage, so that over 90% of cases are less than 5 cm in diameter and 40% less than 1 cm at presentation (Hanson, 1960). Ninety-five per cent of insulinomas are associated with a discrete neoplasm, while 5% have adenomatosis.

Although insulinomas tend to be very small, some surgeons favour exploration and palpation for localization (Daggett et al, 1981). In a review of 772 insulinomas, one series reported finding 76.3% of the tumours during the initial operation (Steffani et al, 1974). A high incidence of second surgical procedures makes accurate preoperative localization attractive (Mengoli and LeQuesne, 1967; Steffani et al, 1974; Edis et al, 1976).

Insulinomas are usually hypervascular tumours, such that arteriography

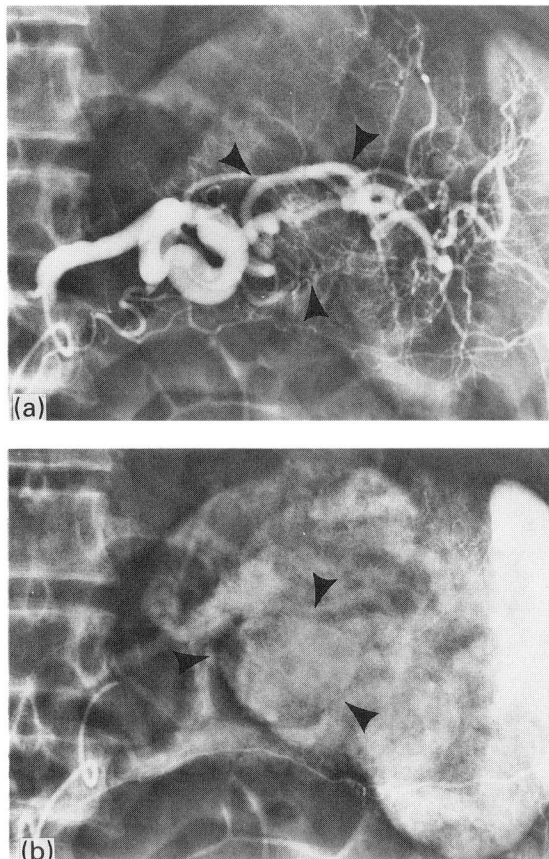

Figure 4. Islet cell tumour: splenic arteriography. (a) Arterial phase. (b) Venous phase; opacifies a hypervascular islet cell tumour of the tail of the pancreas (arrowheads).

with magnification technique has been regarded as the optimal localization technique. Insulinoma generally demonstrates a homogeneous 'well defined blush' during the capillary phase of the arteriogram. The reported sensitivity of angiography varies. However, with good radiographic technique and superselective catheterization, approximately 80% of insulinomas can be localized with angiography alone. Superselective arteriography of the gastroduodenal, dorsal pancreatic and splenic arteries is much more likely to

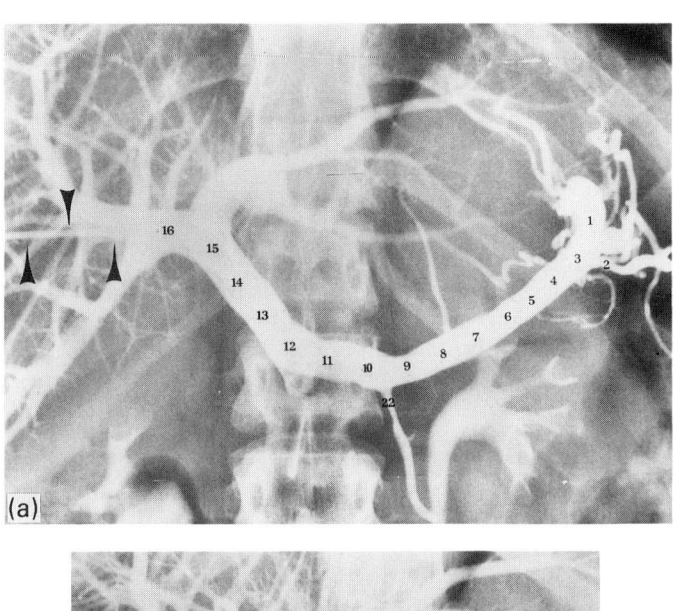

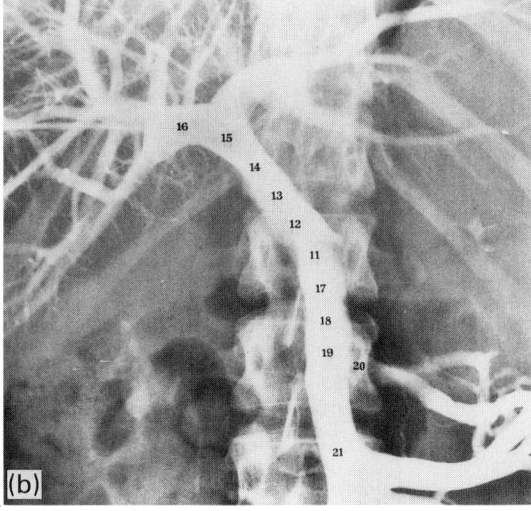

Figure 5. Pancreatic venous sampling (PVS). (a) Percutaneous transhepatic catheterization of the portal and splenic veins with venous samples taken at each site enumerated. Note the position of the catheter in the liver (arrowheads). (b) Venous sampling in the portal and superior mesenteric veins.

localize a small insulinoma than is coeliac and superior mesenteric arteriography (Figure 4) (Epstein et al, 1969; McGarity et al, 1971; Dunnick et al,
1980).

Transhepatic pancreatic venous sampling (PVS) provides a very sensitive
method for localization of insulinomas. In addition, this technique is the
only one available which is capable of localizing sites of islet cell hyperplasia.
The success rate with PVS approaches 100%. Because of the technical
demands of the procedure, PVS is generally reserved for those patients who
have a high clinical suspicion for insulinomas, but a negative CT scan and
arteriogram (Figure 5) (Ingemansson et al, 1975; Ingemansson et al, 1978;
Cho et al, 1982; Roche et al, 1982; Krudy et al, 1984; Carrasco, 1985).

Sonography is not sensitive as a primary modality for investigating the
patient with a suspected insulinoma (Shawker et al, 1982; Siegel et al, 1983).
Shawker and colleagues (1982) were only able to identify three of ten
pancreatic insulinomas with ultrasound. On sonography, insulinomas are
rounded, hypoechoic, well circumscribed lesions. Most insulinomas identified by transabdominal sonography will lie in the head of the pancreas,
simply emphasizing the technical limitations of sonography in imaging the
body and tail of the pancreas. Intraoperative ultrasound, however, appears
to be a promising modality. Most, if not all, insulinomas can be identified by
high resolution (7.5–10.0 MHz) intraoperative ultrasound. Intraoperative
ultrasound is not only useful for tumour localization, but has also proved
valuable in the identification of the relationship between the tumour and the
pancreatic duct (Siegel et al, 1983).

Computed tomography (CT) has virtually supplanted angiography as the
initial investigative modality in the evaluation of the patient with a suspected
insulinoma (Krudy et al, 1984; Stark et al, 1984; Carrasco, 1985; Rossi et al,
1985). It is important to pay attention to the CT technique. The examination
should be performed with 3–5 mm thin slices through the pancreas with a
rapid bolus intravenous injection of 50–150 cm^3 of 60% iodinated contrast
material through a large bore line during dynamic incremental CT. On the
precontrast scans, insulinomas have the same density as normal pancreatic
tissue. Postcontrast, a well circumscribed enhanced mass is identified. CT
has also been useful in demonstrating metastases to peripancreatic lymph
nodes and the liver.

CT can also be performed during arteriography (CT-angio) with the
catheter tip in the coeliac, gastroduodenal, splenic or dorsal pancreatic
artery. After placement of the catheter in the angiographic suite, the patient
is transported to the CT scanner. During the injection of 2 cm^3/s of 30%
contrast material, 3 mm dynamic incremental scans are done through the
pancreas (Figure 6). CT-angio improves the detection of smaller neoplasms.

CT and arteriography are complementary modalities in the investigation of
the patient with a suspected insulinoma. The patient should first be evaluated
with a dynamic intravenous-bolus enhanced CT scan. If this is unrewarding,
superselective arteriography should be the next step. This can be performed
in conjunction with CT-angio if more precise anatomic localization is
required. If both of these investigations are negative, PVS should be
performed. Exploratory surgery, with or without intraoperative ultrasound,

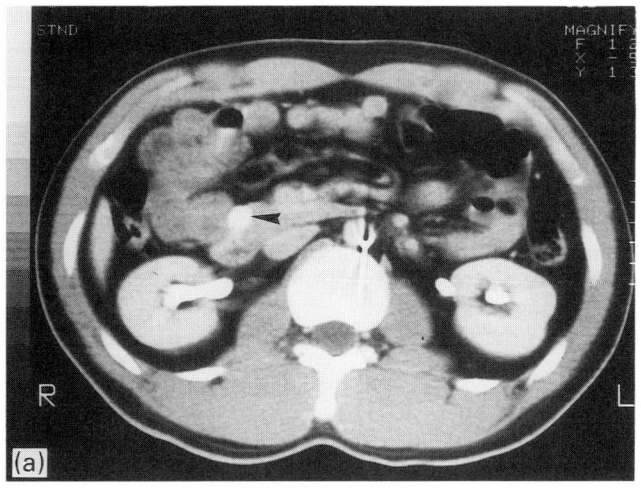

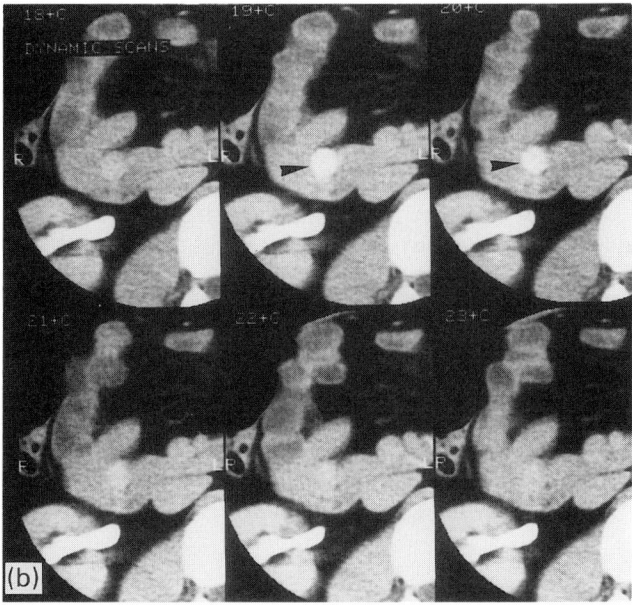

Figure 6. 29-year-old man with insulinoma in the head of pancreas. (a) CT-angio demonstrates the markedly enhanced 1-cm diameter tumour (arrowhead). (b) Series of dynamic scans taken at 5-s intervals on CT-angio without table incrementation reveal that the tumour enhancement (arrowhead) is evident for only 5–10 s after contrast injection. Appropriate timing of CT scanning may be necessary for optimal detection of the insulinoma. Case provided by F. L. Chan, Hong Kong.

should therefore be limited to those few cases where clinical suspicion is high while CT, angiography and PVS are negative, or where for technical reasons, adequate PVS cannot be performed. The use of magnetic resonance imaging (MRI) has not yet been investigated in this disease, but it probably will not add greatly to the already favourable diagnostic armamentarium.

Gastrinoma

The Zollinger–Ellison syndrome consists of the triad of peptic ulcer disease, gastric hypersecretion, and a gastrin producing non-beta islet cell tumour of the pancreas. The syndrome usually becomes manifest in middle age, affects males more commonly than females (65% vs. 35%), and may occur (30%) as a part of the MEN I syndrome (Marshall and Settles, 1980). Approximately 60% of the patients will have a malignant tumour, 30% a benign adenoma, and 10% glandular hyperplasia. Most gastrinomas are multifocal, making surgical resection for cure very difficult (Zollinger and Ellison, 1955; Modlin, 1979). Malignant gastrinomas usually metastasize to the regional lymph node and the liver. Distant metastases are unusual.

The conventional radiographic evaluation of a patient with a suspected gastrinoma usually begins with a standard upper gastrointestinal series. The scout film obtained prior to the ingestion of barium is usually unremarkable, but may reveal tumour-calcifications, in which case, the tumour is usually malignant (Bozymski et al, 1973; Jahnke et al, 1977).

Gastrointestinal barium examination classically reveals enlarged gastric folds, hypersecretion of gastric contents (making gastric mucosal coating with the barium suspension difficult), and peptic ulceration. The most common location for the peptic ulcer is duodenal bulb, with the classic post-bulbar ulcer being found in only 25% of cases (Amberg et al, 1964) (Figure 7). In addition, the duodenum may be dilated and atonic. The duodenal mucosal pattern may be blunted, small bowel folds thickened and

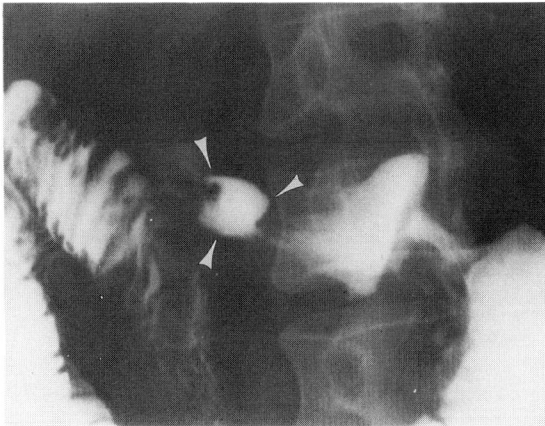

Figure 7. Zollinger–Ellison syndrome. Barium study demonstrates postbulbar ulcer (arrowheads) as a manifestation of a malignant gastrinoma.

small bowel transit time may be very short. Approximately one third of patients will exhibit a concomittant oesophagitis, which may be severe (Dodds et al, 1971; Richter et al, 1980).

Arteriography has not been very successful in localizing the site of gastrinomas, with a reported sensitivity of 20–30% (McGarity et al, 1971; Roche et al, 1982; Collen et al, 1984; Carrasco, 1985). The arteriographic appearance of gastrinomas varies with tumour size. Small (less than 3 cm) lesions usually demonstrate a homogeneous discrete blush, much like that seen in insulinomas. Larger gastrinomas may demonstrate neovascularity, vascular encasement, and arteriovenous shunting. While the primary lesion frequently escapes detection by arteriographic examination, the liver metastasis are generally hypervascular and easily detected by angiographic means. In addition to tumour identification, arteriography in patients with gastrinomas may show an intense blush to the gastric mucosa. PVS has not proven to be very successful for the localization of gastrinomas (Burcharth et al, 1979; Roche et al, 1982). Foremost among the reasons for this is that differential gastrin gradients tend to be lower than those found in insulinoma. This is further complicated by the multifocal nature of the disease and the relatively high incidence of metastasis.

CT has become the imaging modality of choice in attempts to localize these tumours. Stark et al (1984) were able to localize seven of nine gastrinomas using what is now considered out-of-date equipment. With current abdominal CT scanning units, at least similar results, and possibly improved results can be anticipated. CT can also occasionally demonstrate gastric wall thickening, fluid filled loops of small bowel, peripancreatic, and liver metastasis. On non-contrast CT scans, gastrinomas are generally hypodense compared to normal pancreatic tissue. The lesions became hyperdense after the intravenous infusion of contrast material. Punctate or nodular calcifications may also be seen (Figure 8). Secondary findings

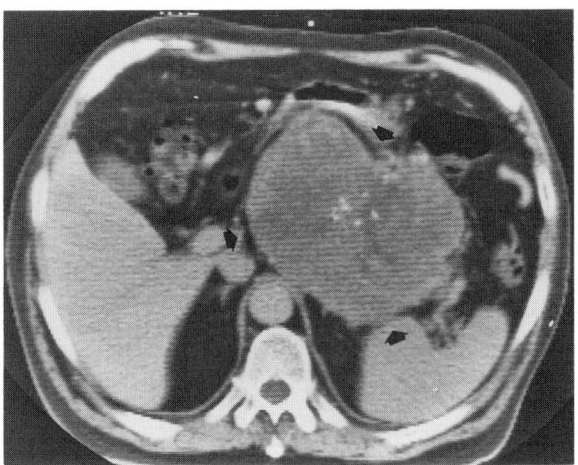

Figure 8. Gastrinoma. CT of abdomen: calcification in a malignant islet cell carcinoma of the body and tail of the pancreas (arrows).

include gastric wall thickening and increased fluid within the bowel.

Ultrasound has likewise not been very successful in the localization of these tumours. This is in part attributed to the difficulty encountered in attempting to image the pancreas in a patient with multiple dilated loops of bowel. Of 25 patients with gastrinomas, sonography was capable of identifying 14 (Shawker et al, 1982). Eight of these were located in the pancreatic head. However, sonography is useful for evaluating liver metastasis. Also, once a lesion has been identified by sonography, it provides a rapid and inexpensive means for follow-up evaluation. Sonography demonstrates a pancreatic mass of low echogenicity. Calcifications may be present. The hepatic metastases tend to be echogenic.

Gastrinomas, therefore, continue to be elusive to the radiologist. Currently, CT and angiography, and possibly PVS, appear to be complementary. The ultimate goal is to identify the 10–15% of patients who have solitary lesions, and who are therefore amenable to surgical cure. A logical radiological approach would start with CT and if negative, PVS and surgical exploration with intraoperative sonography as a last resort.

Verner-Morrison syndrome

This syndrome is also known as the WDHA syndrome, (watery diarrhoea, hypokalaemia, and achlorhydria). Females are affected approximately 70% of the time, and the mean age at diagnosis is 47 years (Inamoto et al, 1980). Vasoactive inhibitory polypeptide (VIP) has most frequently been implicated as the causative hormone in this syndrome (Said and Faloon, 1975). However, some patients with this syndrome do not secrete detectable VIP. The tumour responsible for this syndrome is usually solitary, and found within the body or tail of the pancreas. Fifty percent of the patients will be found to have metastasis at the time of diagnosis (Martin and Potet, 1974).

Conventional radiographic evaluation of the upper gastrointestinal tract will occasionally demonstrate dilated fluid-filled small bowel loops and a distended colon. Barium examination reveals a normal oesophagus and stomach, while small bowel loops demonstrate a delayed transit time with a dilated 'wet' appearance (McGill et al, 1980). The gall bladder may be dilated, but is characteristically without stones. This is in contrast to the findings with somatostatinoma.

While cumulative data is as yet lacking, a prudent current radiological approach to the localization of these lesions would begin with CT. Because of the larger size of these lesions at presentation, both CT and sonography should be capable of diagnosing the pancreatic primary and the metastasis. Angiography will reveal a hypervascular tumour nodule with a reticular network of vessels, or irregular neovascularity with microaneurysms (Inamoto et al, 1980). The tumour stain in patients with this syndrome is generally intense and may last for up to 15–20s after contrast injection. Arteries supplying the tumour are frequently enlarged and early venous filling is seen.

Glucagonoma

Glucagon-producing tumours of the pancreas usually present in the fourth and fifth decades of life. Men and women are affected with equal frequency (Prinz et al, 1981). Most of the lesions occur in the distal pancreas as solitary, relatively large lesions. A pancreatic alpha-cell tumour can be identified and stained by immunocytochemistry with glucagon antibodies. Seventy-five per cent of the tumours are malignant, with peripancreatic and liver metastases being frequent (Prinz et al, 1981). The glucagonoma syndrome is characterized by a necrolytic migratory erythematous rash, angular stomatosis, painful glossitis, normocytic normochromic anaemia, mild diabetes mellitus, weight loss, a tendency to thrombosis and neuropsychosomatic disturbances (Bloom and Polak, 1987).

Radiographically, small bowel folds may be thickened, and show a fine nodularity (Jones et al, 1983). Small bowel transit may be prolonged. Angiography almost invariably demonstrates the tumour. At presentation, glucagonomas are usually large (>3 cm) and hypervascular, and a tumour blush with or without adjacent venous invasion is common (Cho et al, 1977; Prinz et al, 1979). The liver metastases are also hypervascular and best demonstrated by arteriography. Thromboembolism, manifest as deep venous thrombosis and pulmonary embolism, is seen in up to 25% of patients with glucagonoma.

Both CT and ultrasound should be capable of demonstrating the primary tumour. CT is probably the diagnostic modality of choice, because of its capability not only to demonstrate the pancreatic primary, but also more adequately visualize the peripancreatic tissues.

Somatostatinoma

Somatostatin is elaborated by the pancreatic D cells. The syndrome produced by this tumour consists of diabetes, steatorrhoea, weight loss, gastric hypersecretion, and diarrhoea (Gerlock et al, 1979; Krejs et al, 1979). The gall bladder is frequently dilated, and may have calculi. These large lesions (greater than 3 cm) are most frequently found in the tail of the pancreas, and are usually malignant. Because of their large size at the time of diagnosis, angiography, CT and sonography should all be capable of demonstrating the lesion. Sonography, in addition, is quite capable of demonstrating the dilated gall bladder with its calculi.

Non-functioning tumours

The non-functioning islet-cell tumour generally comes to clinical attention as a large tumour mass. These tumours grow slowly, and are generally solitary (Kent et al, 1981). Due to their size at presentation, most available radiographic examinations can demonstrate the lesions. CT, in particular, is valuable in the demonstration of the primary tumour, local invasion, and metastasis (Figure 9) (Eelkema et al, 1984). CT can also be useful in distinguishing between islet-cell tumour and non-endocrine adenocarcinoma

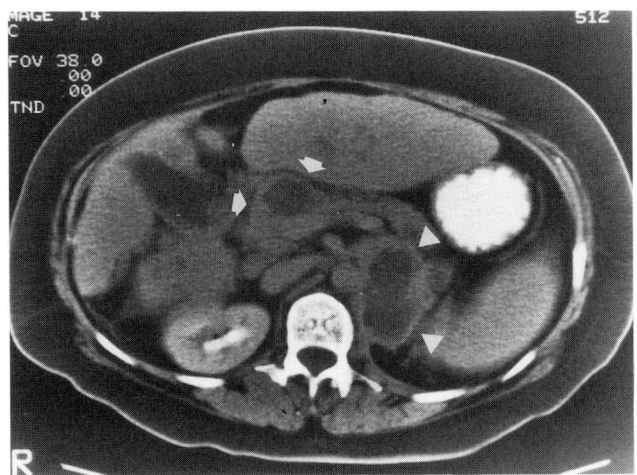

Figure 9. Islet cell carcinoma with lymph node metastases. Both the primary tumour of the head and proximal body (arrows) and the retroperitoneal lymph node metastases (arrowheads) were relatively low in attenuation coefficient. The diagnosis was established by percutaneous fine needle biopsy.

by demonstration of calcifications, which are distinctly unusual in the non-endocrine pancreatic adenocarcinoma. Those non-functioning tumours tend to be hypervascular, as do their metastases. Such being the case, angiography can also be useful in demonstrating both the primary lesion and its metastases. Angiography plays an additional role in evaluating for tumour resectability, and should therefore be considered complementary to CT. Experience with MRI is limited but thus far the pancreatic neoplasm is of intermediate signal intensity on T1- and increased on T2-weighted images (Figure 10).

METASTASES

The size of the primary carcinoid correlates with the likelihood of metastases (Moertel, 1973; Godwin, 1975). Only 2% of the tumours smaller than 1 cm in diameter evidenced metastases, while 80% of tumours larger than 2 cm in diameter were associated with metastatic disease. By the time of diagnosis, metastatic disease is common, as high as 90% in some series (Moertel et al, 1961; Ostermiller and Joergenson, 1966; Brennan and MacDonald, 1985). The major sites of metastases from neuroendocrine tumours are liver, lymph nodes in the mesentery, bone, lung and the peritoneum, whereas skin and nervous system metastases are less frequent (Figures 11 and 12). Metastatic carcinoid tumour has an unusual predilection for the eye and orbital region.

The diagnosis of the presence, nature and location of hepatic metastases is the responsibility of the diagnostic radiologist. The diagnostic armamentarium includes conventional radiography, scintigraphy, sonography, CT, CT-angio, angiography, MRI and percutaneous biopsy (Haaga, 1979, Bernardino et al, 1986; Mittelstaedt, 1987; Ferruci et al, 1988; Foley, 1988; Freeny, 1988; Stark, 1988). The sequence of studies is dictated by the patient's clinical status and habitus, the available facilities, the personnel, the technical and professional expertise as well as the financial burden. Undoubtedly, the diagnosis must be established with a minimum of discomfort and expense to the patient. The rewards must warrant the risks and cost. Solution of the patient's clinical problem seldom necessitates performing all the examinations available.

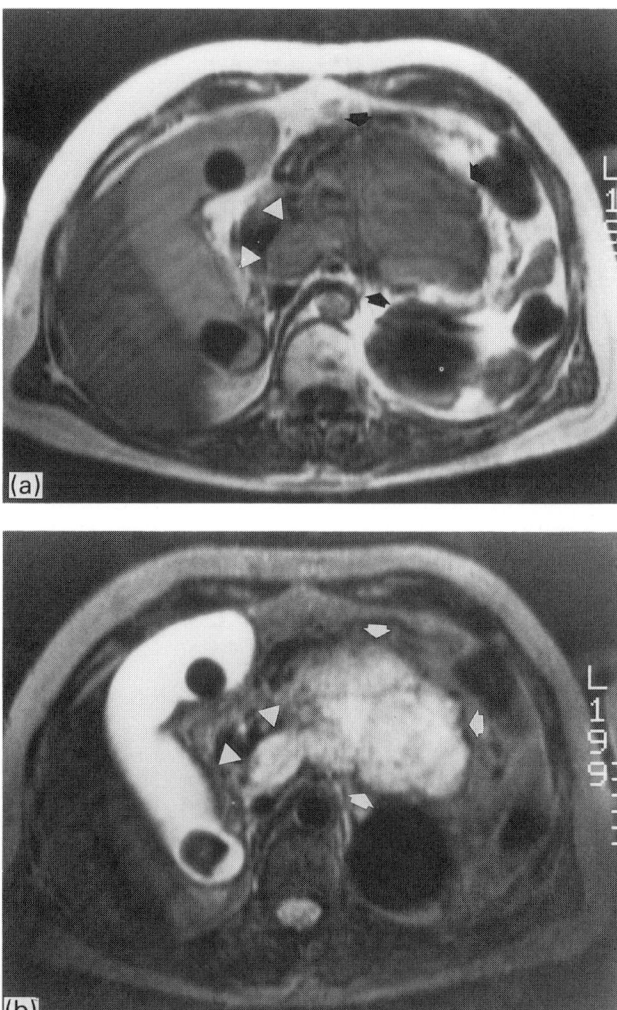

Figure 10. Non-functioning islet cell carcinoma. (a) T1-weighted and (b) T2-weighted images define a mass in the body and tail of the pancreas (arrows). The tumour extended into the splenic vein (arrowheads). Note the gall stones.

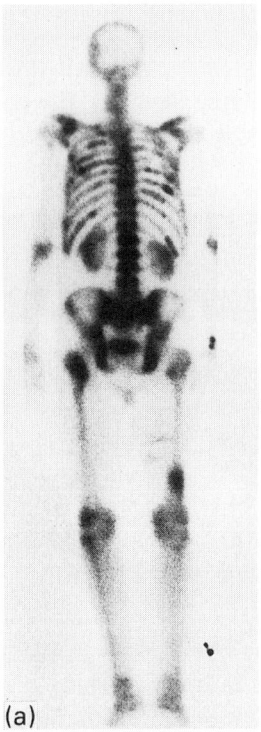

(a)

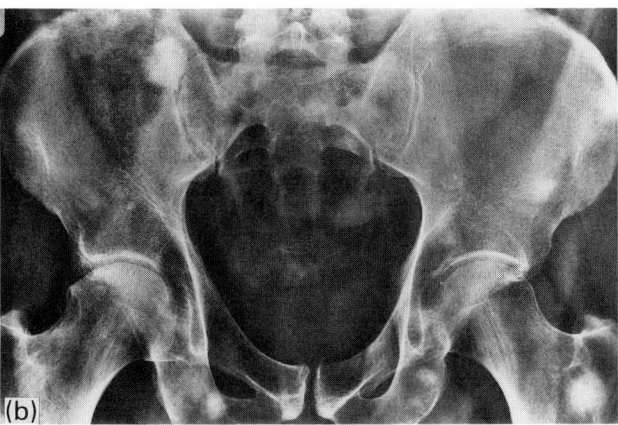

(b)

Figure 11. Osteoblastic metastases from a bronchial carcinoid. (a) Radionuclide bone scan shows multiple hot spots in the skeleton. (b) Radiography reveals blastic metastases to the pelvis.

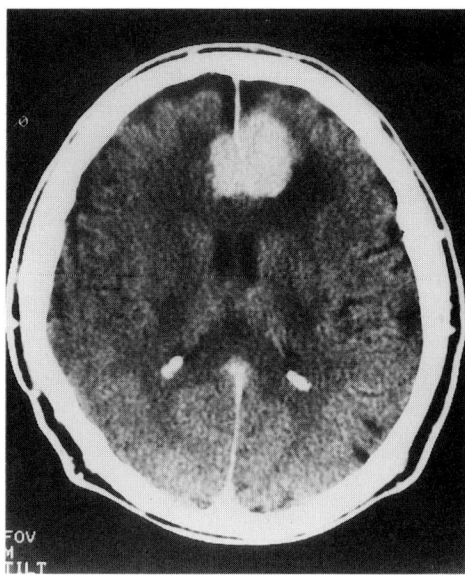

Figure 12. Brain metastases from carcinoid. CT scan demonstrates a markedly contrast-enhanced metastasis simulating a meningioma.

Despite the high sensitivity of these techniques, each has difficulty in differentiating diffuse from unilobar disease. The non-specificity of the screening methods, even in combination, is demonstrated by their inability to differentiate some benign, especially hypervascular lesions (hepatic adenoma, focal nodular hyperplasia, cavernous haemangioma) from hypervascular neuroendocrine metastases. This non-specificity may be resolved by angiography but at times only by histological evaluation, which is now most frequently accomplished by fine needle percutaneous aspiration biopsy guided by the modality that best defines the neoplasm (Haaga, 1979; Goldberg et al, 1980).

In a comparison between scintigraphy, sonography, CT and MRI, CT is still considered the best single examination to determine the presence and extent of a hepatic involvement. Recent reports suggest that MRI is competitive or may in fact surpass CT in accuracy, specificity and sensitivity in the detection of hepatic metastases; more experience is still necessary to define its place. In general, hepatic metastases exhibit a decreased or intermediate signal intensity on T1- and increased signal intensity on T2-weighted sequences. Utilizing spin–echo sequences, hepatic metastases are best demonstrated on T1-weighted images with midfield strength units (0.3–0.6 T) and T2-weighted images on high field strength units (1.0 and 1.5 T) (Figure 13) (Foley, 1988; Stark, 1988).

At our institute, CT is the modality of choice in the detection of hepatic metastases. Especially in hypervascular neoplasms, a precontrast scan is essential. This is optimally followed by rapid bolus injection at 1.3–1.6 cm³/s of $150\,\text{cm}^3$ of contrast material containing $45\,\text{g}$ of iodine during dynamic incremental CT (Freeny, 1988). Delayed iodine CT (DICT) obtained 4–6 hours following intravenous contrast has been reported to improve detection in 58% of cases and detected additional lesions not seen with bolus dynamic CT in 27% of patients (Bernardino et al, 1986).

Hepatic angiography is now reserved for problem solving or in preparation for therapeutic management (Wallace and Chuang, 1982; Chuang et al, 1983). Arteriography must include superselective catheterization and magnification techniques. Secondary neoplasms usually mimic the vascularity of their primary. Although the desmoplastic manifestation of carcinoid tumour is low in vascularity, its nodal as well as the hepatic metastases are almost

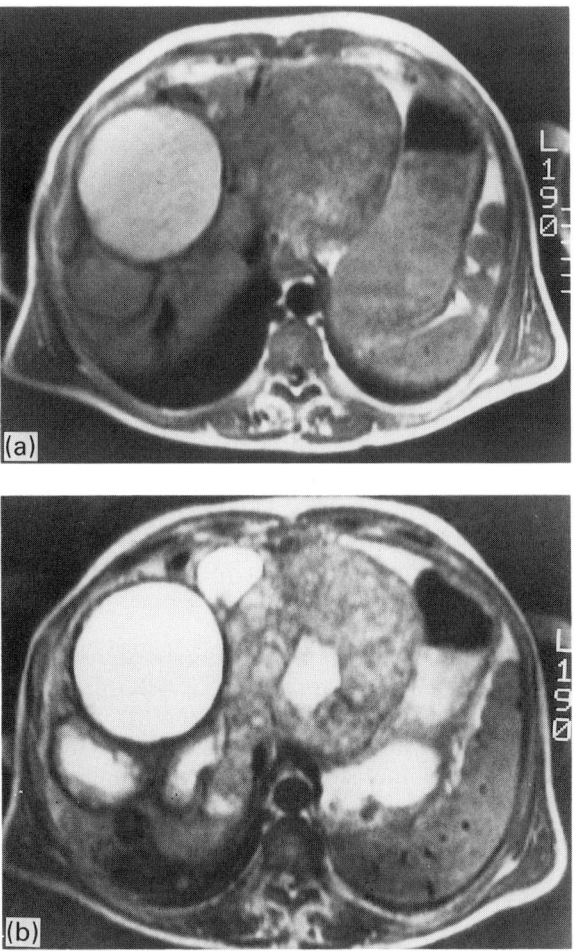

Figure 13. Hepatic metastases on MRI. (a) T1-weighted image defines the heterogeneous signal intensity of the metastases from an islet cell tumour. (b) T2-weighted image demonstrates these lesions to be of increased signal intensity.

invariably hypervascular and therefore best defined by arteriography (Figure 14) (Goldstein and Miller, 1975; Wallace and Chuang, 1982).

CT-angio performed with a catheter in the superior mesenteric artery defines metastases as non-specific low attenuation lesions during the enhanced portal venous parenchymal phase, or in the hepatic artery as enhanced lesions during the tumour capillary phase, is our 'gold' standard. Arteriography and CT-angio done at the same sitting are the most invasive, most expensive but most rewarding (Freeny, 1988).

INTERVENTIONAL MANAGEMENT OF HEPATIC METASTASES

Management of liver metastasis constitutes an important factor in the patient with an endocrine tumour (Wilson H, 1970; Moertel, 1973, 1983; Steffani et al, 1974; Edis et al, 1976; Wilson SD, 1978; Brennan and MacDonald, 1985). Significant improvement in clinical symptomatology may be derived with the control of the hormonally-active liver metastases. Surgical management includes enucleation of the liver metastases and partial hepatectomy (Wilson H and Butterick, 1959; Kune and Goldstein,

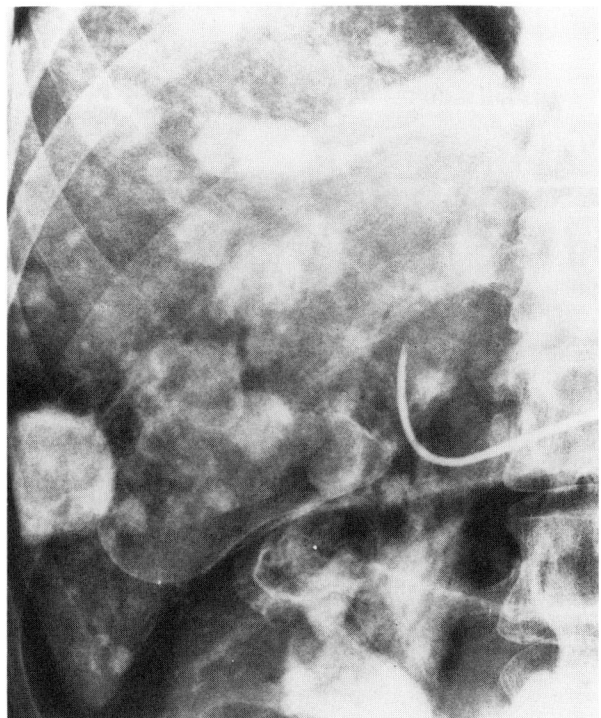

Figure 14. Hepatic metastases. Hepatic arteriography is most revealing in hepatic metastases which are usually hypervascular.

1974). Surgical devascularization of the liver has also been shown to achieve decrease in size of liver metastasis with a concomitant palliation of the hormonal syndrome (Murray-Lyon et al, 1970; Sparks et al, 1975).

The normal hepatic parenchyma receive 20–25% of its blood supply from the hepatic artery and 75–80% of its blood supply from the portal vein. Hepatic neoplasms, however, derive almost all of their blood supply from the hepatic artery (Bierman et al, 1951; Breedis and Young, 1954; Healey and Sheena, 1963; Lin et al, 1984). Occlusion of the hepatic arterial tree will therefore result in varying degrees of necrosis of the neoplasm, while preserving the normal hepatic parenchyma.

Proximal occlusion of the hepatic artery accomplished as the result of ligation or coil occlusion, is less effective than peripheral occlusion in decreasing hepatic arterial flow (Chuang and Wallace, 1981; Soo et al, 1983). This is due, in large part, to the effective collateral circulation which develops following hepatic artery occlusion. The more peripheral the occlusion, the less effective the collateral circulation will be in reconstituting flow. Peripheral occlusion also allows for repeat examinations and repeat occlusion (embolization) (Allison et al, 1977; Pueyo et al, 1978; Lunderquist et al, 1982; Carrasco et al, 1983, 1986; Mitty et al, 1985; Ajani et al, 1988). As experience accrues, peripheral occlusion by percutaneous catheterization is becoming the method of choice in the management of these liver metastases from neuroendocrine tumours.

Hepatic artery embolization

Technique

Our method of hepatic artery catheterization has been previously described (Chuang and Wallace, 1981; Soo et al, 1983). Hepatic artery embolization (HAE) is performed primarily with Ivalon (Unipoint Laboratories, High Point, NC) particles measuring 150–590 μm, Gelfoam powder or Gelfoam cubes (3 mm^3) (Upjohn, Kalamazoo, MI). Gelfoam segments and stainless steel coils are used to occlude collateral vessels. The main hepatic artery is not occluded, to allow for repeated embolization. The first embolization is generally limited to one hepatic artery. Subsequent HAE, usually of both lobes, are then spaced from 1 to 3 months. Usually, the patients are embolized at monthly intervals for a total of three embolizations. The interval between treatments is then prolonged and reflects the patient's imaging status at 3 and 6 months, as well as the recurrence of symptoms. The patients can be re-embolized as long as their vessels remain patent. Occlusion of the common hepatic artery does not preclude future embolizations as collateral circulation develops, and these collaterals can serve as access vessels for further embolization (Figures 15 and 16) (Soo et al, 1983).

Contraindications

There are a few contraindications to HAE (Carrasco et al, 1986). Embolization is contraindicated when *all* of the following coexist: (i)

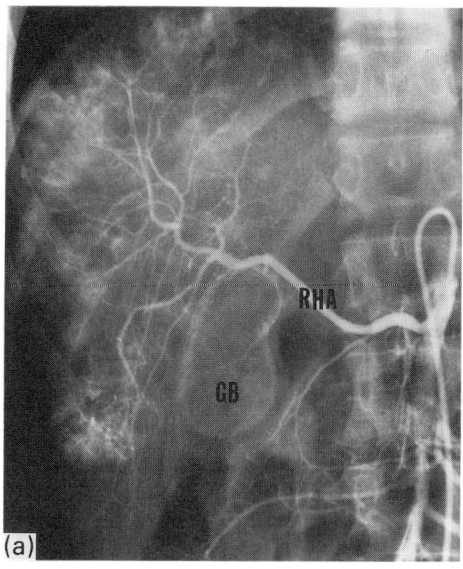

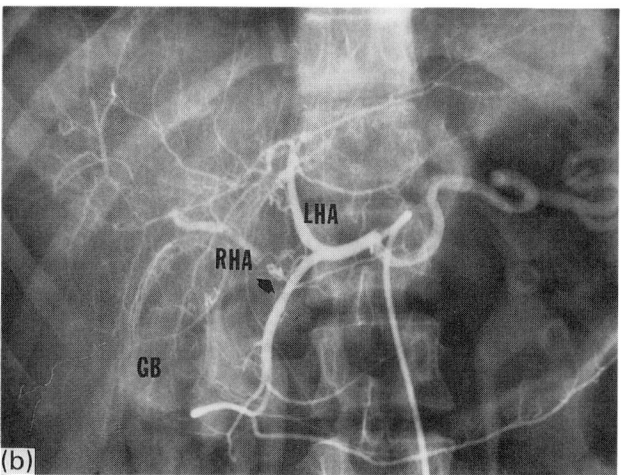

Figure 15. Sequential hepatic artery embolization (HAE). (a) The right hepatic artery (RHA) originates from the superior mesenteric artery. The hypervascular metastases are opacified. The cystic artery to the gallbladder (GB) arises from the RHA. The left hepatic artery (LHA) originates from the coeliac artery. The RHA was embolized with polyvinyl alcohol foam (Ivalon) particles and a stainless steel coil. (b) Coeliac arteriography one month later demonstrates the supply to the RHA and GB now arises from the LHA through collateral circulation. Note the retrograde opacification of the RHA and the steel coil (arrow). The LHA was subsequently embolized with Ivalon particles.

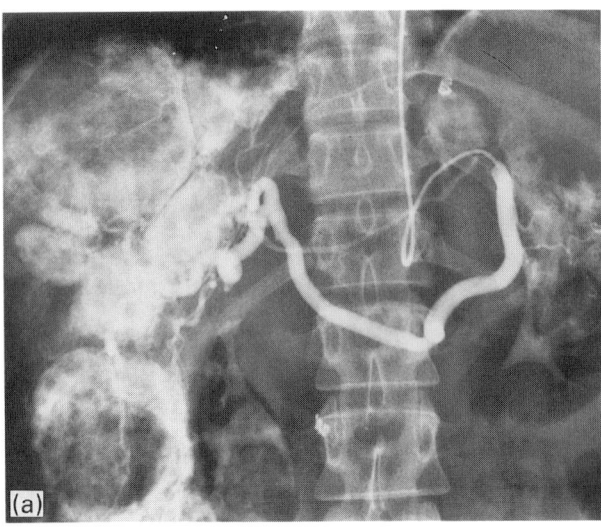

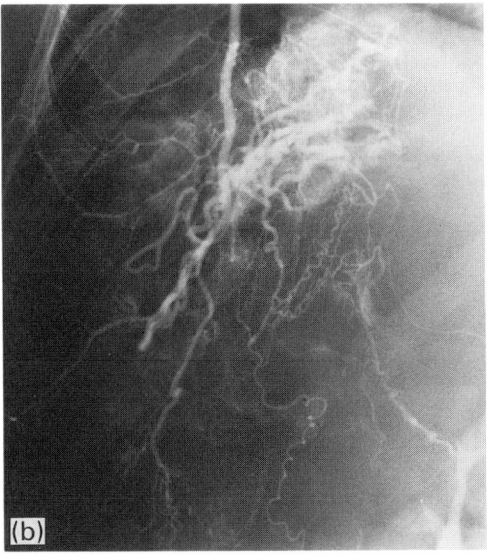

Figure 16. Collateral supply to the liver after HAE. (a) These hypervascular hepatic metastases from a gastrinoma are supplied by the left gastric artery to the right gastric artery to the hepatic artery. This vessel was embolized. (b) The internal mammary artery supplied the hypervascular hepatic metastases in the same patient with a gastrinoma. Embolization followed the arteriogram.

replacement of more than 50% of the liver by tumour, (ii) serum LDH above 425 mu/ml, (iii) serum GOT above 100 mu/ml, and (iv) serum bilirubin above 2 mg/dl. In a review of 310 patients treated with hepatic artery embolization at M. D. Anderson Cancer Center, 18 patients died of hepatorenal failure in the immediate postembolization period (within 1 month). All 18 patients were distinguished by fulfilling all of the above four criteria. Only two of the 292 patients who survived fit into this category. We are also reluctant to embolize patients who have portal venous occlusion with reversal of flow away from liver. Portal vein occlusion with abundant portal venous collaterals (cavernous transformation) to the liver is not a contra-indication to HAE (Carrasco et al, 1983).

Results

Percutaneous transcatheter liver devascularization has been most extensively evaluated in patients with the carcinoid syndrome. From The University of Texas M. D. Anderson Cancer Center, Carrasco et al (1986) reported 20 of 23 evaluable patients (87%) responded to sequential embolization, with a median response duration of 11+ months, one (4%) did not respond, and two (9%) died of complications from the embolization. The symptomatic responses correlated with two variables: (i) a decrease in the extent of the hepatic metastases in 17 of the 18 patients who had follow-up hepatic angiogram and (ii) a decrease in the urine 5-hydroxyindoleacetic acid values to a mean of 41% of pretreatment levels in the 18 patients for whom this test was available. HAE provides the most effective treatment for the carcinoid syndrome and the hepatic metastases. Periodic embolizations will maintain clinical remissions for prolonged periods of time.

While the carcinoid tumour has been most extensively studied, other endocrine tumours are also amenable to transcatheter embolization (Ajani et al, 1988). A recent review from our institution evaluated HAE in 22 patients with metastatic islet-cell tumours. Nine patients had gastrinomas, two had glucagonomas, and 11 had non-functioning tumours. Seventeen of these 22 patients had failed previous chemotherapy. One patient had also failed somatostatin analogue. Twenty patients were available for analysis for response. Twelve of the 20 patients achieved a partial remission (greater than 50% reduction in tumour volume), while four had only a minor reduction in tumour volume. Three of the remaining four patients experienced subjective improvement, while one patient experienced no benefit from the embolization. The projected median survival from the time of initiation of embolization is 33.7 months. Twenty of the total 22 patients underwent serial embolizations (Figure 17).

In summary, the management of liver metastasis in patients with endocrine tumours requires a multidisciplinary approach. Surgical debulking procedures, antineoplastic chemotherapy, and hormone suppression therapy remain important and first-line modalities in these patients. HAE may offer palliation by both reducing the bulk of tumour and by decreasing the secretion of metabolically active substances. Prolongation of life may also be a benefit of HAE, although this is difficult to prove. Patients who fail systemic therapy may benefit from HAE coupled with hepatic arterial chemotherapy infusion. The use of somatostatin analogue prior to HAE to control the carcinoid syndrome is now being investigated (Maton et al, 1985; Kvols et al, 1987; Cruetzfeldt et al, 1987).

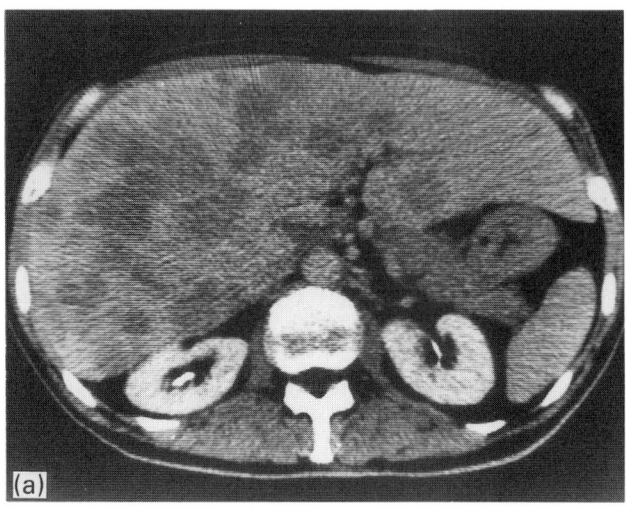

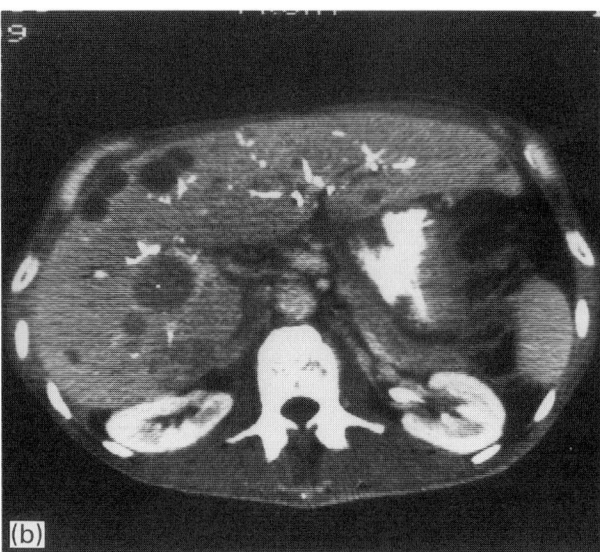

Figure 17. HAE of hepatic metastases from neuroendocrine tumours. (a) CT of the abdomen defines multiple metastases with decreased attenuation. (b) Following embolization, these metastases are necrotic, i.e. lower in attenuation coefficient and more sharply marginated.

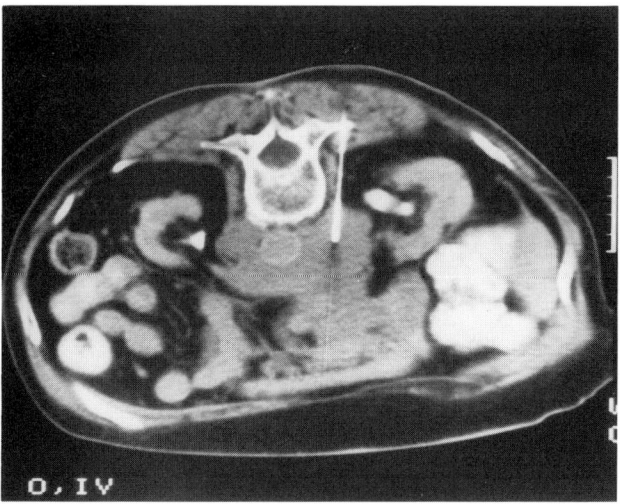

Figure 18. Percutaneous biopsy. Pancreatic islet cell carcinoma with retroperitoneal metastases.

Biopsy and other techniques

Other interventional radiological procedures find application in the abdomen and gastrointestinal tract of patients with neuroendocrine tumours. These include percutaneous biopsy of the primary or metastatic neoplasm (Figure 18), percutaneous drainage of abscesses and the obstructed biliary ducts and ureters, and percutaneous gastrostomy.

SUMMARY

The radiological diagnosis and interventional management of neuroendocrine tumours of the gastrointestinal tract and pancreas are challenging, demanding the complete gamut of available resources.

Carcinoid tumours are most commonly found in the appendix and small bowel. Barium studies usually disclose a small solitary mucosal or submucosal mass in the distal ileum at times associated with smooth muscle hypertrophy and thickening of the mucosal folds. Intussusception and bowel obstruction may be the presenting finding. Mesenteric involvement may evoke a desmoplastic reaction with rigidity, fixation, angulation and tethering of small bowel loops. Angiography may demonstrate a hypervascular primary neoplasm but more frequently reveals vascular encasement and distortion from the mesenteric desmoplastic reaction.

Pancreatic islet cell tumour is best defined radiologically by angiography and computed tomography as a well circumscribed hypervascular mass which enhances with contrast material. Portal venous sampling is of considerable assistance in localizing insulinoma.

Metastases from neuroendocrine tumours to lymph nodes and to the liver are usually hypervascular. In the evaluation of the liver by CT scanning prior to contrast as well as dynamic scanning during the bolus intravenous injection of contrast material are necessary. At times the precontrast scan is more revealing. Computed tomography with the catheter in the superior mesenteric artery followed by selective hepatic arteriography is the most accurate combination for the detection of hepatic metastases.

Interventional radiological management by sequential hepatic arterial embolization is the treatment of choice for multiple hepatic metastases from neuroendocrine tumours. Thus far, the maximum number of embolic episodes in a single patient has been 13. The carcinoid syndrome has been controlled in 87% while 79% of islet cell tumour hepatic metastases have responded.

Contraindications to HAE includes a combination of *all* of the following: (i) replacement of more than 50% of the liver by tumour, (ii) serum lactic dehydrogenase above 425 mU/ml, (iii) serum glutamic oxaloacetic transaminase above 100 mU/ml, and (iv) bilirubin above 2 mg/dl. In the face of occlusion of the portal vein by intravascular neoplasm, HAE is contraindicated only if portal flow through collateral vein is away from the liver.

REFERENCES

Ajani JA, Carrasco CH, Charnsangavej C et al (1988) Islet cell tumors metastatic to the liver: effective palliation by sequential hepatic artery embolization. *Annals of Internal Medicine* **180:** 340–344.

Allison DJ, Modlin IM & Jenkins WJ (1977) Treatment of carcinoid liver metastases by hepatic artery embolization. *Lancet* **ii:** 1323–1325.

Amberg JR, Ellison EH, Wilson SD et al (1964) Roentgenographic observations in the Zollinger–Ellison syndrome. *Journal of the American Medical Association* **190:** 185–187.

Ballard HS, Frame B & Hartsock RJ (1964) Familial multiple endocrine adenoma-peptic ulcer complex. *Medicine* **43:** 481–516.

Bancks NH, Goldstein HM & Dodd GD (1975) The roentgenologic spectrum of small intestinal carcinoid tumors. *American Journal of Roentgenology* **123:** 274–280.

Bernardino ME, Erwin BC, Steinberg HV et al (1986) Delayed hepatic CT scanning: increased confidence and improved detection of hepatic metastases. *Radiology* **159:** 71–74.

Bierman HR, Byron RL, Kelley RH & Grady A (1951) Studies on the blood supply of tumors in man: vascular patterns of the liver by hepatic angiography in vivo. *Journal of the National Cancer Institute* **12:** 107–131.

Bloom SR & Polak JM (1987) Glucagonoma syndrome. *American Journal of Medicine* **82** [supplement 5B]: 25–36.

Bluth I (1960) Gastrointestinal carcinoid tumors: roentgen features. *Radiology* **74:** 573–580.

Boijsen E, Kaude J & Tulem U (1974) Radiologic diagnosis of ileal carcinoid tumors. *Acta Radiologica* (Diagnosis) **15:** 65–82.

Bozymski EM, Woodruff K & Sessions JT Jr (1973) Zollinger–Ellison syndrome with hypoglycemia associated with calcification of the tumor and its metastasis. *Gastroenterology* **65:** 658–661.

Breedis C & Young G (1954) The blood supply for neoplasms in the liver. *American Journal of Pathology* **30:** 969–985.

Brennan MF & MacDonald JS (1985) Cancer of the endocrine system. In De Vita Jr VT, Hellman S & Rosenberg SA (eds) *Cancer Principles and Practice of Oncology*, pp 1179–1241. Philadelphia: JB Lippincott.

Burcharth F, Stage JG, Stadil F, Ingemann L, Fischermann K (1979) Localizations of gastrinomas by transhepatic portal catheterization and gastrin assay. *Gastroenterology* **77:** 444–450.

Carrasco CH (1985) Localization of neuroendocrine tumors of the pancreas. *Seminars in Surgical Oncology* **1:** 196–199.

Carrasco CH, Chuang VP & Wallace S (1983) Apudomas metastatic to the liver: treatment by hepatic artery embolization. *Radiology* **149:** 79–83.

Carrasco CH, Charnsangavej C, Ajani J et al (1986) The carcinoid syndrome: palliation by hepatic artery embolization. *American Journal of Roentgenology* **147:** 149–154.

Cho KJ, Wilcox CW & Reuter SR (1977) Glucagon producing islet cell tumor of the pancreas. *American Journal of Roentgenology* **129:** 159–161.

Cho KJ, Vink AI, Thompson NW et al (1982) Localization of the source of hyperinsulism: percutancous transhepatic portal and pancreatic vein catheterization with hormone assay. *American Journal of Roentgenology* **139:** 237–245.

Chuang VP & Wallace S (1981) Hepatic artery embolization in the treatment of hepatic neoplasms. *Radiology* **140:** 51–58.

Chuang VP, Soo C-S, Carrasco CH & Wallace S (1983) Superselective catheterization technique in hepatic angiography. *American Journal of Roentgenology* **141:** 803–811.

Collen MJ, Doppman JL, Krudy AGA et al (1984) Assessment of the ability of angiography to localize gastrinoma in patients with Zollinger–Ellison syndrome (ZES). *Gastroenterology* **86:** 1015.

Cruetzfeldt W & Stockman F (1987) Carcinoids and carcinoid syndrome. *American Journal of Medicine* **82** [supplement 5B]: 4–16.

Creutzfeldt W, Lembcke B, Folsch VR, Schleser S & Koop I (1987) Effect of somatostatin analogue (SMS 201-995, Sandostatin) on pancreatic secretion in humans. *American Journal of Medicine* **82** [supplement 5B]: 49–54.

Daggett PR, Kurtz AB, Morris DV et al (1981) Is preoperative localization of insulinomas necessary? *Lancet* **i:** 483–486.

Davis Z, Moertel CG & McIlrath DC (1973) Malignant carcinoid syndrome. *Surgery, Gynecology and Obstetrics* **137:** 637–644.

DiBisceglie AM, Segal I, Mannell A et al (1984) Pancreatic endocrine tumor presenting with obstructive jaundice. *American Journal of Gastroenterology* **79:** 43–45.

Dodd GD (1978) Carcinoid tumors of the gastrointestinal tract. In Margulis AR & Gooding CA (eds) *Diagnostic Radiology*, pp 265–278. University of California at San Francisco Extended Programs in Medical Education.

Dodd GD (1985) The radiologic features of multiple endocrine neoplasia types IIA and IIB. *Seminars in Roentgenology* **20:** 64–90.

Dodds WJ, Dehn TG, Hogan WH et al (1971) Severe peptic esophagitis in a patient with Zollinger–Ellison syndrome. *American Journal of Roentgenology* **113:** 237–240.

Dodds WJ, Wilson SD, Thorsen M et al (1985) MEN I syndrome and islet cell lesions of the pancreas. *Seminars in Roentgenology* **20:** 17–63.

Doppman JL (1985) Multiple endocrine syndromes: A nightmare for the endocrine radiologist. *Seminars in Roentgenology* **20:** 7–15.

Dunnick NR, Long JA Jr, Drudy AG, Shawker TH & Doppman JL (1980) Localizing insulinomas with combined radiographic methods. *American Journal of Roentgenology* **135:** 747–752.

Edis AJ, McIlrath DC, van Heerden JA et al (1976) Insulinoma: current diagnosis and surgical management. *Current Problems in Surgery* **13:** 1–45.

Eelkema EA, Stephens DH, Ward EM & Sheedy PF (1984) CT features of non-functioning islet cell carcinoma. *American Journal of Roentgenology* **143:** 943–948.

Epstein HY, Abrams RM, Berandaum ER et al (1969) Angiographic localization of insulinomas: High reported success rate and two additional cases. *Annals of Surgery* **169:** 349–354.

Ferrucci JT, Freeny PC, Stark DD et al (1988) Advances in hepatobiliary radiology. *Radiology* **168:** 319–323.

Foley WD (1988) Hepatic MR imaging at 1.5T. *Radiology* **168:** 326–328.

Freeny PC (1988) Hepatic CT: state of the art. *Radiology* **168:** 319–323.

Friesen SR (1982) Tumors of the endocrine pancreas. *New England Journal of Medicine* **306:** 580–590.

Friesen SR, Tomita R & Kimmel JR (1983) Pancreatic polypeptide update: its roles in detection of the trait for multiple endocrine adenopathy syndrome, type I, and pancreatic polypeptide-secreting tumors. *Surgery* **94**: 1028–1037.

Gerlock AJ Jr, Muhletaer CA, Halter S et al (1979) Pancreatic somatostatinoma: histologic, clinical and angiographic features. *American Journal of Roentgenology* **133**: 939–943.

Godwin DJ (1975) Carcinoid tumors: an analysis of 2,837. *Cancer* **36**: 560–569.

Goldberg BB, Cole-Beuglet C, Kurtz AB et al (1980) Real time aspiration-biopsy transducer. *Journal of Clinical Ultrasound* **8**: 107.

Goldstein HM & Miller M (1975) Angiographic evaluation of small intestinal carcinoid tumors. *Radiology* **115**: 23–25.

Haaga JR (1979) New techniques for CT guided biopsies. *American Journal of Roentgenology* **133**: 633.

Hanson JJ (1960) Hypoglycemia associated with pancreatic islet cell tumors. Review of the literature and case report of a malignant tumor. *American Journal of Medicine* **28**: 468–475.

Healey JE Jr & Sheena KS (1963) Vascular pattern in metastatic liver tumors. *Surgical Forum* **14**: 121–122.

Hill CS Jr, Ibanez ML, Samaan NA et al (1973) Medullary (solid) carcinoma of the thyroid gland: an analysis of the M. D. Anderson experience with patients with the tumor. Its special features and its histogenesis. *Medicine* **52**: 141–171.

Hudson HL & Margulis AR (1964) Roentgen findings of carcinoid tumors of gastrointestinal tract: report of 12 recent cases. *American Journal of Roentgenology* **91**: 833–839.

Hutcheon DF, Bayless TM, Cameron JL & Baylin SB (1979) Hormone-mediated watery diarrhea in a family with multiple endocrine neoplasms. *Annals of Internal Medicine* **90**: 932–934.

Inamoto K, Yoshino F, Nakoa N et al (1980) Angiographic diagnosis of a pancreatic islet tumor in a patient with the WDHA syndrome. *Gastrointestinal Radiology* **5**: 259–261.

Ingemansson S, Lunderquist A, Lunderquist I, Luodahl R & Tibblin S (1975) Portal and pancreatic vein catheterization with radioimmunologic determination of insulin. *Surgery Gynecology and Obstetrics* **14**: 705–711.

Ingemansson S, Kuhl C, Larsson LI et al (1978) Localization of insulinomas and islet cell hyperplasia by pancreatic vein catheterization and insulin assay. *Surgery, Gynecology and Obstetrics* **146**: 724–734.

Jager RM & Polk HC (1977) Carcinoid apudomas. *Current Problems in Cancer* **1**: 1–53.

Jahnke RW, Gnekow W & Harrel GS (1977) Non-beta islet-cell tumor calcification associated with Zollinger–Ellison syndrome and multiple endocrine adenomatosis. *Gastrointestinal Radiology* **1**: 345–347.

Jones B, Fishman EK, Bayless TM et al (1983) Villous hypertrophy of the small bowel in a patient with glucagonoma. *Journal of Computer Assisted Tomography* **7**: 334–337.

Kent RB, van Heerden JA & Weiland LH (1981) Nonfunctioning islet cell tumors. *Annals of Surgery* **193**: 185–190.

Krejs GJ (1987) Gastrointestinal endocrine tumors. *American Journal of Medicine* **82**: 2–3.

Krejs GJ, Ora L, Conlon J et al (1979) Somatostatinoma syndrome. *New England Journal of Medicine* **301**: 285–292.

Krudy AG, Doppman JL, Jensen RT et al (1984) Localization of islet cell tumors by dynamic CT: comparison with plain CT, arteriography, sonography and venous sampling. *American Journal of Roentgenology* **143**: 585–589.

Kune GA & Goldstein J (1974) Malignant liver carcinoid: the case of surgery and chemotherapy. Review and case presentation. *Medical Journal of Australia* **2**: 777–780.

Kvols Lk, Buck M, Moertel CG et al (1987) Treatment of metastatic islet cell carcinoma with somatostatin analogue (SMS 201-995). *Annals of Internal Medicine* **107**: 162–168.

Larsson LI, Grimelius L, Haksanson R et al (1975) Mixed endocrine pancreatic tumors producing several peptide hormones. *American Journal of Pathology* **79**: 271–284.

Launay JM, Tabuteau F, Haimart M et al (1983) The diffuse neuroendocrine (APUD) system. *Biomedicine and Pharmacotherapy* **37**: 322–328.

Lin G, Hagerstrand I & Lunderquist A (1984) Portal blood supply of liver metastases. *American Journal of Roentgenology* **143**: 53–55.

Linnell F & Mansson K (1966) On the prevalence and incidence of carcinoid in Malmo. *Acta Medica Scandinavia* **445** [supplement]: 377.

Lunderquist A, Ericsson M, Nobin A & Sander G (1982) Gelfoam powder embolization of the hepatic artery in liver metastases of carcinoid tumors. *Radiology* **22**: 65–70.

McGarity WC, Miles AE & Hoffman JC (1971) Angiographic diagnosis and localization of endocrine tumors. *Annals of Surgery* **173**: 583–592.

McGill DB, Carney JA, Phillips JF et al (1980) Hormonal diarrhea due to pancreatic tumor. *Gastroenterology* **79**: 571–582.

Marshall JB & Settles RH (1980) Zollinger–Ellison syndrome: a clinical update. *Postgraduate Medicine* **68**: 38–50.

Martin EN & Potet F (1974) Pathology of endocrine tumors of the GI tract. *Clinics in Gastroenterology* **3**: 511–532.

Maton PN, O'Dorisio TM, Brent AH et al (1985) Effect of a long acting somatostatin analogue (SMS 201-995) in a patient with pancreatic cholera. *New England Journal of Medicine* **312**: 17–21.

Mengoli L & LeQuesne LP (1967) Blind pancreatic resection for suspected insulinoma: a review of the problem. *British Journal of Surgery* **54**: 749–756.

Mittelstaedt C (1987) *Abdominal ultrasound.* New York: Churchill Livingstone.

Mitty HA, Warner RRP, Newman LH, Train JS & Parnes IH (1985) Control of carcinoid syndrome with hepatic artery embolization. *Radiology* **155**: 623–626.

Modlin IM (1979) Endocrine tumors of the pancreas. *Surgery, Gynecology and Obstetrics* **149**: 751–769.

Moertel CG (1973) Small intestine. In Holland JF & Frie E (eds) *Cancer Medicine,* pp 1574–1584. Philadelphia: Lea and Febiger.

Moertel CG (1983) Treatment of carcinoid tumors and the malignant carcinoid syndrome. *Journal of Clinical Oncology* **1**: 727–740.

Moertel CG, Sauer WG, Dockerty MB & Baggenstoss AH (1961) Life history of carcinoid tumor of the small intestine. *Cancer* **14**: 901–912.

Murray-Lyon IM, Parson VA, Blendis LM et al (1970) Treatment of secondary hepatic tumors by ligation of hepatic artery and infusion of cytotoxic drugs. *Lancet* **ii**: 172–175.

O'Berg K, Walinder O, Bostrom H et al (1982) Peptide hormone markers in screening for endocrine tumors in multiple endocrine tumors in multiple endocrine adenomatosis, type I. *American Journal of Medicine* **73**: 619–630.

Oberndorder S (1907) Karzinoide tumoren des dunndarms. *Frankfurt Zeitschrift Fur Pathologe* **1**: 426–439.

Ostermiller WE & Joergenson EJ (1966) Carcinoid tumors of the small bowel. *Archives of Surgery* **93**: 616–619.

Pearse AGE (1968) Common cytochemical and ultrastructural characteristics of cells producing polypeptide hormones (the APUD series) and their relevance to thyroid ultimobronchial c cells and calcitonin. *Proceedings of the Royal Society of London* (Biol) **170**: 71–80.

Pearse AGE (1977) The diffuse neuroendocrine system and the APUD concept: related 'endocrine' peptides in brain, intestine, pituitary, placenta and anuran cutaneous glands. *Medical Biology* **55**: 115–125.

Pearse AGE, Polak HM & Heath CM (1974) Polypeptide hormone production by 'carcinoid' apudomas and their relevant cytochemistry. *Virchows Archiv (Cell Pathology)* **16**: 95–109.

Prinz RA, Parenti AJ, Dorsch TR et al (1979) Glucagon producing islet cell tumors of the pancreas. *Proceedings of the Institute of Medicine of Chicago* **32**: 133–135.

Prinz RA, Dorsch TR & Lawrence AM (1981) Clinical aspects of glucagon producing islet cell tumors. *American Journal of Gastroenterology* **76**: 125–131.

Pueyo I, Jimenez JR, Hernandez J et al (1978) Carcinoid syndrome treated by hepatic embolization. *American Journal of Roentgenology* **131**: 511–513.

Richter JE, Pandol SJ, Castell DO et al (1980) Esophageal abnormalities are frequent in the Zollinger–Ellison syndrome (ZES). *Clinics of Radiology* **28**: 726A (abstract).

Rivier J, Spiess J, Thorner M & Vale W (1982) Characterization of a growth hormone releasing factor from a human pancreatic islet tumour. *Nature* **300**: 276–278.

Roche A, Raissonnier A & Gillion-Savouret MC (1982) Pancreatic venous sampling and arteriography in localizing insulinomas and gastrinomas: procedure and results in 55 cases. *Radiology* **145**: 621–627.

Rossi P, Baert A, Passariello R et al (1985) CT of functioning tumors of the pancreas. *American Journal of Roentgenology* **144**: 57–60.

Said SI & Faloon GR (1975) Elevated plasma and tissue levels of vasoactive intestinal polypeptides in the watery diarrhea syndrome due to pancreatic, bronchogenic and other tumors. *New England Journal of Medicine* **293:** 155–160.

Schein PS, De Lellis RA, Kahn CR et al (1973) Islet cell tumors. Current concepts and management. *Annals of Internal Medicine* **79:** 239–257.

Shawker TH, Doppman JL, Dunnick NR et al (1982) Ultrasonic investigation of pancreatic islet cell tumors. *Journal of Clinical Ultrasound* **10:** 173–175.

Siegel B, Duarte B, Coelho JCU et al (1983) Localization of insulinomas of the pancreas at operation by real-time ultrasound scanning. *Surgery, Gynecology and Obstetrics* **156:** 145–147.

Soo C-S, Chuang VP, Wallace S, Charnsangavej C & Carrasco CH (1983) Treatment of hepatic neoplasms through extrahepatic collaterals. *Radiology* **147:** 45–49.

Sparks FC, Mosher MB, Hallauer WC et al (1975) Hepatic artery ligation and postoperative chemotherapy for hepatic metastases: clinical and pathophysiological results. *Cancer* **35:** 1074–1082.

Stark DD (1988) MR imaging of focal liver masses. *Radiology* **168:** 323–326.

Stark DD, Moss AA, Goldberg HI & Deveney CW (1984) CT of pancreatic islet cell tumors. *Radiology* **150:** 491–494.

Steffani P, Carboni M, Patrassi N et al (1974) Beta-islet cell tumors of the pancreas: results of a study of 1067 cases. *Surgery* **75:** 597–609.

Thorson A, Bjork G, Bjerkman G, Waldenstrom J (1954) Malignant carcinoid of the small intestine with metastases to the liver, valvular disease of the right heart (pulmonary stenosis and tricuspid regurgitation without septal defect), peripheral vasometer symptoms, bronchoconstriction and an unusual type of cyanosis. *American Heart Journal* **47:** 795–817.

Wallace S & Chuang VP (1982) The radiologic diagnosis and management of hepatic metastases. *Radiologe* **22:** 56–64.

Wilson H (1970) Carcinoid syndrome. *Current Problems in Surgery* **11:** 36–41.

Wilson H & Butterick OD (1959) Massive liver resection for control of severe vasomotor reaction secondary to malignant carcinoid. *Annals of Surgery* **149:** 641–647.

Wilson SD (1978) Wermer's syndrome: multiple endocrine adenopathy, type I. In Friesen S (ed.) *Surgical Endocrinology and Clinical Syndromes*, pp 285–286. Philadelphia: JB Lippincott.

Wolf JH, Long RJ, Miller FJ et al (1977) Pancreatic islet cell tumor presenting as bleeding gastric varices secondary to splenic vein occlusion. *American Journal of Digestive Diseases* **22:** 652–655.

Zollinger RM & Ellison EH (1955) Primary peptic ulcerations of jejunum associated with islet cell tumors of the pancreas. *Annals of Surgery* **142:** 709–728.

6

Imaging for adrenal tumours

F. L. CHAN
CHRISTINA WANG

The effective investigation of a patient with an endocrine disorder is based on a thorough clinical history and physical examination, coupled with relevant biochemical tests required to establish the diagnosis. A search for the hormone-induced pathology is only justifiable in the presence of firm clinical and biochemical evidence. This basic philosophy is applicable to disorders of the adrenal glands, many of which can be surgically cured with low mortality and morbidity. After biochemical confirmation of the diagnosis, imaging plays a primary role in the lateralization, localization and presurgical planning of the suspected functioning tumour. It can also define and evaluate non-functioning tumours. The imaging modality of choice and the desirable sequence of investigations should be tailored to the individual patient and his problem. The level of diagnostic accuracy to be pursued has to be considered in the light of the preferred therapeutic approach, and balanced against the invasiveness of the intended imaging studies.

THE IMAGING MODALITIES

The localization of adrenal tumours has evolved rapidly in the past twenty years with the development of both functional and anatomic imaging techniques. The advance of medical imaging is highlighted by a review on the trends of adrenal surgery during the 1970s: accurate preoperative localization was achieved in 50% of patients in the early 1970s, 80% by the mid-1970s and 98% during the latter part of the decade (Hamburger et al, 1982). Modern imaging aims at direct visualization of the pathology, and its success will vary with the anatomic topography, multiplicity, dimensions, biological behaviour and vascularity of the tumour. The modalities will be considered in the context of presently available techniques.

Computed tomography (CT)

The steady advance in instrumentation and electronic computation has resulted in high-resolution CT scanners being widely available. Most scanners can now obtain scans with a scanning time of less than 3 s and a bed incrementation interval in the millimetre range. The resultant thin slices with high spatial resolution allow both adrenal glands to be consistently visualized on abdominal CT in virtually all adults (Reynes et al, 1979), and detailed study of their relationship to neighbouring structures.

In view of the constant position of the adrenal glands within the cone of renal fascia and surrounded by abundant perirenal fat they are easily imaged by CT without the application of contrast media, making CT one of the least invasive procedures. Imaging may be difficult only in the thinnest and youngest patients or in those who cannot cooperate in holding breath to roughly the same extent with each scan. Depending on the clinical indication, 1-cm contiguous abdominal scans are usually obtained initially to cover the entire glands, and these may suffice for large adrenal masses. For smaller masses, thinner (e.g. 3 mm) scans, with an appropriate smaller display field of view over a range as directed by the initial thick scans, are necessary to provide large adrenal images with excellent resolution. Oral contrast to opacify the bowels is required for investigations of extra-adrenal phaeochromocytomas and in patients with prior nephrectomy. Intravenous contrast is used only in situations where distinction from vascular structures or enhancement characterization of the lesion is preferred.

Detection of calcification, contour alteration of the gland and size of mass is reliably achieved by CT. False-negative examinations may be due to a tumour smaller than 1 cm buried in the substance of the gland. False-positive examinations are frequently due to interpretative errors from mistaking varices, splenic vessels, gastric fundus, splenic lobulations or pancreas for adrenal masses (Johnson et al, 1985). However, the CT appearance of an adrenal mass is non-specific apart from adrenal cyst and myelolipoma. The administration of intravenous contrast media contributes lesion characterization, but is not uniformly successful in distinguishing malignancy from benignity in every case.

Alternative non-invasive techniques

Conventional radiography

The diagnostic work-up of patients suspected of having an adrenal tumour has been radically altered with the introduction of CT. At present, there is very little practical role for plain abdominal radiographs or excretory urography. Although large adrenal masses are sometimes identified by these examinations, especially with nephrotomogram, they are not sufficiently sensitive or specific without the back-up by other imaging modalities. They also provide little information on the extent or relationship of the adrenal mass to surrounding organs.

Ultrasonography

With the introduction of better real-time ultrasound equipment and specific high-frequency transducers, normal adrenals can now be routinely visualized in neonates and small children (Oppenheimer et al, 1983). In adults, however, even in the hands of an expert with advanced equipment, imaging is successful in 92% of cases for the right adrenal gland and in only 71% for the left one (Marchal et al, 1986). Experienced workers have pointed out the technical difficulty of consistently producing accurate ultrasound images of the adrenals. Visualization varies with the size of the patient, the position of the bowels, and the experience of the examiner (Sample, 1978; Yeh, 1982). Apart from aldosteronomas, the overall detection rate of adrenal masses by ultrasonography is above 90%. Nevertheless, the high false-positive rate of 27–39% as cited by Abrams et al (1982), and the demand on examination time and technical expertise make this an unpopular technique and ensure a preference for CT as an initial diagnostic test for adrenal tumours. Once an adrenal mass has been identified, ultrasonography may be employed to differentiate adrenal cysts from soft tissue masses, to evaluate the status of the large vessels and liver, and to follow up after surgical resection of the mass.

Adrenal scintigraphy

Scintigraphy allows a non-invasive, functional approach to the localization of hyperactive adrenal glands. The study is, however, often difficult to perform or interpret. The ideal radiopharmaceuticals are not widely available. The findings offer much less anatomical information than other imaging modalities. Radiopharmaceuticals have been developed to scan either the cortex or the medulla.

The most commonly used radionuclide for scanning the adrenal cortex is ^{131}I-6β-iodomethyl-19-norcholesterol (NP59). Other agents include ^{131}I-19 iodocholesterol (19-IC) and selenium-75 selenomethyl cholesterol. The use of dexamethasone suppression during adrenal scintigraphy may increase its accuracy. The investigation has been reported to be efficacious in the localization of adrenal tumours in Cushing's syndrome (Barbarino et al, 1979) and primary aldosteronism (Gross et al, 1984), but carries some degree of false-positives and false-negatives. CT was found to cost less, take less time to perform and bear smaller doses of radiation compared to scintigraphy (Guerin et al, 1983).

Meta-iodobenzylguanidine (MIBG) has been used to image the adrenal medulla and extra-adrenal phaeochromocytomas. The MIBG molecules compete with adrenaline for cellular uptake and thus can be employed to localize such tumours. The ^{123}I radiopharmaceutical has been found to be more accurate than ^{131}I, with better detection efficiency and dosimetry, and permits single photon emission computed tomography (Lynn et al, 1985; Bomanji et al, 1988). This agent, however, is even more difficult to obtain than the others. MIBG scans have been very useful in localizing phaeochromocytomas (Sisson et al, 1981) but carry a high radiation dose and a significant false-negative rate (Swensen et al, 1985).

Magnetic resonance imaging (MRI)

At present the availability of this recently developed modality is still limited in many places. Compared with CT, current MRI has good contrast resolution but less spatial resolution, can scan directly in any planes, does not involve ionizing radiation, can visualize vascular structures without intravenous contrast media, and can serve as functional imaging to some extent. The study is, however, more affected by respiratory motion, more time-consuming and has difficulty in detecting areas of calcification (Moon et al, 1983; Schultz et al, 1985). As clinical experience accumulates the exact role of MRI and its optimal techniques in the work-up of adrenal disorders will become clearer.

More invasive techniques

Arteriography

The information obtained from aortography and selective arteriography varies and depends on the type of adrenal lesion. Before the advent of better, non-invasive imaging modalities, this technique has yielded good results and was the diagnostic method of choice in the evaluation of adrenal masses (Colapinto and Steed, 1971). It is invasive, requires considerable expertise and may be hazardous especially for patients with phaeochromocytomas (Rossi et al, 1968). Currently it is reserved for more selective situations after non-invasive imaging to evaluate the blood supply to large masses when the origin remains obscure after CT, or to secure more definitive information of therapeutic significance.

Adrenal venography and venous sampling

Selective catheterization of the adrenal veins is a sophisticated technique. It can be performed successfully in nearly all cases for the left adrenal but in a much lower percentage for the right adrenal. Adrenal venography is now largely replaced by high-resolution CT, but previously it had been used to detect small adrenal tumours with a wide range of reported accuracy (Mitty et al, 1973; Dunnick et al, 1982a). The procedure is not without risk, and about 5% have complications consisting of contrast extravasation, haematoma and venous thrombosis of the adrenals (Bayliss et al, 1970). Use of non-ionic contrast and digital subtraction technique is advisable.

Adrenal venous sampling consists of obtaining blood samples from each catheterized adrenal vein for hormonal assay. It is safer and more accurate than adrenal venography. Almost all functioning adrenal tumours can be lateralized by this method, so much so that it has been regarded by some as the 'gold standard'. In view of its invasiveness, the technique is currently reserved for cases who have equivocal findings on non-invasive imaging. Besides the adrenal veins, blood sampling for chemical analysis from various other sites of the venous system has also been applied in the search for ectopic ACTH-producing tumours and extra-adrenal phaeochromocytomas.

Adrenal biopsy

In recent years, CT-guided percutaneous needle biopsy of the adrenal has been selectively applied to obtain definitive diagnosis especially for non-functioning or metastatic adrenal tumours. It has been found to be an accurate and safe alternative to the more expensive and invasive surgical biopsy (Bernardino et al, 1985). However, the possibility of phaeochromocytoma should be excluded prior to adrenal biopsy because percutaneous biopsy of such tumours can result in hypertensive crisis, haemorrhage and death (McCorkell and Niles, 1985).

Since CT is the most reliable, widely available and non-invasive examination for evaluation of adrenal pathology, the following discussion on medical imaging of the adrenal glands and various related endocrine tumours in the adults will be focused on CT as the initial and sometimes the definitive diagnostic test, supplemented by the application of other modalities in an attempt to solve the clinical problems specific to individual adrenal disorder. The current status of MRI as applied to the adrenals will also be addressed because of its potential as the imaging modality of choice in the future.

THE NORMAL ADRENAL GLANDS

The anatomical relationships of the adrenal glands permit their ready identification on medical imaging. The right adrenal gland is usually suprarenal in position, lying posterior to the inferior vena cava, between the right lobe of the liver and the right crus of the diaphragm. The left adrenal gland is

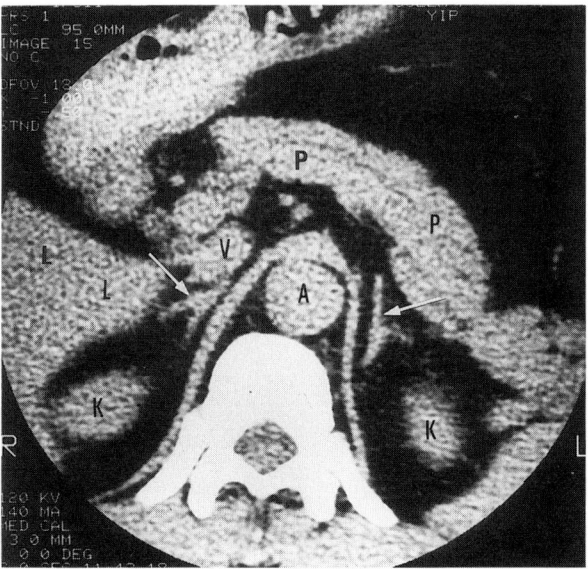

Figure 1. Normal adrenal glands. Non-contrast thin CT section in a 48-year-old man demonstrates inverted-Y shaped adrenal glands (white arrows) surrounded by abundant fat in front of the upper pole of each kidney. A, aorta; V, inferior vena cava; K, kidney; L, liver; P, pancreas.

located anteromedial to the upper pole of the left kidney, lying medial to the spleen, posterior to the pancreatic tail and the splenic vessels, and lateral to the left crus of the diaphragm. The left adrenal normally extends more caudally than the right gland. Both adrenal glands are retroperitoneal structures surrounded by abundant fat (Figure 1) at the apex of the perirenal space, allowing them to be precisely and consistently delineated by CT in all persons except the thinnest, unless obscured by interference factors like movement artefacts or presence of metallic clips. In most instances, the visualization of normal glands by CT should be sufficient to negate further investigations for adrenal tumours.

The transverse sectional configuration of the glands on CT varies with the craniocaudal level (Figure 2) and depends on the relative prominence of either the medial or lateral limb at that particular level, the varying angle between the two limbs and the torsion of the gland along its longitudinal or transverse axis. The shape of the right adrenal gland is most often an inverted V or Y. Its lateral limb may merge with the edge of the liver, especially in thin patients, so that the gland may appear as a vertical line. The gland is sometimes seen as a horizontal line. The left adrenal gland often appears triangular or as an inverted V or Y. The normal adrenal gland has a smooth outline, with homogeneous attenuation similar to that of liver. The cortex and medulla of the adrenal cannot be differentiated on CT scans. The limbs are of uniform thickness, usually 5–6 mm, and thinner than the apex. Absolute measurements of adrenal size, about 2.0–3.5 cm in length, 2–3 cm

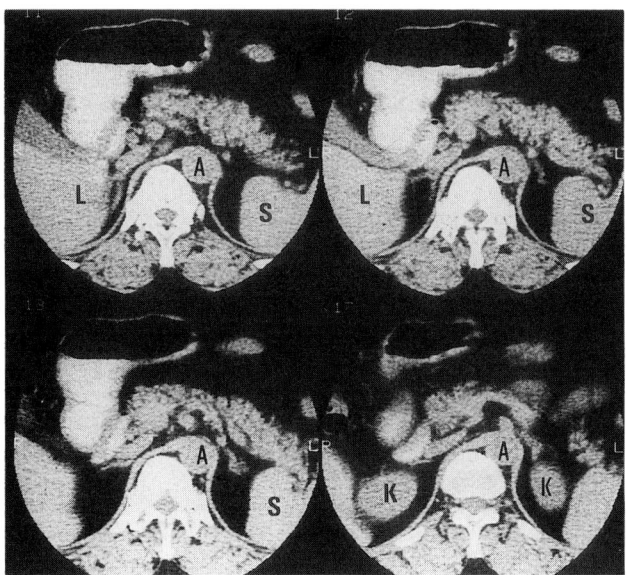

Figure 2. Variations in the configuration of normal adrenal glands. CT sections at four different levels in the same patient show the change in the CT appearance of the normal gland depending on the relation of the sectional plane to the various portions of the gland. A, aorta; K, kidney; L, liver; S, spleen.

in width and less than 1.0 cm thick (Montagne et al, 1978), have not proved clinically helpful. A visual appreciation of the overall uniformity and symmetry of size and configuration is more accurate. Thus a rounded gland is never normal, whereas convexity of one surface of gland sometimes occurs in normal subjects especially on the left side. The lobulated contour should be considered with more care, since it may represent normal accessory cortical bodies or multiple small adenomas or nodular hyperplasia (El-Sherief and Hemmingsson, 1982).

CUSHING'S SYNDROME

Clinical features and diagnosis

The clinical features of Cushing's syndrome are easily recognized. The biochemical confirmation of diagnosis rests on the finding of elevated plasma cortisol levels with loss of diurnal variation and non-suppressibility by overnight 1 mg (Crapo et al, 1979; Aron et al, 1981) or 2-day, 2 mg dexamethasone tests (Liddle, 1960). Twenty-four hour and spot urinary free-cortisol tests reflect the plasma levels of biologically active cortisol and are thus a sensitive indication of endogenous glucocorticoid excess (Moore et al, 1985; Contreras et al, 1986). The diagnosis of Cushing's syndrome is usually made from the clinical features and screening tests. Falsely high results can occur in patients with acute stress, depression, renal failure and alcoholic pseudo-Cushing's syndrome (Aron et al, 1988).

After the diagnosis of Cushing's syndrome has been made, the next question is to determine whether the disease is adrenocorticotrophic hormone (ACTH)-dependent (pituitary adenoma, ectopic ACTH syndrome, ectopic corticotropin releasing hormone (CRH) syndrome) or ACTH-independent (iatrogenic, adrenal neoplasm or adrenocortical nodular dysplasia). The differentiation of the causes depends on hormonal tests including high dose (8 mg) dexamethasone suppression test, plasma ACTH level, CRH test and petrosal sinus ACTH sampling. Plasma ACTH levels are uniformly suppressed in patients with ACTH-independent Cushing's syndrome e.g. adrenal adenoma/carcinoma and exogenous glucocorticoid administration. However plasma ACTH levels do not help to distinguish clearly between pituitary adenoma and ectopic ACTH syndrome. In these conditions, ACTH levels ranged from normal to markedly elevated (Besser and Edwards, 1972). The 8 mg, high-dose dexamethasone test helps to distinguish most patients with pituitary-dependent Cushing's syndrome from the ectopic ACTH-related form. A distinct suppression (over 50% of basal levels) suggests pituitary disease. Recently the CRH test has been investigated for the differential diagnosis of Cushing's syndrome (Chrousos et al, 1984) since patients with Cushing's disease due to pituitary adenoma showed normal or exaggerated responses to CRH whereas patients with ectopic ACTH usually showed no increase in ACTH levels. Many exceptions to this responsiveness are seen and sampling for ACTH from the petrosal sinuses with CRH stimulation may be a more

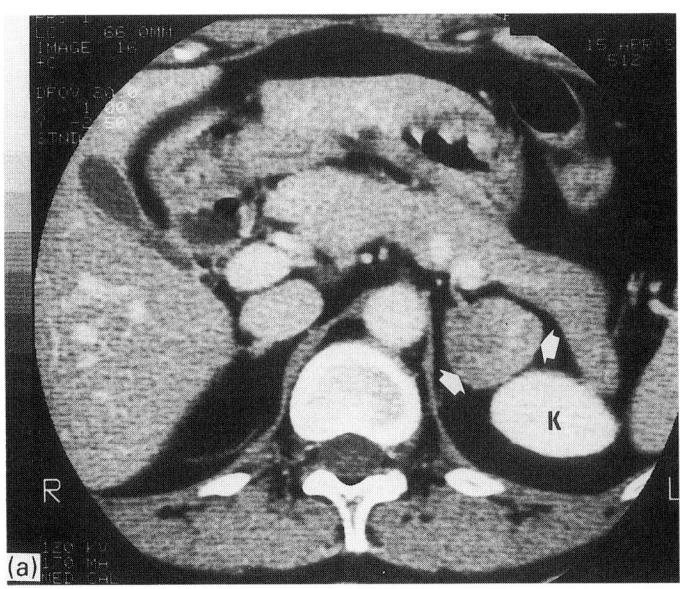

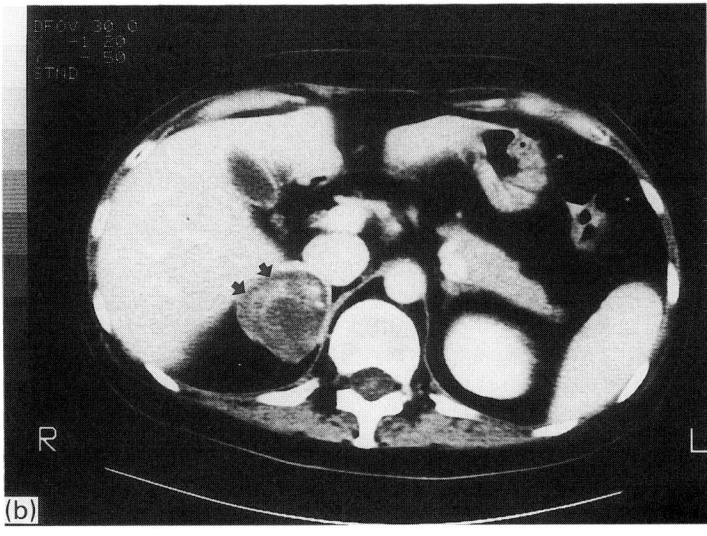

Figure 3. Cushing's syndrome—adrenal adenoma. Postcontrast CT in two patients. (a) Large left adrenal tumour (white arrows) without contrast enhancement. Note the abundant retroperitoneal fat. K, left kidney. (b) A well-demarcated right adrenal tumour (arrows) with areas of contrast-enhancement inside.

useful diagnostic test to distinguish and lateralize them (Findling et al, 1981; Oldfield et al, 1985).

Adrenal CT

The primary function of imaging in Cushing's syndrome is localization of the abnormal adrenal gland, and this is indicated in patients with suspected tumours and those with equivocal laboratory results. This function is often clearly achieved by abdominal CT scans with 10-mm collimation because the large amount of retroperitoneal fat in patients with this disorder facilitates easy identification of the adrenal glands.

Most adrenal adenomas causing the syndrome are 2–5 cm in size, so that CT detection approaches 100% (White FE et al, 1982). The adenoma may

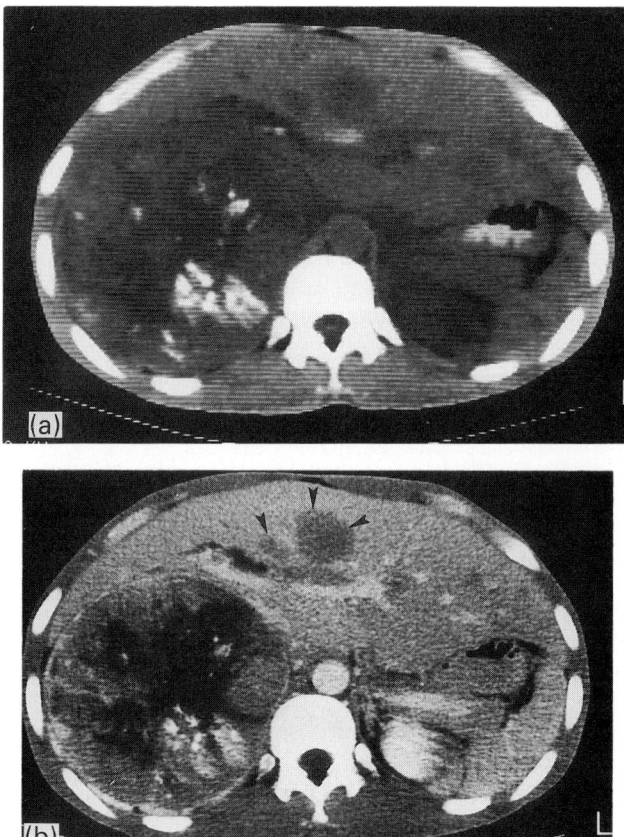

Figure 4. Cushing's syndrome—adrenal carcinoma. (a) Non-contrast CT shows a huge right adrenal tumour with inhomogeneous attenuation and irregular calcification. Metastases are present in the liver. (b) There is irregular internal enhancement plus rim enhancement of the tumour after intravenous contrast injection. The hepatic metastases (arrowheads) are more evident.

arise in any portion of the gland. The density is variable, mostly similar to the soft tissue density of the rest of the adrenal gland but some adenomas demonstrate decreased attenuation. Contrast medium administration by rapid intravenous injection may assist differentiation of eccentrically situated adenomas from vascular structures, and a few adenomas may show contrast enhancement (Figure 3). Although functional atrophy should occur in the contralateral gland this is infrequently discernible on CT.

Approximately 35% of adrenocortical tumours producing Cushing's syndrome in adults are carcinomas. They are large tumours readily detected by CT. Most are heterogeneous with central areas of low density due to necrosis or haemorrhage, and some show scattered calcification (Figure 4) (Dunnick et al, 1982b). Irregular contrast enhancement is present especially in the periphery. The CT features however are not absolute evidence of malignancy, and may not be present in small carcinomas. The definitive diagnosis of adrenal malignancy by CT is consequent upon the detection of local invasion of adjacent structures or metastases in the liver, lungs or lymph nodes. Preoperative staging will help to monitor the subsequent therapy. In the absence of metastases, nevertheless, the distinction between functioning adenoma and carcinoma by imaging may not be totally important since these tumours will be surgically resected and pathology obtained. Patients with adrenocortical tumours may present a mixed form of androgen and cortisol excess, or predominantly androgen excess. These virilizing tumours are large and are detected easily by CT (Figure 5).

In addition to adrenocortical tumours CT may also be helpful in the evaluation of adrenal hyperplasia. Only about half of patients with ACTH-

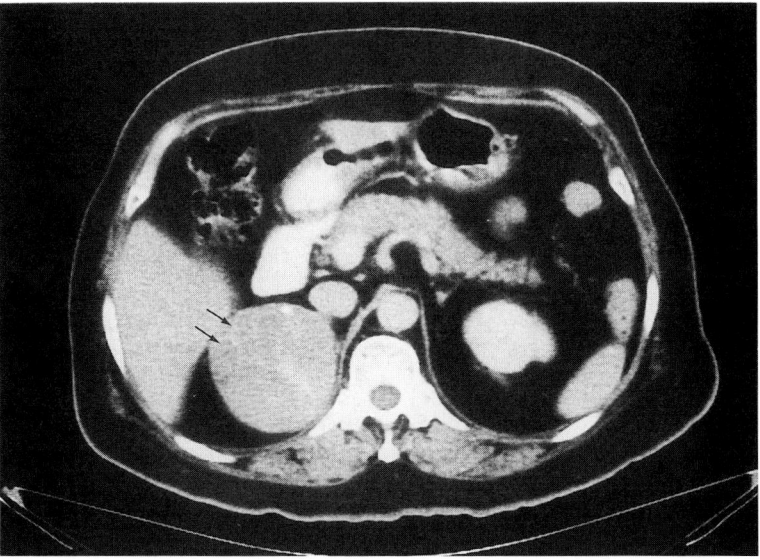

Figure 5. Virilizing adrenal adenoma. CT in a 28-year-old female presenting with hirsutism shows a large right adrenal tumour (arrows) containing a peripheral fleck of calcification.

dependent Cushing's syndrome will show enlarged adrenal glands with diffuse, uniform thickening of both limbs on CT (Adams et al, 1983). Ectopic ACTH syndrome tends to lead to more massive adrenal hyperplasia than Cushing's disease. CT is unable to demonstrate any morphological changes in 50% or more of patients despite the presence of microscopic hyperplasia. This inability of CT to distinguish between normal and hyperplastic glands is not clinically critical since the absence of an adrenal tumour on CT in a patient with clinically proven Cushing's syndrome already indicates adrenal hyperplasia. Most enlarged hyperplastic glands retain their normal configuration, but macronodular hyperplasia may present with nodules as large as 2–3 cm (Figure 6), usually bilateral and multiple. Caution should be exercised in examining the whole gland to distinguish a single dominant macronodule from an autonomous adenoma (Doppman et al, 1988). CT can demonstrate the return to normal of diffusely enlarged adrenals after removal of the source of excessive ACTH production.

Pituitary CT

In contrast to adrenal CT, despite the application of the most sensitive CT techniques, pituitary CT has only a low sensitivity of 30% in detecting ACTH-producing pituitary tumours. It is often unhelpful to differentiate patients with Cushing's disease from those with ectopic ACTH syndrome (Saris et al, 1987). In general, in a patient with positive high-dose dexamethasone suppression and normal adrenal CT a well-defined hypo-

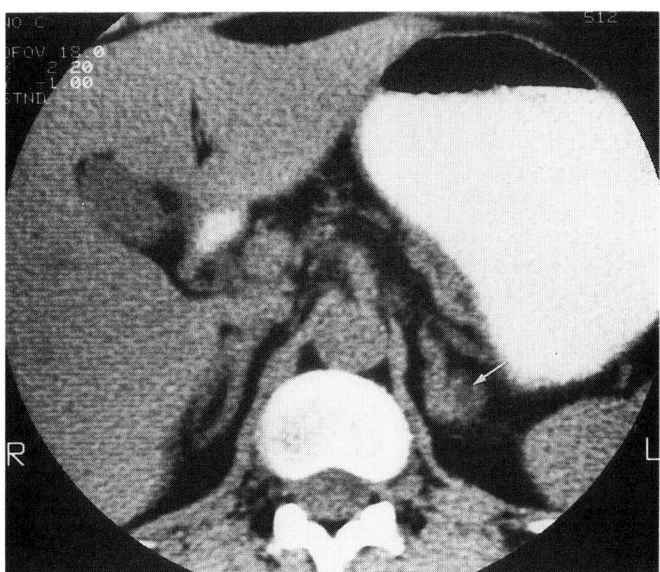

Figure 6. Adrenal hyperplasia. A 53-year-old woman who presented with Cushing's syndrome. CT scan shows bilateral enlargement of the adrenal glands with thick limbs. A 8-mm hypodense hyperplastic nodule (white arrow) is also present in the left adrenal gland.

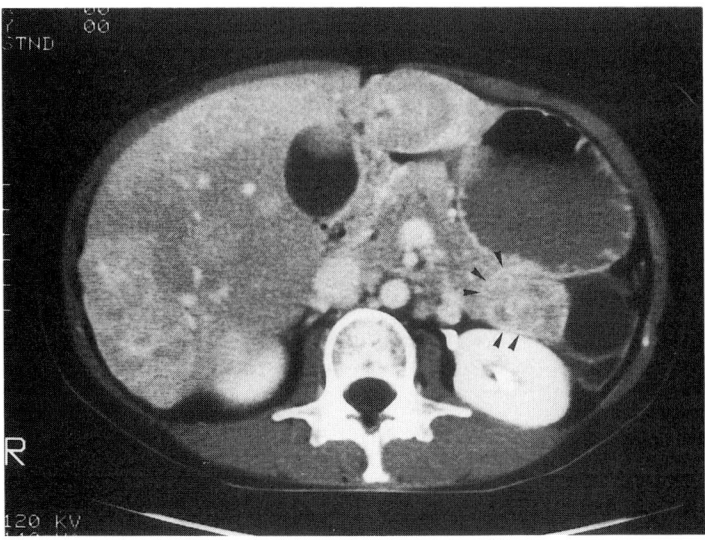

Figure 7. Ectopic ACTH syndrome. A 30-year-old female who presented with Cushing's syndrome. Abdominal CT reveals a partly enhanced tumour (arrowheads) in the tail of the pancreas. The liver shows fatty infiltration and metastases.

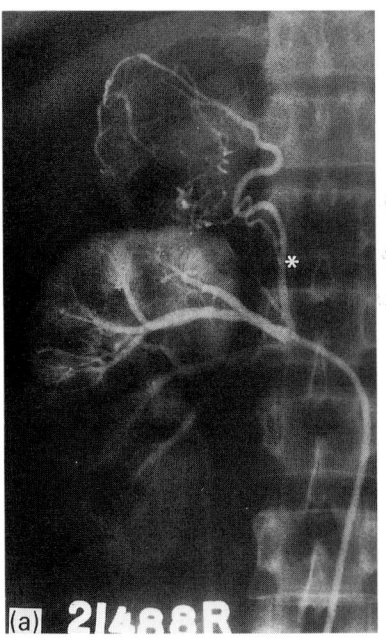
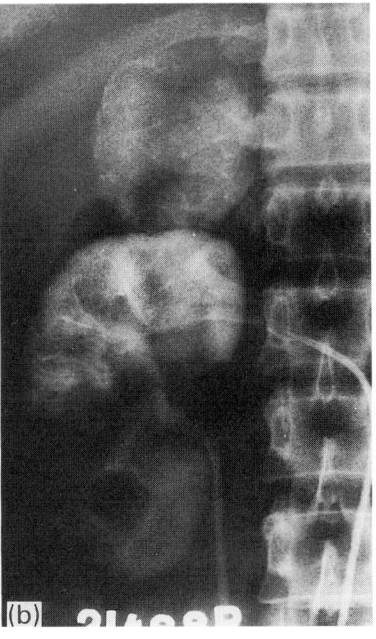

Figure 8. Arteriography in adrenal adenoma: (a) arterial phase, (b) capillary phase. Hypertrophied tortuous vessels supply a right adrenal tumour, which also shows a dense stain in the capillary phase. *, right inferior adrenal artery.

density within the pituitary gland should be interpreted as a microadenoma, while a normal pituitary CT should not be a contraindication to trans-phenoidal exploration if the clinical diagnosis is appropriate (Pojunas et al, 1986). Similarly, although CT of the thorax and abdomen (Figure 7) may be effective in detecting the site of the tumour causing ectopic ACTH syndrome (Brown et al, 1982; White FE et al, 1982), many patients need other studies to locate the responsible tumour.

Other imaging modalities and diagnostic approaches

The truncal obesity typical of patients with Cushing's syndrome renders abdominal ultrasonography difficult. Although ultrasonography can detect most of the large adrenal tumours it will not be an effective imaging modality to evaluate the adrenal glands in adults with Cushing's syndrome.

The role of adrenal arteriography decreases dramatically with the advent of CT and it is rarely used in current evaluation of the adrenal glands. Hypovascular adenomas present displacement of vessels while vascular ones demonstrate a fine reticular arterial network and a localized blush (Figure 8). Angiographic signs of malignancy, including irregular tortuous neo-vascularity, vascular invasion, focal encasement and contrast pooling, may also be found in adenoma and are therefore not strictly specific in differen-tiating between carcinoma and adenoma. On the other hand, adrenal arter-ial embolization may play an effective role in the palliation of pain and reduction of hormone production for inoperable adrenal lesions (O'Keeffe et al, 1988).

Adrenocortical scintigraphy with iodocholesterol has an overall accuracy around 90% in the detection of tumours. Symmetric visualization of the adrenals in patients with documented Cushing's disease indicates hyper-plasia. Unilateral radionuclide uptake is typical of a functioning adenoma suppressing the opposite gland. Bilateral non-uptake of the adrenals (if technical factors like elevated serum cholesterol or prior glucocorticoid administration are excluded) indicates adrenal carcinoma because the con-centration of radionuclide in the carcinoma is usually insufficient to permit visualization while the contralateral gland is suppressed (Herwig and Sonda, 1979). The place of scintigraphy is limited since these tumours are easily identified by CT.

Another approach to CT-negative cases is venous sampling for ACTH. It is especially useful in establishing the source of excessive ACTH secretion in ACTH-dependent Cushing's syndrome. A catheter introduced via the femoral vein and manipulated into various great veins allows samples to be obtained for plasma ACTH estimation from different sites of the body, including the internal jugular veins and the inferior petrosal sinuses (Figure 9). The procedure is tedious and requires reliable biochemical support. Pituitary-dependent disease is confirmed by a gradient of secretion into the inferior petrosal sinus or high internal jugular compared with peripheral samples (Doppman et al, 1984; Oldfield et al, 1985). The test may be further enhanced by stimulation of CRH. Bilateral simultaneous inferior petrosal sinus sampling may correctly identify for the neurosurgeon the side of the

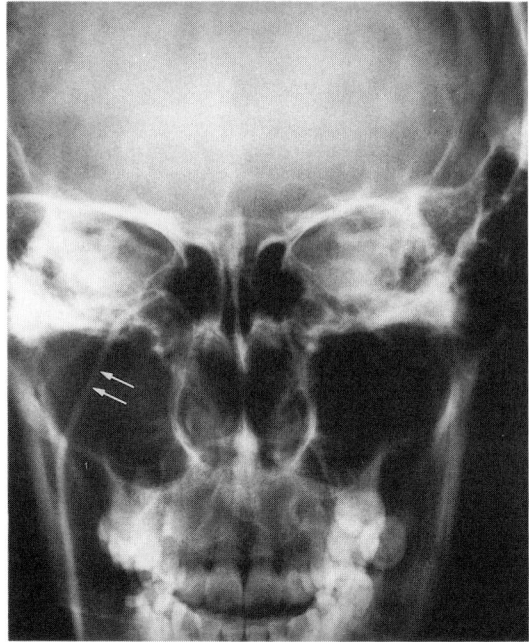

Figure 9. Inferior petrosal sinus sampling. Frontal radiograph of the skull demonstrates the catheter (white arrows) positioned in the right sinus for venous samples.

pituitary gland containing the microadenoma. For ectopic ACTH syndrome, a gradient of secretion may be established at other sites of venous samples; but absence of any gradient is more common with ectopic ACTH production since many of the ectopic tumours do not drain directly into the central great veins available for sampling.

PRIMARY HYPERALDOSTERONISM

Clinical features and diagnosis

Primary hyperaldosteronism is characterized by hypertension and hypo-kalaemia. Other clinical presentations include headaches, muscle weakness, polyuria and polydipsia (Conn et al, 1964). In Orientals, periodic paralysis may often be a presenting feature (Ma et al, 1986). The commonest cause of primary hyperaldosteronism is an adenoma (aldosteronoma). Bilateral aldosteronomas or aldosterone-producing carcinomas are uncommon. Adenomas producing excessive mineralocorticoids have to be distinguished from idiopathic hyperaldosteronism (Weinberger et al, 1979) and dexamethasone suppressible hyperaldosteronism (Ganguly, 1982).

Biochemical diagnosis of primary hyperaldosteronism depends on the finding of persistent hypokalaemia with inappropriate kaluresis. Confirmation of primary hyperaldosteronism is by the finding of elevated and non-suppressible urine and plasma aldosterone in the presence of suppressed plasma urine activity (Drury, 1985; Young and Klee, 1988). Studying the patients after sodium-loading increases the accuracy of these diagnostic tests (Weinberger et al, 1979; Bravo et al, 1982).

The importance of distinction between unilateral aldosteronoma and bilateral hyperplasia is evident from a therapeutic standpoint. Sixty-six per cent of patients who have had aldosteronomas removed will be cured of their hypertension, whereas surgical intervention in idiopathic hyperaldosteronism, even with bilateral adrenalectomy, is seldom curative and is therefore abandoned (Auda et al, 1980). In general, the clinical features of patients with aldosteronoma differ from those with idiopathic hyperaldosteronism because of the more severe hypertension, more profound hypokalaemia and higher plasma aldosterone level, but these features are not totally reliable in the distinction.

CT imaging

Unlike the large tumours producing Cushing's syndrome, aldosteronomas are mostly small—0.5–2 cm in diamater. Their detection by CT therefore demands thinner section, for instance with 3-mm collimation contiguous slices, with an appropriate field of view, through the entire adrenal glands. Cooperation of the patient is essential in holding equal respiratory excursion for each section, otherwise small tumours may be missed. Non-contrast studies are sufficient: contrast medium administration being utilized only occasionally to differentiate small adenomas from adjacent vascular structures. In earlier series using 10-mm thick slices the CT detection rate is only 60–70% (White EA et al, 1980; Geisinger et al, 1983), but the application of thin sections on a high-resolution CT scanner has improved it to over 95% (Ma et al, 1986), picking up small adenomas between 5 and 10-mm. The most easily missed adenomas are those small and isodense tumours buried in the gland near the apex where the gland is thickest. Macroadenomas are easily detected even with 10-mm thick CT scans. CT should be the initial imaging study. Carcinomas or bilateral adenomas are rare, but the patient with an adrenal mass greater than 3 cm should be suspected of having an aldosterone-producing adrenocortical carcinoma (Isles et al, 1987).

Aldosteronomas often appear well-marginated, round or oval, isodense or less dense than the adjacent adrenal parenchyma (Figure 10). The reduced CT attenuation, although more frequently seen in aldosteronoma, is not specific for the pathology and has been attributed to a high lipid content. These adenomas are not enhanced after contrast administration. Preoperative CT localization allows the surgeon to employ a unilateral loin approach instead of a midline transabdominal exploratory procedure which is associated with greater discomfort and morbidity. The CT accuracy is high enough to locate the site of the tumour for partial adrenalectomy in patients with coexistent adrenal dysfunction of the contralateral gland (Figure 11). To assist the retroperitoneal approach to the adrenal tumour, CT also sheds information on the depth of the tumour from the posterior body surface, the presence of adjacent large vascular structures, and the relation of the tumour to the 12th rib, the liver and the kidneys.

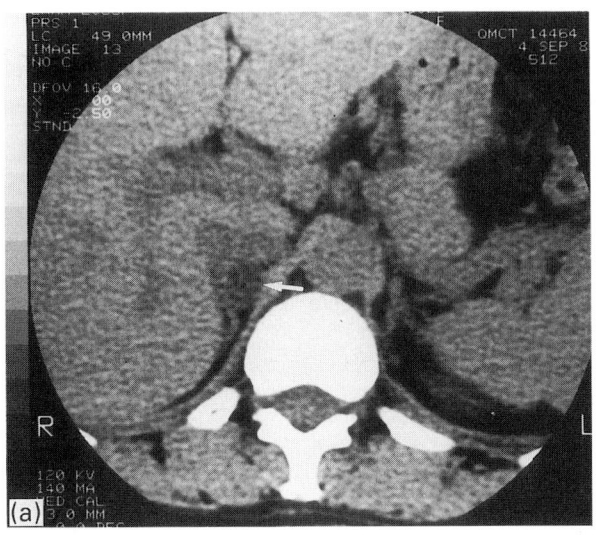

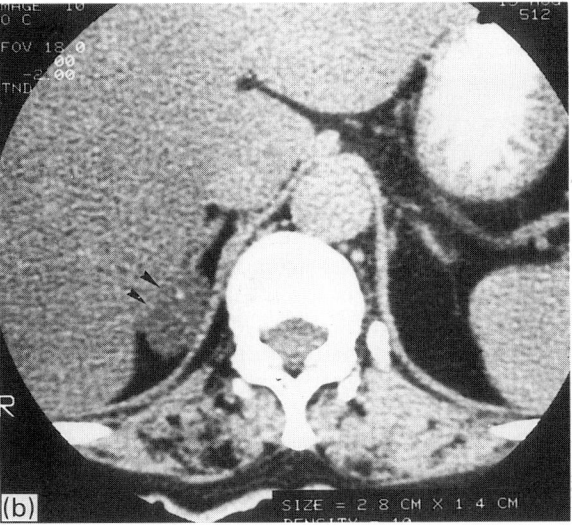

Figure 10. Variations in the appearance of aldosteronomas on non-contrast CT. (a) An oval low attenuation 12-mm adenoma (white arrow) lies on the medial surface of the right adrenal gland which is displaced laterally. (b) A pedunculated oval 22-mm macroadenoma (arrowheads) arises from the tip of the medial limb of the right adrenal gland. A small speck of calcification is present in the adenoma. (c) A round, hypoattenuated 8-mm adenoma (white arrow) lies on the inferior surface of the left adrenal gland. (d) An oval 10-mm adenoma (white arrow) arises from the medial limb of the left adrenal gland.

Patients with idiopathic hyperplasia have either normal-looking adrenal glands or changes consistent with bilateral nodular hyperplasia on CT (Roberts et al, 1985). The CT appearance does not permit differentiation from bilateral aldosteronomas or unilateral aldosteronoma plus contralateral non-functioning adenoma.

Other imaging modalities and diagnostic approaches

The usually small and hypovascular aldosteronomas render excretory urography, nephrotomography and arteriography very insensitive and

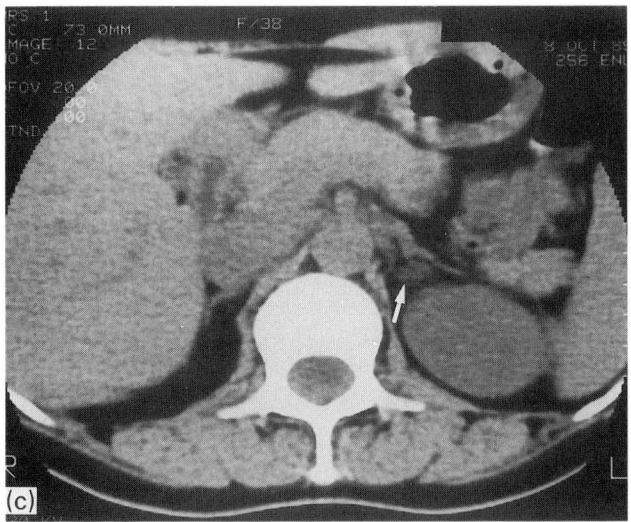

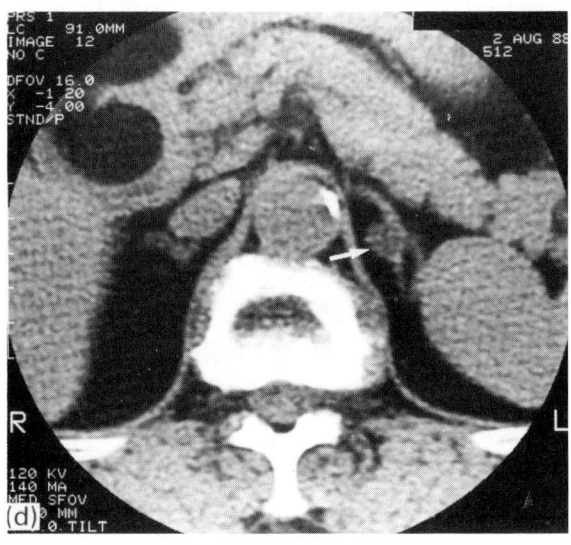

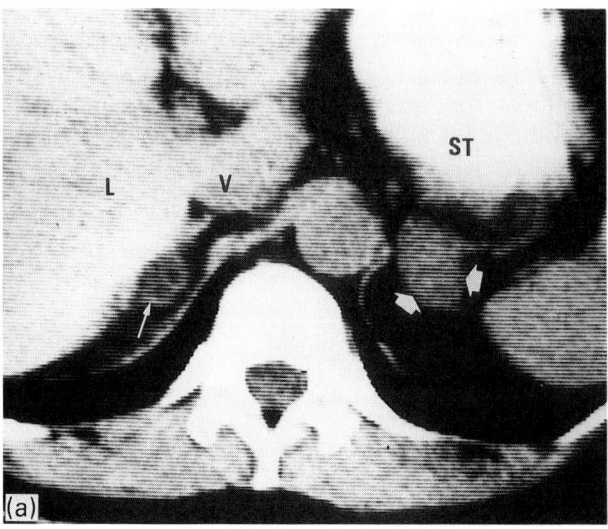

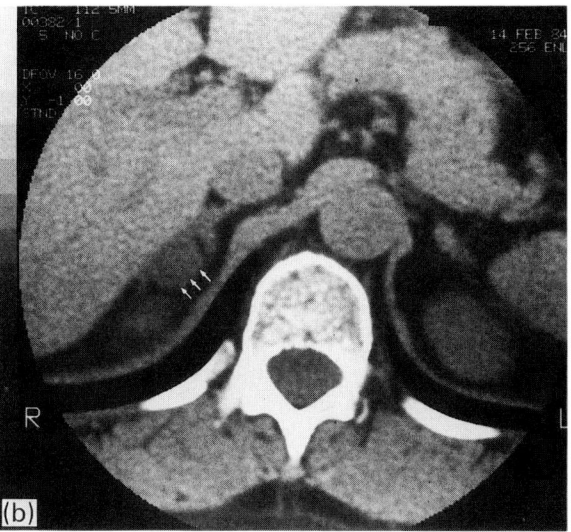

Figure 11. A 51-year-old woman presented aldosteronism for investigation. She experienced left abdominal pain after a left adrenal venus sampling study. (a) CT scan immediately afterwards shows a left adrenal haematoma (large white arrows). An adenoma (small white arrow) is present in the right adrenal gland. L, liver; ST, stomach; V, inferior vena cava. (b) CT scan 4 months later shows resolution of the left haematoma. The right adrenal adenoma (white arrows) is again evident, arising from the medial surface of the lateral limb. In view of the possibility of left adrenal dysfunction from previous haematoma, a partial right adrenalectomy with removal of the adenoma was performed.

therefore useless in their detection. Ultrasonography is also not sufficiently sensitive to be used as a primary method for localization of small aldosteronomas or to define hyperplasia.

The single draining vein of each adrenal gland presents the unique chance of obtaining blood samples for analysis as well as opacifying the gland by venography. Theoretically the former should provide functional lateralization while the latter serves as morphological documentation of the aldosteronomas in the same sitting. Catheterization of the adrenal veins, however, requires a skilful angiographer, while aldosterone assay of blood samples may not be available in every hospital. The procedure must be regarded as invasive because of the risk of complications and possible infarct of the gland. The complication rate is much higher with venography than simple venous sampling. The right adrenal vein, because of its more variable anatomy and insertion, may not be catheterized in about 30% of patients, making complete adrenal venography unsuccessful. Venography alone detects the small cortical adenomas by demonstration of filling defects or a puddling effect in glands with enlarged sinusoids (Figure 12). Accurate detection is achieved in only 40–70% (Nicolis et al, 1972). Thus a negative venogram does not rule out the presence of an adenoma. On the other hand, venous sampling is very accurate by itself. Lateralization is achieved by calculation of the ratio of adrenal venous to inferior vena cava aldosterone. For bilateral venous sampling the aldosterone–cortisol ratio helps to correct for the variation in the degree of selectivity of the catheterization study. Usually the ratio of ipsilateral to contralateral aldosterone concentration in patients with aldosteronoma is greater than 10:1. In the lack of a right adrenal venous sample, a left adrenal vein to inferior vena cava (IVC) aldosterone ratio can be used and is also sensitive for lateralization of a tumour (Lund et al, 1980). Adrenal venography is no longer performed because of the lower accuracy and greater hazard compared to sampling alone.

The sensitivity of NP59 scanning varies greatly with different series, with reported accuracy ranging from 50% to over 90% (Gross et al, 1984; Herd et al, 1987). Dexamethasone pretreatment improves the accuracy, and the test should be performed after diuretics and other antihypertensive medications have been discontinued for two weeks. In patients with aldosteronoma the NP59 scan shows an asymmetric pattern in the first 48–72 hours, with radionuclide uptake in the adenoma. Patients with idiopathic hyperplasia show mild bilateral adrenal uptake at 72–120 hours. Bilateral uptake seen after 5 days is considered non-diagnostic. The test is time-consuming and more costly than CT. The sensitivity of scintigraphy depends heavily on the size of adenoma, and it is unlikely to obtain additional information if the adrenal CT is normal (Guerin et al, 1983). It is therefore not a practical alternative to CT.

For practical purposes, if CT scan shows a unilateral tumour and the biochemical data are diagnostic, no further imaging is necessary. If the CT is normal, equivocal or showing bilateral adrenal masses, adrenal venous sampling can be considered (Lim et al, 1986). There are two other approaches for this latter group. Some clinicians rely on posture study and

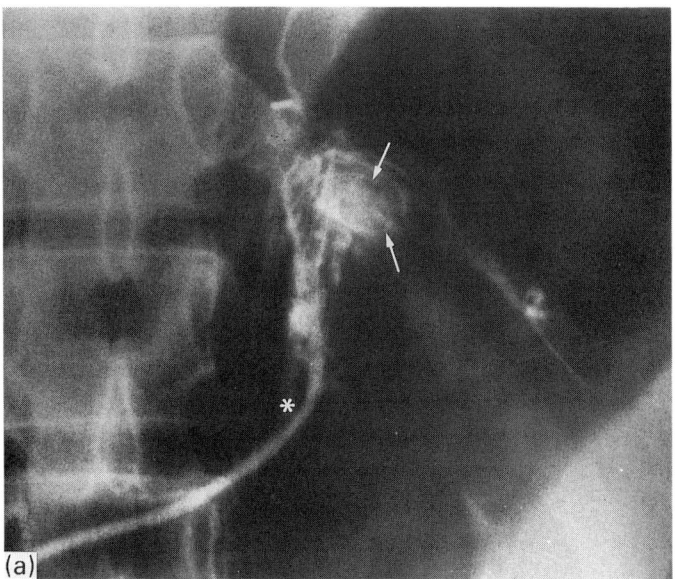

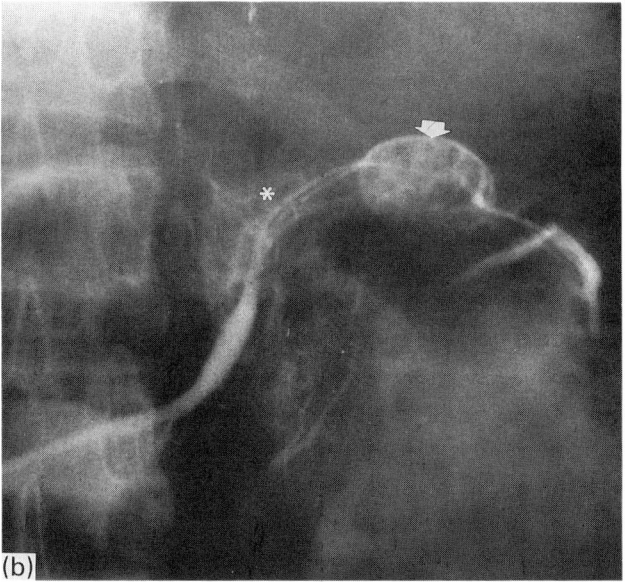

Figure 12. Adrenal venogram demonstrating adenomas. (a) A small space-occupying lesion (arrows) is present in the left adrenal gland with displacement of the intraglandular veins around it, and puddling of contrast within the tumour. (b) An oval adenoma (arrow) lies very laterally as a filling defect in the venous sinusoids. *, left adrenal vein.

measurement of 18–hydroxycorticosterone to differentiate between aldosteronoma and idiopathic hyperaldosteronism (Grant et al, 1984; Young and Klee, 1988). In response to upright posture, patients with idiopathic hyperaldosteronism show a rise in plasma aldosterone whereas there is a fall in the majority of patients with adenomas (Espiner and Donald, 1980). The 18-hydroxycorticosterone levels are high in adenomas and normal in idiopathic hyperaldosteronism (Biglieri and Schambelan, 1979). Others prefer a period of medical management with repeat CT at a later date if such therapy fails.

PHAEOCHROMOCYTOMA

Clinical features and biochemical diagnosis

The diagnosis of phaeochromocytoma should be suspected in patients with paroxysmal, labile or resistant hypertension. Episodic symptoms such as headaches, palpitations, pallor and sweating with rapid onset and slower offset are characteristic. Over a third of the patients have persistent elevation of blood pressure. Family history of phaeochromocytoma suggests multiple endocrine neoplasm (MEN) IIa and b (medullary carcinoma of thyroid, parathyroid hyperplasia, phaeochromocytoma). Phaeochromocytomas are also associated with neurocutaneous syndromes e.g. neurofibromatosis, and may secrete other peptides such as vasoactive polypeptides, serotonin and substance P.

Biochemical diagnosis is based on finding raised 24-hour urinary levels of vanillylmandelic acid (VMA), catecholamines (adrenaline, noradrenaline, dopamine) and other metabolites (metanephrine, normetanephrine) and/or plasma concentrations of catecholamines. Urine and blood sampling frequently have to be repeated and collected during the symptomatic episodes. Fluorometric or spectrophometric measurements of catecholamines and metabolites are the traditional methods to diagnose phaeochromocytomas (Cryer, 1985). These methods are subjected to interferences by a large number of drugs (especially in patients on antihypertensive drug therapy) and urinary pigments. These methods have been replaced by radio-enzymatic assays (Bravo et al, 1979) and high-pressure liquid chromatography (HPLC) (Bravo and Gillford, 1984; Sheps et al, 1988). The HPLC method determines the levels of fractionated catecholamines and has the advantage that drugs appear as separate peaks and do not interfere with the measurement of catecholamines. The sensitivity is high. Higher cut-off levels give good clinical specificity. Usually in patients with tumours, either adrenaline or noradrenaline and one of their metabolites are elevated. Mild increases in levels are seen in patients without tumours. In situations where endogenous catecholamines are increased such as stress, surgery, hypoglycaemia, theophylline, alcohol withdrawal, clonidine withdrawal and vasodilator therapy, values are often above the normal range. Interpretation of the results may be difficult in patients taking monoamine oxidase inhibitors, phenothiazines and beta-blockers. Sampling for plasma catecholamines, in particular, is very labile and affected by the same physiological and pharmacological states described above. Nowadays, provocative tests with glucagon or histamine are rarely necessary for the diagnosis of phaeochromocytomas.

If levels of noradrenaline and its metabolites are elevated, this may be indicative of extra-adrenal phaeochromocytomas. Extra-adrenal tumours comprise 10% of phaeochromocytomas, and can occur where nests of the primitive neural crest cells have survived. They may be found anywhere from the base of skull to the epididymis, including posterior mediastinum, lungs, heart and bladder, but the commonest ectopic site is a collection of neural crest cells along the sympathetic chain adjacent to the abdominal aorta and near the origin of the inferior mesenteric artery (organ of Zuckerlandl). In adults, approximately 10% of phaeochromocytomas are multicentric (including bilateral intra-adrenal), and 10% malignant. There is an increased frequency of ectopia, bilaterality, multicentricity and malignancy when phaeochromocytomas are associated with the neuroectodermal disorders or the MEN syndromes (Figure 13). While the extratumoral adrenal medulla is normal in sporadic adrenal phaeochromocytomas, there is medullary hyperplasia in MEN syndromes. Examination of the extratumoral medulla in resected adrenal glands is therefore recommended to identify previously unsuspected patients with MEN in view of the difference in management (Webb et al, 1980).

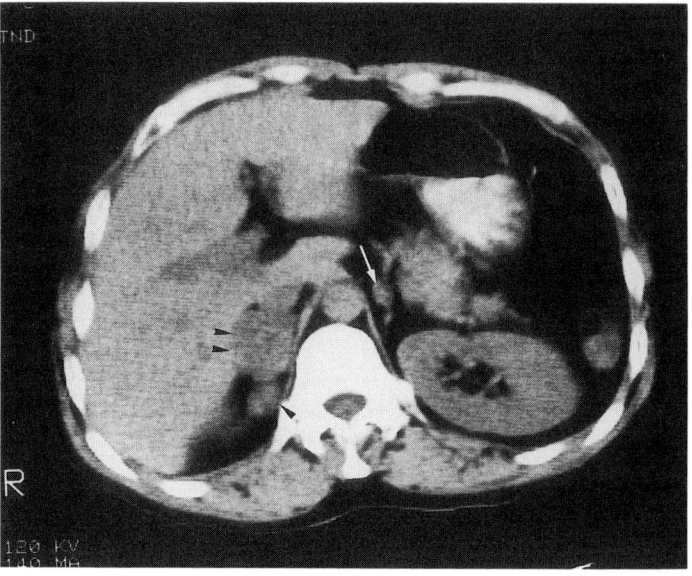

Figure 13. Multiple phaeochromocytomas. A 39-year-old man with multiple endocrine neoplasia syndrome. CT scan of the adrenal region shows bilobed right phaeochromocytoma (arrowheads) and a small left phaeochromocytoma (white arrow).

CT imaging

Since over 95% of all phaeochromocytomas are located within the abdomen, an abdominal CT after peroral contrast preparation of the bowels, with contiguous 10-mm thick slices, from the level of the diaphragm down to the region of the aortic bifurcation, should be the initial imaging. Direct

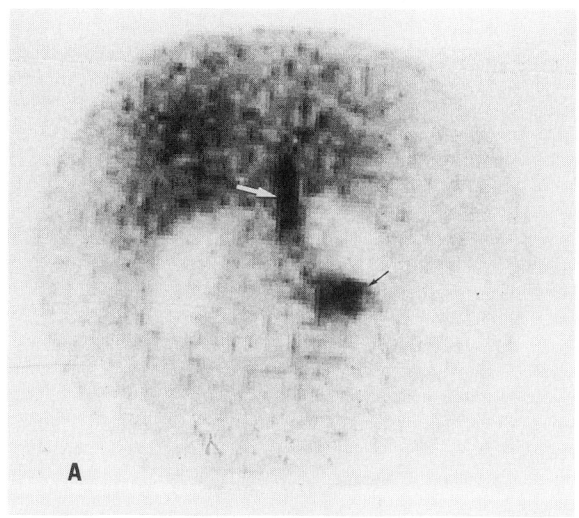

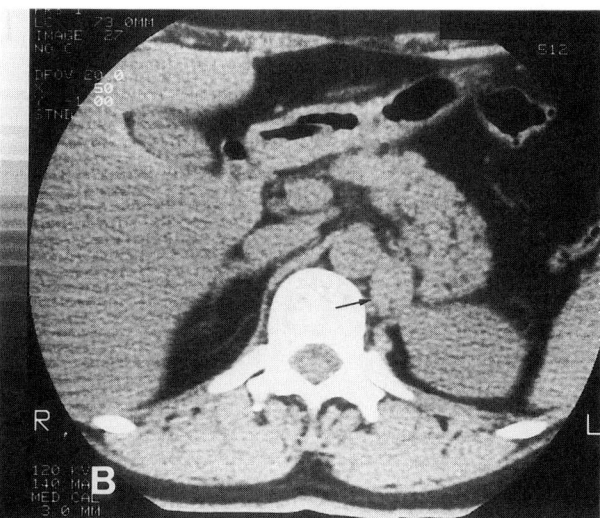

Figure 14. Recurrent phaeochromocytoma. (a) MIBG scan in the follow-up investigation of recurrent hypertension in a patient with previous resection of a left adrenal phaeochromocytoma shows increased radionuclide uptake over the region of the left diaphragmatic crux (white arrow) and the lower part of the left kidney (black arrow). (b) The recurrent tumour (arrow) arising from the left crux is clearly demonstrated on the non-contrast CT.

supervision of the entire examination by a radiologist is essential. Non-contrast CT is recommended to avoid the small but definite risk of hypertensive crisis associated with intravenous contrast administration (Radin et al, 1986). Occasionally, intravenous contrast is required to improve the quality of scans in patients with paucity of retroperitoneal fat, and to clarify equivocal or confusing areas encountered during the non-contrast study.

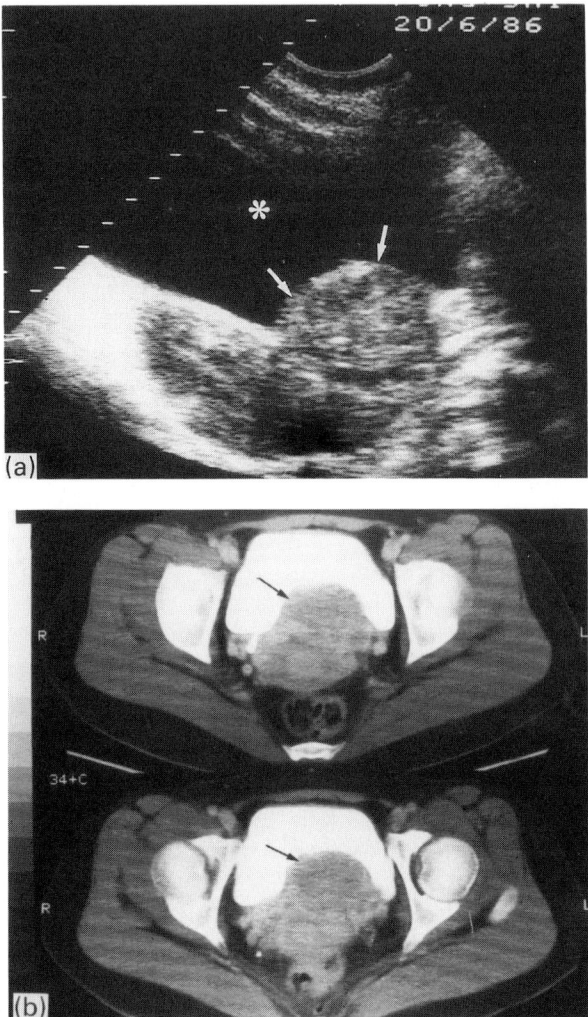

Figure 15. Pelvic phaeochromocytoma in a 23-year-old female. (a) Sagittal ultrasonography images a 5-cm mass (white arrows) lying between the bladder (marked *) and the uterus, bulging into the posterior wall of the bladder. (b) Two sections of the postcontrast CT of pelvis demonstrate the partially enhanced tumour (arrows) lying behind the bladder. (c) Selective arteriography of the supplying branch of the left internal iliac artery shows the hypervascular tumour. Preoperative embolization via the catheter was performed.

For localization of ectopic phaeochromocytomas, large areas of the body may have to be covered by CT, so that the examination must be carefully monitored to reserve appropriate contrast administration for areas of least clarity. When contrast-enhanced CT is performed, we would recommend pretreatment with appropriate alpha and beta blockade since a variable, unpredictable but significant rise in plasma catecholamine levels had been observed after giving contrast intravenously (Raisanen et al, 1984). Another consideration after the intravenous contrast is the effect on biochemical measurements: contrast containing methylglucamine may cause false urinary metanephrine values up to 72 hours after its administration.

CT detection of adrenal phaeochromocytomas, mostly larger than 2 cm, should approach 100% with proper examination techniques utilizing the modern high-resolution scanners (Welch et al, 1983). The CT appearance varies. Most are discrete round or oval masses, occasionally protruding from the adrenal glands as pedunculated tumours, with homogeneous density slightly less than that of the adjacent liver or pancreas. Central hypodense necrotic, haemorrhagic or cystic changes, or calcification may be present. On postcontrast CT the degree of enhancement of the phaeochromocytoma varies but the periphery of the tumour will be more intensely enhanced. Contrast enhancement also exaggerates the presence of hypodense areas. Diagnosis of malignancy on the CT appearance of the phaeochromocytoma is unreliable.

CT can also detect extra-adrenal, recurrent and metastatic phaeochromocytomas in most cases, although the sensitivity is inferior to that for intra-adrenal tumours. Recurrent tumours vary in appearance, as solid intra-adrenal masses, destructive bone lesions, solid soft-tissue masses, or multiple small nodules in the area of the resection (Figure 14b) (Welch et al, 1983). CT detection of these recurrent tumours may be hampered by their small size, scarring at operative sites, artefacts created by surgical clips and postoperative distortion of normal anatomy. Ectopic phaeochromocytomas need tedious and meticulous examination for localization. Reynes et al

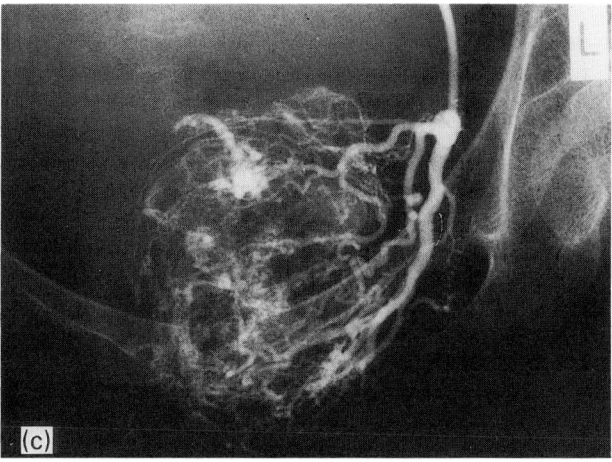
(c)

(1979) recommended extension of the CT examination to include the rest of the abdomen, pelvis and thorax; but most would consider MIBG scanning or selective venous sampling if the initial abdominal CT is negative (Dunnick et al, 1982a; Adams et al, 1983). After an approximate localization of the ectopic tumour by these methods, further careful CT scanning of the relevant region will be performed. These ectopic tumours appear as unremarkable soft tissue masses that may enhance with contrast (Figure 15b).

Other imaging modalities and diagnostic approaches

Ultrasonography can locate some phaeochromocytomas including adrenal, pelvic and bladder ones (Figure 15a) (Bowerman et al, 1981). The sonographic spectrum varies from solid to cystic masses, but most are large, sharply marginated and complex in echogenicity. Success of the method is very dependent upon the anatomy and position of the tumour and the overlying structures. It is therefore not suitable as a regular initial test. Similarly arteriography does not play an important role in the routine diagnosis of phaeochromocytoma, although it used to be applied for the ultimate diagnosis. It has been mainly replaced by CT because of its invasiveness and the possible risk of acute hypertensive crisis (Kader and Robinette, 1981); nevertheless small vascular tumours may be detected with arteriography but not CT (Tisnado et al, 1980). Hypervascular phaeochromocytoma shows a dominant feeding artery which supplies radiating branches converging towards the centre or a fine reticular pattern, with a dense capillary stain. About 15% of phaeochromocytomas, however, are hypovascular. Vascular mapping for very large tumours and preoperative arteriographic embolization of phaeochromocytomas may also be performed (Figure 15c). All these procedures are done after preparation of the patient with alpha and beta blocking agents, together with careful intraprocedural monitoring of the blood pressure. Improvements in the contrast media and the application of digital vascular imaging will make arteriography safer and more accurate.

MIBG scans are sensitive and serve as functional imaging (Figure 16). The advantages of this agent include the possibility of localizing tumours throughout the body, identification of small tumours, reliability unpromised by postoperative scarring or clips, and demonstration of adrenal medullary hyperplasia (Swensen et al, 1985). However, the method has limited availability, poor resolution, higher radiation dose and takes 1–3 days to complete. It is useful in the detection of coexistent extra-adrenal disease, unsuspected multicentricity and recurrence of tumour (Figure 14a). Screening for recurrent and metastatic disease is probably best achieved with MIBG scans, with more precise anatomic locations subsequently obtained with CT (Quint et al, 1987). It is also the examination of choice for imaging patients with MEN syndromes (Valk et al, 1981). The method cannot detect 10% of phaeochromocytomas, but the cause of false negatives is not yet documented.

Selective venous sampling for catecholamines from the superior and inferior vena cavae and their major contributing veins provides help in localization when the other tests are non-diagnostic, especially for ectopic and multiple phaeochromocytomas (Palubinskas et al, 1980; Allison et al, 1983). The procedure is rather time-consuming and demands reliable laboratory support for assay of adrenaline and noradrenaline. A positive result accurately identifies the presence of the tumour, and locates the specific region for further effective morphologic imaging. It is a reliable means of refuting the diagnosis of phaeochromocytoma when the clinical and biochemical evidence is conflicting.

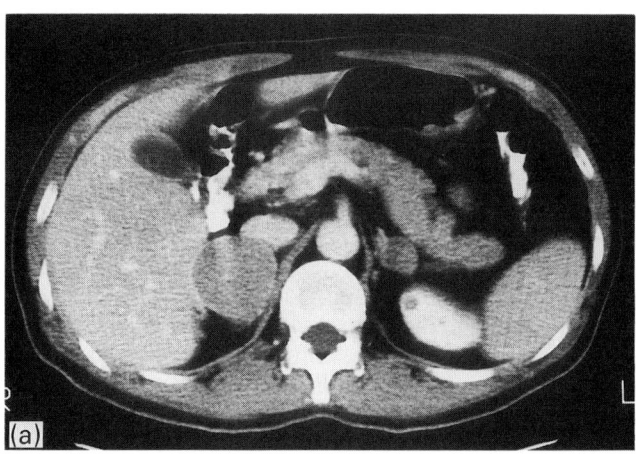

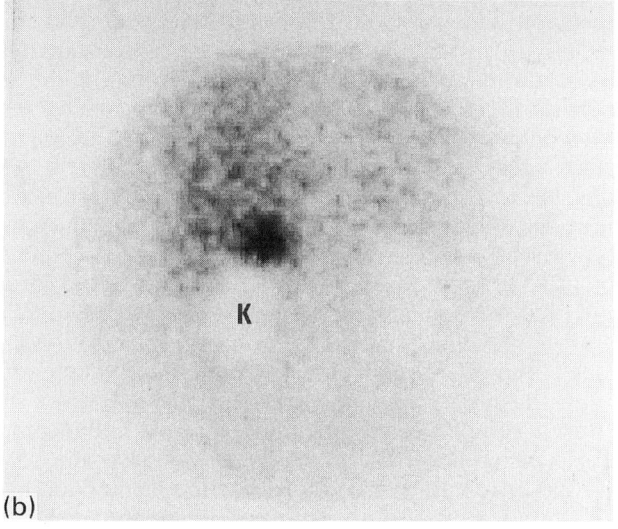

Figure 16. Bilateral adrenal tumours. A 58-year-old man presented with clinical and bio-chemical symptoms of phaeochromocytoma. (a) CT scan shows bilateral adrenal tumours. (b) MIBG scan reveals radionuclide uptake only over the right adrenal region (K, right kidney). At surgery, a right phaeochromocytoma and a left non-functioning adenoma were documented.

At present, the initial imaging examination for a patient who may have a phaeochromocytoma should be an abdominal CT scan, the extent of this initial study being guided by the available clinical and laboratory data. Further investigation with MIBG scan is pursued if the CT is negative. On the other hand, MIBG may be the preferred initial test, in centres with such facility (Bomanji et al, 1988), for patients with the MEN syndromes, or suspected recurrent or metastatic disease. If the results of these investigations are equivocal or negative while the clinical evidence is quite definite, venous sampling is the complementary study. Where phaeochromocytomas are only roughly located by scintigraphy or venous sampling, further documentation by CT or arteriography of the specific region may be necessary before operative resection. The application of MRI is under investigation, and shows promise of becoming the method of choice for extra-adrenal phaeochromocytomas.

THE 'INCIDENTALOMA'

The widespread use of CT has created a problem of a different nature. The excellent visualization of the adrenal glands on routine abdominal CT has resulted in the incidental discovery of adrenal masses in about 1% of patients (Glazer HS et al, 1982). Such tumours have been coined 'incidental-omas' and the prevalence corresponds to reported autopsy studies demonstrating grossly visible non-functioning adenomas in 1–9% of adults (Hedeland et al, 1968). Apart from adrenal cysts and myelolipomas, tissue characterization by CT is too limited to permit reliable diagnosis of the nature of the mass. This poses a significant diagnostic and management problem especially in patients harbouring known primary malignancy.

In patients without existing cancer, evaluation should attempt to determine whether there is hypersecretion of adrenal cortical or medullary hormones and whether the mass represents a primary adrenal malignancy. In both circumstances, the adrenal mass needs to be resected. After clinical history and physical examination to exclude adrenal hyperfunction, laboratory assessment discussed previously should be performed as appropriate.

In patients without cancer and without laboratory evidence of adrenal hyperfunction most of these masses are adenomas. Adrenal carcinomas are rarer since half of all adrenal carcinomas cause adrenal dysfunction, including Cushing's syndrome, precocious puberty, virilization and mixed syndrome. Size is the most important discriminant between adenoma and carcinoma, with the latter extremely unlikely to be 4 cm or smaller. For other CT features, tumour consistency and contrast enhancement characteristic may also be relative discriminants in assessing the probability of malignancy (Hussain et al, 1985). Non-functioning adenomas appear as homogeneous, round or oval masses with well-delineated margins, probably with punctate enhancement. Adrenal carcinomas tend to have poorly defined irregular or lobulated margins, large central area or multiple scattered areas of decreased attenuation representing tumour necrosis, and irregular contrast enhancement. The predictive value of these CT features is

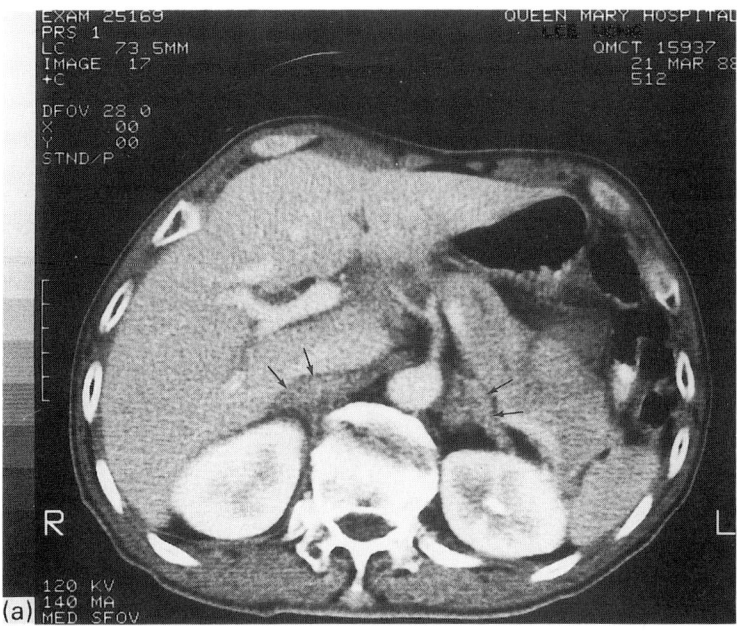

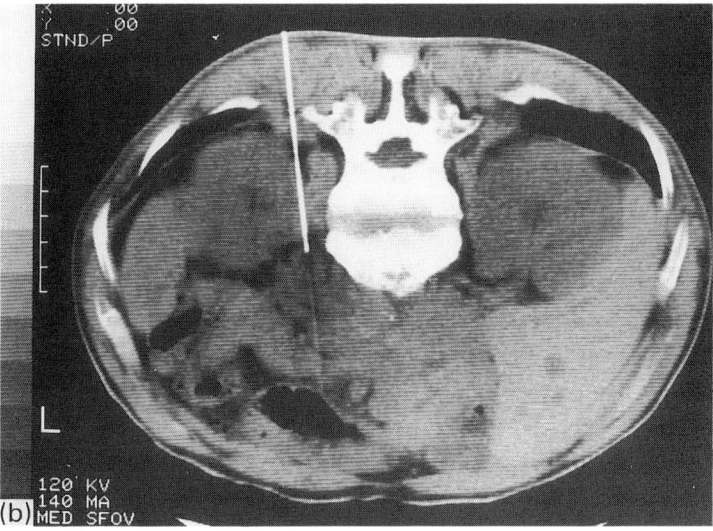

Figure 17. CT-guided biopsy of adrenal mass. (a) Bilateral adrenal masses (arrows) are discovered on the CT scan. (b) With the patient lying prone, a CT-guided percutaneous aspiration needle biopsy was performed for the left adrenal mass, documenting metastatic malignancy.

further enhanced by experienced workers using dynamic incremental CT technique (Berland et al, 1988). Nevertheless, none of these discriminants can consistently confer precise diagnosis (Fishman et al, 1987). Copeland (1983) recommended resection of all lesions of 6 cm or larger (others set the limiting value differently at 3 or 5 cm) and following smaller lesions with sequential scans at 2, 6 and 18 months. Any mass without interval change in size is assumed to be a benign non-functioning adenoma.

Incidental non-functioning adrenal masses in patients with cancer may need a more aggressive approach. Bilateral masses are usually assumed to be metastases except in patients with phaeochromocytoma. For unilateral masses, MRI has been applied to characterize the lesion at some institutions. More recently, NP59 scintigraphy has been used to identify the 'non-hyperfunctioning' adenomas and the results appear promising (Francis et al, 1988). The indeterminate spread is, however, usually undesirably large with these techniques. In view of the need to decide on surgery or chemotherapeutic treatment, many authorities advocate CT-guided biopsy (Figure 17) of all such masses to obtain tissue diagnosis (Katz and Shirkhoda, 1985; Bernardino, 1988).

MAGNETIC RESONANCE IMAGING OF THE ADRENAL GLANDS

When magnetic resonance imaging (MRI) was introduced, CT had already been well established with its high sensitivity albeit limited specificity to image nearly all adrenal masses. Work on MRI of the adrenal glands thus concentrates on exploration of its potential to characterize the morphology and functional activities of the adrenal lesions.

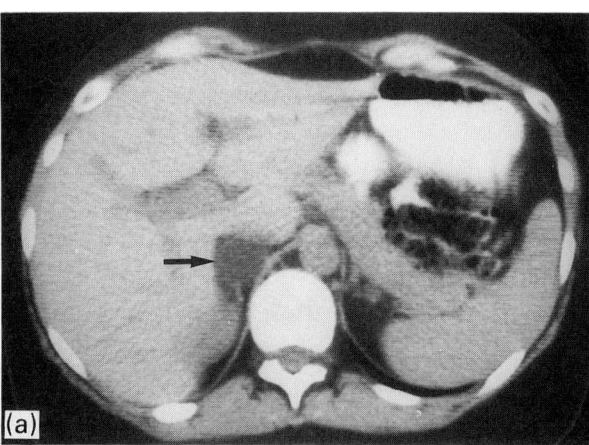

Figure 18. Non-functioning adrenal adenoma. (a) CT scan demonstrates a homogeneous low attenuation mass in the right adrenal gland (arrow). On TR 500/TE 35 (b), TR 500/TE 70 (c), and TR 2100/TE 90 (d) images the adenoma (arrow) is similar in signal intensity to liver, and much lower intensity than fat (mass/fat ratio 0.46 at TR 2100/TE 90). From Chang et al (1987), with permission.

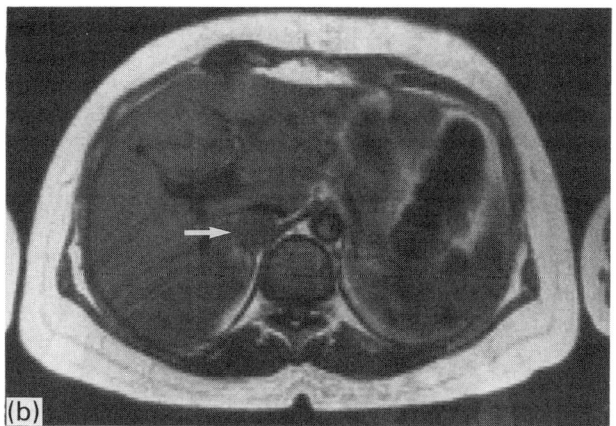

(b)

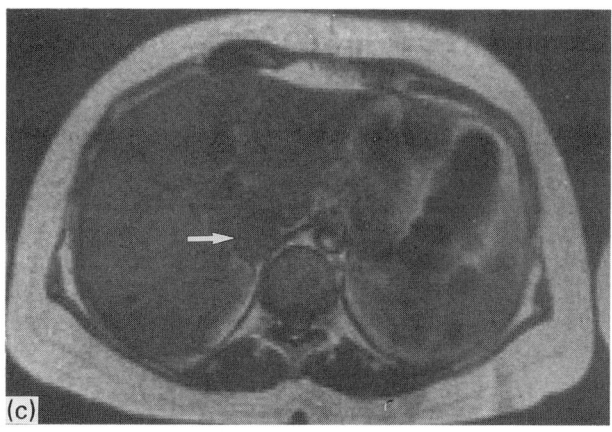

(c)

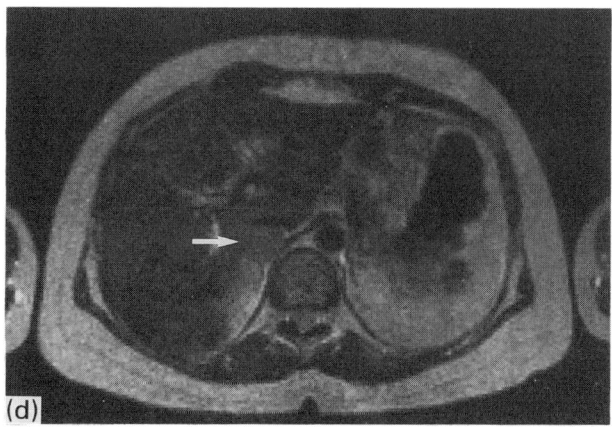

(d)

The normal adrenal glands can be clearly delineated by MRI in over 95% of cases, especially with the T1-weighted spin–echo pulse sequences. The left gland is often better visualized than the right. The surrounding vascular structures can be easily distinguished from any adrenal nodules (Brady et al, 1985). Early expectation of differentiation between adrenal cortex and medulla with MRI, however, has not been fully documented (Chang et al, 1987). Compared with CT, the overall sensitivity for adrenal masses is slightly lower: sensitivity is nearly equivalent for masses larger than 1.0–1.5 cm in diameter but CT is much better for masses smaller than 1 cm (Schultz, 1986). The advantage of superior contrast and optimal plane selection enables MRI better to evaluate tumour extent in relation to surrounding structures. In general, MRI has a greater specificity for mass lesions and may be useful to differentiate non-functioning adenomas from functioning tumours, metastases, phaeochromocytomas, cysts and intra-adrenal haemorrhage. Taking its limitations into consideration, the present role of MRI in the evaluation of adrenal disease is believed to be comple-mentary to CT (Falke et al, 1986).

For adrenal cortical hyperfunction MRI can detect the adrenal tumours accounting for Cushing's syndrome with a sensitivity comparable to CT. However, the aldosteronomas and nodular hyperplasia in primary hyper-aldosteronism are small and poorly resolved on MRI, and thus much better assessed by thin-section CT. At the current stage of development there is no consistent relationship between MRI characteristics and the adrenal cortical function (Glazer GM, 1988).

In the evaluation of phaeochromoctyomas MRI enjoys higher sensitivity than CT in the detection of extra-adrenal, recurrent or metastatic lesions owing to its superior soft tissue contrast resolution and its capability of direct imaging in the coronal or sagittal planes. MRI also permits distinction between phaeochromocytomas and non-functioning adenomas because of the marked hyperintensity of phaeochromocytomas on T2-weighted pulse sequences (Quint et al, 1987).

The application of MRI to 'incidentalomas' has been most extensively investigated, focusing on the distinction between benign adenomas and adrenal metastases. Several studies have shown that non-functioning adenomas typically possess significantly lower MRI signal intensities than adrenal metastases on T2-weighted sequences. Such distinction can be achieved by comparing the intensity of the adrenal mass to that of liver or body fat (Figures 18 and 19). Although cut-off points (which vary with the instrumentation and technique used) of quantitative intensity data could be established, below which the lesions are adenomas and above which the lesions are metastases, there is considerable overlap and 21–31% of adrenal masses are in the indeterminate range (Reinig et al, 1986; Chang et al, 1987). Furthermore, a significant number of low intensity metastases simulate adenomas. Similarly, significant overlap in signal intensities also occurs with T1-weighted sequences (Chezmar et al, 1988). At present MRI character-ization is pending larger series to identify the optimal pulse sequence for such differentiation, and is still not sufficiently accurate to dispense with biopsy in every individual patient presenting an 'incidentaloma'.

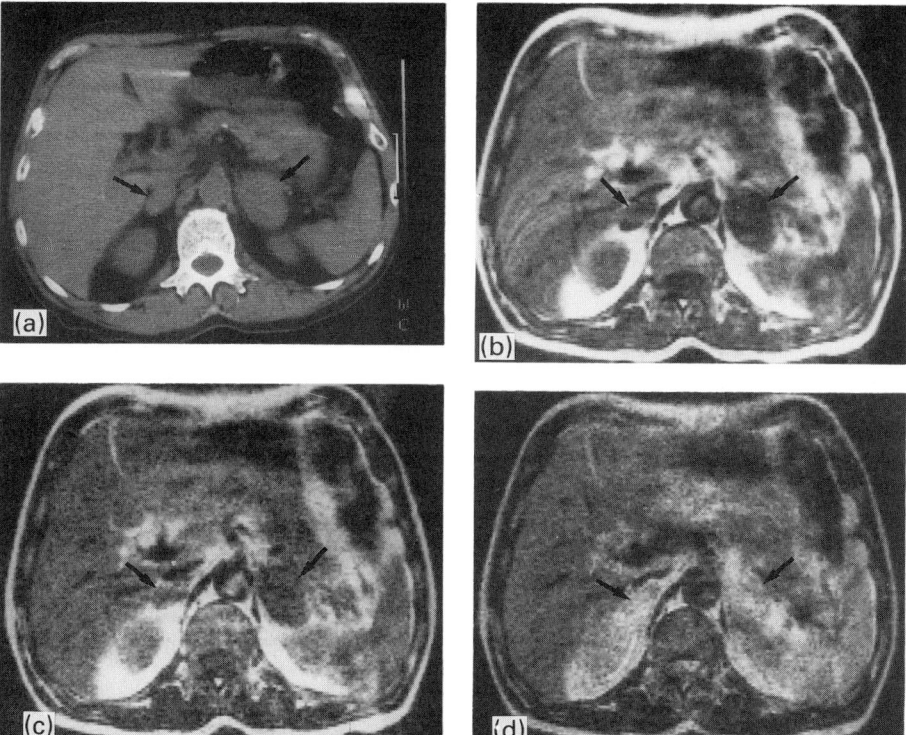

Figure 19. Bilateral adrenal metastases from bronchogenic carcinoma. (a) CT scan shows bilateral soft tissue density adrenal masses (arrows). (b) On TR 500/TE 35 image the masses (arrows) are hypointense to liver. (c) On TR 500/TE 70 image the left adrenal mass is slightly lower in signal intensity than liver, whereas the right adrenal mass is similar in signal intensity to liver. (d) On TR 2100/TE 90 image both masses (arrows) are hyperintense compared to liver and approach the signal intensity of fat making them difficult to see (mass/fat ratio 0.92 at TR 2100/TE 90). From Chang et al (1987), with permission.

SUMMARY

Modern medical imaging has transformed the diagnosis and management of adrenal disease. The various types of adrenal tumours bear different aspects of problems in diagnostic imaging. The investigation used must be determined and monitored individually, as directed by the clinical and biochemical findings. CT plays a central role in the localization of the functioning adrenal tumours. It is regarded as the imaging modality of choice because it combines safety with a high rate of detection. It is highly sensitive in the localization of the large adrenal tumours that account for Cushing's syndrome and phaeochromocytomas, as well as the small tumours that account for primary hyperaldosteronism. It is, however, not reliable for the detection of adrenal hyperplasia, and does not yield functional imaging information. For small tumours not detectable by CT, and for ectopic tumours, complementary investigations with appropriate application of venous sampling, radionuclide scintigraphy and occasionally arteriography, will be very useful. CT-guided percutaneous biopsy is employed for the incidentalomas in oncologic patients. MRI appears to hold a great potential for the diagnosis of adrenal disorders, but this modality is awaiting wider availability of instrumentation and clearer documentation of techniques.

Acknowledgements

The authors are grateful to Dr Joseph K. T. Lee, Mallinckrodt Institute of Radiology, St Louis, for permission to publish figures 18 and 19; to Dr David W. C. Yeung, Queen Mary Hospital, Hong Kong, for figures 14a and 16b, and to Dr John Boey for the surgical findings of our patients. We thank Miss Kitty Kwok for her secretarial assistance in the preparation of the manuscript.

REFERENCES

Abrams HL, Siegelman SS, Adams DF et al (1982) Computed tomography versus ultrasound of the adrenal glands: a prospective study. *Radiology* **143:** 121–128.

Adams JE, Johnson RJ, Rickards D & Isherwood I (1983) Computed tomography in adrenal disease. *Clinical Radiology* **34:** 39–49.

Allison DJ, Brown MJ, Jones DH & Timmis JB (1983) Role of venous sampling in locating a pheochromocytoma. *British Medical Journal* **286:** 1122–1124.

Aron DC, Tyrrell JB, Fitzgerald PA et al (1981) Cushing's syndrome: problems in diagnosis. *Medicine* (Baltimore) **60:** 25–35.

Aron DC, Findling JW & Tyrrell JB (1988) Cushing's disease. *Endocrinology and Metabolism Clinics of North America* **16:** 705–730.

Auda SP, Brennan MF & Gill JR Jr (1980) Evolution of the surgical management of primary aldosteronism. *Annals of Surgery* **191:** 1–7.

Barbarino A, DeMarinis L, Liberale I & Mincini E (1979) Evaluation of steroid laboratory tests and adrenal gland imaging with radiocholesterol in the aetiological diagnosis of Cushing's syndrome. *Clinical Endocrinology* **10:** 107–121.

Bayliss RIS, Edwards OM & Starer F (1970) Complications of adrenal venography. *British Journal of Radiology* **43:** 531–533.

Berland LL, Koslin DB, Kenney PJ, Stanley RJ & Lee JY (1988) Differentiation between small benign and malignant adrenal masses with dynamic incremented CT. *American Journal of Roentgenology* **151:** 95–101.

Bernardino ME (1988) Management of the asymptomatic patient with a unilateral adrenal mass. *Radiology* **166:** 121–123.

Bernardino ME, Walther MM, Phillips VM et al (1985) CT-guided adrenal biopsy: Accuracy, safety, and indications. *American Journal of Roentgenology* **144:** 67–69.

Besser GM & Edwards CRW (1972) Cushing's syndrome. *Clinics in Endocrinology and Metabolism* **1:** 451–490.

Biglieri EG & Schambelan M (1979) The significance of elevated levels of plasma 18-hydroxy-corticosteroid in patients with primary aldosteronism. *Journal of Clinical Endocrinology and Metabolism* **49:** 87–91.

Bomanji J, Conry BG, Britton KE & Reznek RH (1988) Imaging neural crest tumours with ^{123}I-metaiodobenzylguanidine and x-ray computed tomography: a comparative study. *Clinical Radiology* **39:** 502–506.

Bowerman RA, Silver TM, Jaffe MH et al (1981) Sonography of adrenal pheochromocytomas. *American Journal of Roentgenology* **137:** 1227–1231.

Brady TM, Gross BH, Glazer GM & Williams DM (1985) Adrenal pseudomasses due to varices: angiographic–CT–MR–pathologic correlations. *American Journal of Roent-*

genology **145:** 301–304.

Bravo EL & Gillford RW Jr (1984) Pheochromocytoma: diagnosis, localization and management. *New England Journal of Medicine* **11:** 1298–1303.

Bravo EL, Tarazi RC Gifford RW Jr & Steward BH (1979) Circulating and urinary catecholamines in pheochromocytoma. *New England Journal of Medicine* **301:** 682–686.

Bravo EL, Tarazi RC, Fonad FM & Textor SC (1982) A reappraisal of diagnostic criteria for primary aldosteronism. *Clinical Science* **63:** 97–100.

Brown LR, Aughenbaugh GL, Wick MR et al (1982) Roentgenologic diagnosis of primary corticotropin-producing carcinoid tumours of the mediastinum. *Radiology* **142:** 143–148.

Chang A, Glazer HS, Lee JKT, Ling D & Heiken JP (1987) Adrenal gland: MR imaging. *Radiology* **163:** 123–128.

Chezmar JL, Robbins SM, Nelson RC et al (1988) Adrenal masses: characterization with T1-weighted MR imaging. *Radiology* **166:** 357–359.

Chrousos GP, Schulte HM, Oldfield EM et al (1984) The corticotropin-releasing factor stimulation test: an aid in the evaluation of patients with Cushing's syndrome. *New England Journal of Medicine* **310:** 622–626.

Colapinto RF & Steed BL (1971) Arteriography of adrenal tumours. *Radiology* **100:** 343–350.

Conn JW, Knopf RF & Neshit RM (1964) Clinical characteristics of primary aldosteronism from an analysis of 145 cases. *American Journal of Surgery* **107:** 159–172.

Contreras LN, Hane S & Tyrrell JB (1986) Urinary cortisol in the assessment of pituitary-adrenal function: utility of 24-hour and spot determinations. *Journal of Clinical Endocrinology and Metabolism* **62:** 965–969.

Copeland PM (1983) The incidentally discovered adrenal mass. *Annals of Internal Medicine* **98:** 940–945.

Crapo L (1979) Cushing's syndrome. A review of diagnostic tests. *Metabolism* **29:** 955–977.

Cryer PE (1985) Phaeochromocytoma. *Clinics in Endocrinology and Metabolism* **14:** 203–220.

Doppman JL, Oldfield E, Krudy AG et al (1984) Petrosal sinus sampling for Cushing syndrome: anatomical and technical considerations. *Radiology* **150:** 99–103.

Doppman JL, Miller DL, Dwyer AJ et al (1988) Macronodular adrenal hyperplasia in Cushing Disease. *Radiology* **166:** 347–352.

Drury PL (1985) Disorders of mineralocorticoid activity. *Clinics in Endocrinology and Metabolism* **14:** 175–202.

Dunnick NR, Doppman JL, Gill JR Jr et al (1982a) Localization of functional adrenal tumours by computed tomography and venous sampling. *Radiology* **142:** 429–433.

Dunnick NR, Heston D, Halvorsen R et al (1982b) CT appearance of adrenal cortical carcinoma. *Journal of Computer Assisted Tomography* **6:** 978–982.

El-Sherief MA & Hemmingsson A (1982) Computed tomography of the normal adrenal gland. *Acta Radiologica* (Diagnosis) **23:** 433–442.

Espiner EA & Donald RA (1980) Aldosterone regulation in primary aldosteronism: influence of salt balance, posture and ACTH. *Clinical Endocrinology* **12:** 277–286.

Falke THM, Strake L, Shaff MI et al (1986) MR imaging of the adrenals: correlation with computed tomography. *Journal of Computer Assisted Tomography* **10:** 242–253.

Findling JW, Aron DC, Tyrrell JB et al (1981) Selective venous sampling for ACTH in Cushing's syndrome: differentiation between Cushing's disease and the ectopic ACTH syndrome. *Annals of Internal Medicine* **94:** 647–652.

Fishman EK, Deutch BM, Hartman DS et al (1987) Primary adrenocortical carcinoma: CT evaluation with clinical correlation. *American Journal of Roentgenology* **148:** 531–535.

Francis IR, Smid A, Gross MD et al (1988) Adrenal masses in oncologic patients: functional and morphologic evaluation. *Radiology* **166:** 353–356.

Ganguly A (1982) New insight and questions about glucocorticoid-suppressible hyperaldosteronism. *American Journal of Medicine* **72:** 851–854.

Geisinger MA, Zelch MG, Bravo EL et al (1983) Primary hyperaldosteronism: comparison of CT, adrenal venography and venous sampling. *American Journal of Roentgenology* **141:** 299–302.

Glazer GM (1988) MR imaging of liver, kidneys, and adrenal glands. *Radiology* **166:** 303–312.

Glazer HS, Weyman PJ, Sagel SJ et al (1982) Non-functioning adrenal masses: incidental discovery on computed tomography. *American Journal of Roentgenology* **139:** 81–85.

Grant CS, Carpenter P, van Heerden JA & Hamberger B (1984) Primary aldosteronism: clinical management. *Archives of Surgery* **119:** 585–590.

Gross MD, Shapiro B, Grekin RJ et al (1984) Scintigraphic localization of adrenal lesions in primary aldosteronism. *American Journal of Medicine* **77:** 839–844.

Guerin CK, Wahner HW, Gorman CA, Carpenter PC & Sheedy PF II (1983) Computed tomographic scanning versus radioisotope imaging in adrenocortical diagnosis. *American Journal of Medicine* **75:** 653–657.

Hamburger B, Russell CF, van Heerden JA et al (1982) Adrenal surgery: trends during the seventies. *American Journal of Surgery* **144:** 523–526.

Hedeland H, Ostberg G & Hokfelt B (1968) On the prevalence of adrenocortical adenomas in an autopsy material in relation to hypertension and diabetes. *Acta Medicine Scandinavica* **184:** 211–214.

Herd GW, Semple PF, Parker D et al (1987) False localization of an aldosteronoma by dexamethasone-suppressed adrenal scintigraphy. *Clinical Endocrinology* **26:** 699–705.

Herwig KR & Sonda LP III (1979) Usefulness of adrenal venography and iodocholesterol scan in adrenal surgery. *Journal of Urology* **122:** 7–8.

Hussain S, Belldegrun A, Seltzer SE et al (1985) Differentiation of malignant from benign adrenal masses: predictive indices on computed tomography. *American Journal of Roentgenology* **144:** 61–65.

Isles CG, MacDougall IC, Lever AF & Fraser R (1987) Hypermineralocorticoidism due to adrenal carcinoma: plasma corticosteroids and their response to ACTH and angiotensin II. *Clinical Endocrinology* **26:** 239–251.

Johnson CM, Sheedy II PF, Welch TJ & Hattery RR (1985) CT of the adrenal cortex. *Seminars in Ultrasound, CT and MR* **6:** 241–260.

Kader S & Robinette C (1981) Accuracy of angiography in the localization of pheochromocytomas. *Journal of Urology* **126:** 789–793.

Katz RL & Shirkhoda A (1985) Diagnostic approach to incidental adrenal nodules in the cancer patient: results of a clinical, radiologic, and fine-needle aspiration study. *Cancer* **55:** 1995–2000.

Liddle GW (1960) Tests of pituitary adrenal suppressibility in the diagnosis of Cushing's syndrome. *Journal of Clinical Endocrinology and Metabolism* **12:** 1539–1560.

Lim RC Jr, Nakayama DK, Biglieri EG, Schambelan M & Hunt TK (1986) Primary aldosteronism: changing concepts in diagnosis and management. *American Journal of Surgery* **152:** 116–121.

Lund JO, Nielsen MD, Giese J et al (1980) Localization of aldosterone-producing tumours in primary aldosteronism by adrenal and renal vein catheterization. *Acta Medica Scandinavica* **207:** 345–351.

Lynn MD, Shapiro B, Sisson JC et al (1985) Pheochromocytoma and the normal adrenal medulla: improved visualization with I-123 MIBG scintigraphy. *Radiology* **156:** 789–792.

Ma JTC, Wang C, Lam KSL et al (1986) Fifty cases of primary hyperaldosteronism in Hong Kong Chinese with a high frequency of periodic paralysis: evaluation of techniques for tumour localization. *Quarterly Journal of Medicine* **61:** 1021–1037.

McCorkell SJ & Niles NL (1985) Fine-needle aspiration of catecholamine-producing adrenal masses: a possibly fatal mistake. *American Journal of Roentgenology* **145:** 113–114.

Marchal G, Gelin J, Verbeken E, Baert A & Lauwerijns J (1986) High-resolution real-time sonography of the adrenal glands: a routine examination? *Journal of Ultrasound in Medicine* **5:** 65–68.

Mitty HA, Nicolis GL & Gabrilove JL (1973) Adrenal venography: clinico-roentgenographic correlation in 80 patients. *Radiology* **119:** 564–575.

Montagne JP, Kressel HY, Korobkin M & Moss A (1978) Computed tomography of the normal adrenal glands. *American Journal of Roentgenology* **130:** 963–966.

Moon KL, Hricak H, Crooks LE et al (1983) Nuclear magnetic resonance imaging of the adrenal gland: a preliminary report. *Radiology* **147:** 155–160.

Moore A, Aitken R, Burhe C et al (1985) Cortisol assay: guidelines for the provision of a clinical biochemistry service. *Annals of Clinical Biochemistry* **22:** 435–454.

Nicolis GL, Mitty HA, Modlinger RS & Gabrilove JL (1972) Percutaneous adrenal venography: a clinical study of 50 patients. *Annals of Internal Medicine* **76:** 899–909.

O'Keeffe FN, Carrasco CH, Charasangavej C, Richli WR & Wallace S (1988). Arterial embolization of adrenal tumors: results in nine cases. *American Journal of Roentgenology* **151:** 819–822.

Oldfield EH, Chrousos GP, Schulte HM et al (1985) Preoperative lateralization of ACTH-secreting pituitary microadenomas by bilateral and simultaneous inferior petrosal venous sinus sampling. *New England Journal of Medicine* 312: 100–103.

Oppenheimer DA, Carroll BA & Yousem S (1983) Sonography of the normal neonatal adrenal gland. *Radiology* 146: 157–160.

Palubinskas AJ, Roizen MF & Conte FA (1980) Localization of functioning pheochromocytomas by venous sampling and radioenzymatic analysis. *Radiology* 136: 495–496.

Pojunas KW, Daniels DL, Williams AL, Thorsen MK & Haughton VM (1986) Pituitary and adrenal CT of Cushing syndrome. *American Journal of Roentgenology* 146: 1235–1238.

Quint LE, Glazer GM, Francis IR, Shapiro B & Chenevert TL (1987) Pheochromocytoma and paraganglioma: comparison of MR imaging with CT and I-131 MIBG scintigraphy. *Radiology* 165: 89–93.

Radin DR, Ralls PW, Boswell WD Jr et al (1986) Pheochromocytoma: detection by unenhanced CT. *American Journal of Roentgenology* 146: 741–744.

Raisanen J, Shapiro B, Glazer GM et al (1984) Plasma catecholamines in pheochromocytoma: effect of urographic contrast media. *American Journal of Roentgenology* 143: 43–46.

Reinig JW, Doppman JL, Dwyer AJ & Frank J (1986) MRI of indeterminate adrenal masses. *American Journal of Roentgenology* 147: 493–496.

Reynes CJ, Churchill R, Moncada R & Love L (1979) Computed tomography of adrenal glands. *Radiologic Clinics of North America* 17: 91–104.

Roberts L Jr, Dunnick NR, Thompson WM et al (1985) Primary aldosteronism due to bilateral nodular hyperplasia: CT demonstration. *Journal of Computer Assisted Tomography* 9: 1125–1127.

Rossi P, Young IS & Panke WF (1968) Techniques, usefulness and hazards of arteriography of pheochromocytoma. *Journal of American Medical Association* 205: 547–553.

Sample WF (1978) Adrenal ultrasonography. *Radiology* 127: 461–466.

Saris SC, Patronas NJ, Doppman JL et al (1987) Cushing syndrome: pituitary CT scanning. *Radiology* 162: 775–777.

Schultz CL (1986) CT and MR of the adrenal glands. *Seminars in Ultrasound, CT, and MR* 7: 219–233.

Schultz CL, Haaga JR, Fletcher BD et al (1984) MRI of the adrenal gland: a comparison with computed tomography. *American Journal of Roentgenology* 143: 1235–1241.

Sheps SC, Jiang NS & Klee GC (1988) Diagnostic evaluation of phaeochromocytoma. *Endocrinology and Metabolism Clinics of North America* 17: 397–414.

Sisson JC, Frager MS, Valk TW et al (1981) Scintigraphic localization of pheochromocytoma. *New England Journal of Medicine* 305: 12–17.

Swensen SJ, Brown ML, Sheps SG et al (1985) ^{131}I-MIBG in the evaluation of suspected pheochromocytoma. *Mayo Clinic Proceedings* 60: 299–304.

Tisnado J, Amendola MC, Konerding KF, Shirazi KK & Beachley MC (1980) Computed tomography versus angiography in the localization of pheochromocytoma. *Journal of Computer Assisted Tomography* 4: 853–859.

Valk TW, Frager MS, Gross MD et al (1981) Spectrum of pheochromocytoma in multiple endocrine neoplasia: a scintigraphic portrayal using ^{131}I-metaiodobenzylguanidine. *Annals of Internal Medicine* 94: 762–767.

Webb TA, Sheps SG & Carney JA (1980) Difference between sporadic pheochromocytoma and pheochromocytoma in multiple endocrine neoplasia, type 2. *American Journal of Surgical Pathology* 4: 121–126.

Weinberger MH, Grim CE, Hollifield JW et al (1979) Primary aldosteronism: diagnosis, localization and treatment. *Annals of Internal Medicine* 90: 386–395.

Welch TJ, Sheedy PF II, van Heerden JA et al (1983) Pheochromocytoma: value of computed tomography. *Radiology* 148: 501–503.

White EA, Schambelan M, Rost CR et al (1980) Use of computed tomography in diagnosing the cause of primary aldosteronism. *New England Journal of Medicine* 303: 1503–1507.

White FE, White MC, Drury PL et al (1982) Value of computed tomography of the abdomen and chest in investigation of Cushing's syndrome. *British Medical Journal* 284: 771–774.

Yeh HC (1982) Ultrasound and CT of the adrenals. *Seminars in Ultrasound* 3: 97–113.

Young WF Jr & Klee GG (1988) Primary aldosteronism: diagnostic evaluation. *Endocrinology and Metabolism Clinics of North America* 17: 367–395.

7

Imaging paediatric endocrine disorders

KENNETH M. COOKE
CHRISTOPHER COWELL
ALBERT H. LAM
MERL DE SILVA
ROBERT HOWMAN-GILES
KIM DONAGHUE

In paediatric endocrinology, the scope of imaging has been expanded to become a part of the initial evaluation of the patient and can be responsible for primary diagnosis. For example, bone age is used as a measure of biological age in pubertal and growth disorders as it more clearly reflects an individual's maturity than does chronological age. Pelvic ultrasound in the female plays a large part in determining whether puberty is truly precocious or pseudoprecocious (of central or of peripheral origin—gonadotrophin-dependent or gonadotrophin-independent). We will discuss a few selected topics in paediatric endocrinology and attempt to show the place of organ imaging in relation to the clinical setting and the biochemical findings.

PUBERTAL DISORDERS

Introduction and pathophysiology

Precocious puberty is defined as the appearance of secondary sexual traits before 9 years of age in girls and 10 years of age in boys. In true precocious puberty (true PP) or gonadotrophin-dependent puberty, the changes occur under the influence of pituitary gonadotrophin secretion and the hypothalamic–pituitary–gonadal axis is operative in a normal pubertal pattern at an unusually early age. The production of gonadotrophin-like substances (HCG) from chorio-epithelioma, teratoma or hepatoblastoma will also lead to gonadal development as in true PP. True PP is always isosexual, that is, secondary sexual characteristics are appropriate for the gender of the child. It is five times more frequent in girls than boys but a pathological cause is more likely to be present in boys and has been identified in about 50% of reported cases (Rayner, 1981). This is usually due to a central nervous system (CNS) abnormality. Thus, the diagnostic approach in boys should be more aggressive. With true PP, not only is there premature appearance of the secondary sexual characteristics, there is also increase in the size of the gonads and development of mature sperm or ova.

Pseudoprecocious puberty (pseudo PP) or gonadotrophin-independent puberty, is either iso-sexual or heterosexual due to primary gonadal or adrenal dysfunction. It is characterized by the early appearance of secondary sexual characteristics but the gonads do not mature and spermatogenesis or ovulation does not occur. This disorder is generally associated with elevated oestrogen and androgen levels but with normal or suppressed gonadotrophin levels (Salardi et al, 1985). Pseudo PP is differentiated from true PP by the confirmation of clinical findings such as a palpable abdominal mass, failure of gonadotrophin to rise following gonadotrophin releasing hormone (GRH) stimulation and by organ imaging. In the isosexual form, precocious puberty results from ovarian granulosa cell tumour in the female and from adrenal tumour, adrenal hyperplasia or Leydig cell tumour in the male.

The adrenal tumour or adrenal hyperplasia and ovarian adrenal rest or cyst of a female child produce heterosexual precocious puberty (heterosexual PP) with development of male secondary sexual characteristics. In males, feminizing adrenal cortical tumours result in heterosexual PP with development of female secondary sexual characteristics.

Incomplete precocious puberty (incomplete PP) includes premature thelarche and adrenarche which occur independent of gonadal maturation and no treatment is required.

Imaging strategy for diagnosis

The essential problem faced by the clinician when presented with a child with early puberty is to distinguish a significant endocrine (true PP and pseudo PP) from an essentially benign problem (incomplete PP). The diagnosis of precocious puberty is based on clinical history and physical examination, and is generally confirmed by hormonal assay and radiological advancement in bone age. The initial imaging is thus a radiograph of one hand and wrist for bone age. If there is no significant advance in bone age the diagnosis is likely to be incomplete PP (premature thearche or adrenarche). Further imaging evaluation depends on the endocrinological results and sex of the patients. In males, enlarged testes are clinically obvious, easily measured and indicate true precocious puberty. In the female, pelvic ultrasound offers a simple non-invasive method for evaluation of uterine and ovarian size and shape and, with knowledge of normal biometry, differentiation of incomplete PP and true or pseudo PP can usually be made.

Sonographic assessment of the uterus and ovaries

For children who are toilet-trained, the ultrasound examination is performed with conventional full bladder technique, obtained by voluntary urine retention and oral administration of fluid one hour beforehand. For infants, parents are requested to bring with the child a bottle for feeding during the study. The bladder is usually filled shortly after feeding. The frequency of the ultrasound transducer used varies from 5 to 10 MHz, depending on the size of the patient.

Longitudinal (L), antero-posterior (AP) and transverse (T) diameters of the uterus as a whole, the corpus and cervix separately, and of the ovaries are measured. The formula for a prolate ellipsoid is used to calculate the volume of both ovaries ($V = L \times AP \times T \times 0.52333$). The ratio of the length and thickness of corpus to the length and thickness of cervix are determined separately. The number and size of cystic structures in both ovaries are recorded. Adrenals and both kidneys are included in the examination to detect adrenal mass and associated renal abnormality.

Normal biometry of uterus and ovaries

The shape and size of uterus and ovaries change with age. The uterus in the newborn is characterized by the effect of maternal oestrogen—it is large (3.5–5.0 cm in length) and echogenic endometrium may be present (Figure 1a). This is the best time to look for the presence of the uterus in infants with ambiguous genitalia.

After 2 months, the size of the uterus becomes infantile (2.5–3.0 cm in length) and remains unchanged until early puberty. The size of the uterus under 7 years of age is not influenced by age nor can it be correlated with the body size, breast development or hormonal level (Salardi et al, 1985). Cervix and isthmus make up more than half and up to two thirds of the organ (Figure 1b).

There is a rapid growth of the uterus at puberty when it becomes age- and hormone-dependent. Uterine growth is more pronounced in the fundus and corpus, leading to the adult pear-shape, 6–8 cm in length (Figure 1c). At puberty, the echogenicity of the endometrium becomes more prominent and increases considerably during the premenstrual phase.

According to anatomical studies (Peters et al, 1976), both ovaries show morphological and biometric similarities throughout the prepubertal period due to the lack of ovulatory changes. However, antral follicles at different stages of development or degeneration are present, and the increase in number causes a slight increase in ovarian volume with age up to 5 years. As maturity approaches, the ovaries are subjected to gonadotrophic stimulation and contain pre-ovulatory follicles and corpora lutea.

Ultrasound studies have been performed to determine uterine and ovarian size in the prepubertal girls. In the study by Sample et al (1977), uterine length in prepubertal girls over the age of 1 year ranged from 2.0 to 3.3 cm with a mean of 2.8 cm. In another study by Orsini et al (1984), the mean uterine length was 3.3 cm from 2 to 7 years of age and increased from a mean of 3.5 to 4.2 cm by 11 years of age. Ivarrson et al (1983) found a mean uterine length of 2.5 cm. Both Sample and Ivarsson reported that the cervix occupies two thirds to five sixths of the total uterine length. Orsini measured the ratio of the anteroposterior diameters of the corpus to the cervix: a ratio of less than one was typical for the infantile uterus. For ovarian size and morphology, Sample reported prepubertal volume to be less than 1 ml. Both Orsini and Ivarsson reported higher measurement, 1 ml at 2 years, 2 ml at 12 years and 3–4 ml or even 5–6 ml in adult or postpubertal ovaries. The geographical discrepancy of measurements is probably related to the population samples.

We have studied the range of measurements in Sydney. The uterine length for prepubertal girls is under 3.5 cm, with a bulbous fundus and a corpus/cervix ratio of less than one. The upper limit of ovarian volume is 1 ml by 5 years of age, 2 ml by 8 years. The maximal prepubertal follicular size is less than 7 mm in diameter.

A megacystic ovary is defined as one containing more than 4 follicles

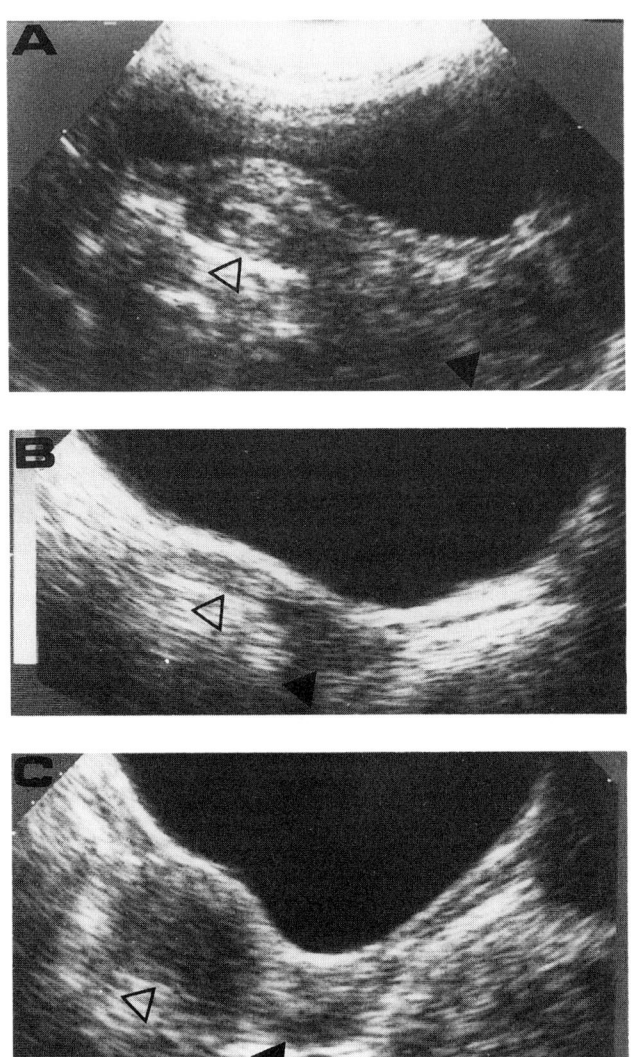

Figure 1. Sagittal ultrasound sections through the uterus showing the configuration and relative sizes of corpus (open arrowhead) and cervix (closed arrowhead) at different ages: (a) at 3 weeks of age there is an echogenic endometrium and bulbous cortex; (b) at 3 years of age the corpus is small and echogenic; (c) at 13 years there is a pear-shaped, postpubertal uterus.

greater than 4 mm in diameter present in each ovary (Stanhope et al, 1985). A megacystic ovary under the age of 8 years is either functional or under hormonal stimulation. However these ovarian changes are not observed in all patients (Salardi et al, 1988) and cannot be considered to be peculiar to precocious puberty. Regression of megacystic ovary and decrease in ovarian size were reported after treatment with synthetic GRH analogues.

Clinical application

The female. The clinical and biochemical findings are used in conjunction with sonographic and other medical imaging findings to arrive at the diagnosis of the cause or type of precocious puberty (Figure 2). If the uterus is prepubertal in size and shape, the ovaries appear normal and adrenal tumour is absent, diagnosis of incomplete PP is assumed and no further test is indicated.

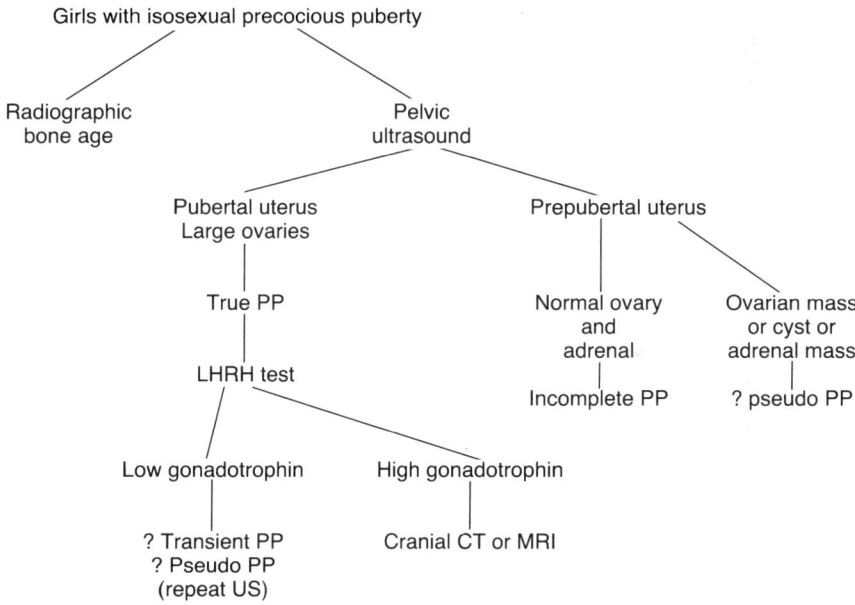

Figure 2. A flow chart outlining the strategy for the diagnosis of precocious puberty in the female.

True PP, whether it be idiopathic or the result of a CNS abnormality or gonadotrophin-like secreting tumour, shows premature development of uterus and ovaries. This can be assessed by pelvic ultrasound. The uterus with a length longer than 3.5 cm and a ratio of corpus to cervix larger than one is consistent with true PP. In addition to the uterine changes the ovaries in true PP are large approaching adult size and are often but not always megalocystic (Shawker et al, 1984; Salardi et al, 1988). An ovarian volume

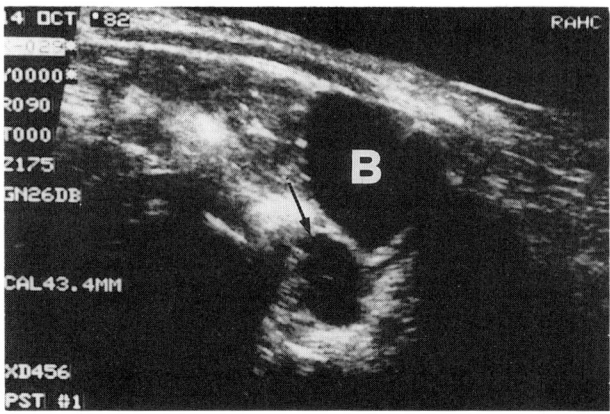

Figure 3. An 8-year-old girl with precocious puberty. A sagittal ultrasound section of the left side of the pelvis through the bladder (B) shows a 2.5 × 4.0 cm cyst (arrow) arising from the left ovary.

greater than 1 ml under the age of 5 years or 2 ml under the age of 8 years is outside the normal range and supports true PP.

A uterus of infantile size and shape is seen in both incomplete PP and many girls with pseudo PP. Ultrasound should be used to define causes of pseudo PP, such as an adrenal or ovarian tumour and cyst. As cysts in the ovary are common prepubertally, we should be cautious before labelling a cyst as the cause of precocious puberty (Figure 3). The adrenal and hypo-thalamic causes should also be evaluated by ultrasound and high resolution CT. If no extra-ovarian cause is found, the ovarian cyst is followed up in 1 month's time. If the same unilateral ovarian cyst persists and is accompanied by advanced bone age, elevated sex steroids and low gonadotrophins, then an ovarian functioning tumour is to be excluded. Ovarian tumour occurs in 1–2% of girls with isosexual PP. Most are oestrogen-producing or feminizing tumours such as granulosa cell tumour, theca cell tumour and theca lutein cyst. Theca cell tumours are among the more commonly reported lesions which occur in older age groups, with only 5% found prepubertally. In our institution, laparoscopy is first performed in suspicious cases and proceed to surgical excision if the findings are confirmed.

For girls with heterosexual PP, androgen-producing tumours of the adrenal and ovary should be searched for by sonography. Adrenal tumours (adenoma, carcinoma) usually present with virilization and may be associated with Cushing's syndrome (Davies and Lam, 1987). Computed tomography (CT) and/or magnetic resonance imaging (MRI) should be used to further define the pathology. Congenital adrenal hyperplasia, the most common cause of adrenarche with advanced bone age in girls, is not easily visualized by sonography and the diagnosis is made biochemically.

The male. True PP must be differentiated from excessive androgen production alone. Examination of testis usually will distinguish the two entities.

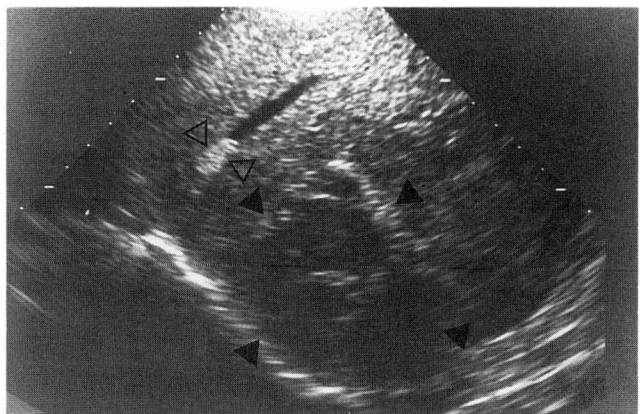

Figure 4. A boy with precocious puberty. A sagittal ultrasound section through the right liver demonstrates a large adrenal adenocarcinoma (closed arrows) with a metastatic tumour thrombus in the inferior vena cava and right hepatic vein (open arrows).

True PP shows bilateral testicular enlargement with testis 2.5 cm or greater in longest diameter or greater than or equal to 4 ml in volume. Boys with androgen excess from adrenal causes (Figure 4) have small, prepubertal size testes. Rarely, boys with congenital adrenal hyperplasia have testicular enlargement because they truly have entered into puberty or because of bilateral hyperplasia of adrenal rests in the testis. There is no reported ultrasound findings of Leydig cell tumour of testis but it is usually unilateral and easily imaged.

CNS abnormalities. Associated with true PP is an increase prevalence of CNS abnormalities. These are best studied with MRI or high resolution CT. Direct coronal or reformatted coronal CT scans or coronal and sagittal MRI scans are valuable in the assessment of suprasellar and midline intracranial lesions.

In the series published by Rieth et al (1987) of 90 children with true PP who were studied with high resolution CT, 32 had cerebral abnormalities and these were demonstrated in equal distribution of girls and boys. These included 17 cases of hypothalamic hamartomas, one hypothalamic astrocytoma, six optic chiasm lesions, eight with ventricular abnormalities, one with arachnoid cyst and one with teratoma.

If the CT or MRI is normal then no additional scanning is necessary. Idiopathic precocious puberty is presumed and confirmed by elevated gonadotrophins and testosterone for age. In those patients in whom a hypothalamic mass is discovered, no additional scans are needed unless a change of symptoms occur. Patients with optic gliomas and hypothalamic astrocytomas require careful follow-up and serial CT examinations to detect tumour growth. Radiosensitive suprasellar germinoma should be isolated from this glioma group when there is elevated serum HCG or associated diabetes insipidus.

Gonadotrophin-like secreting tumours. These are rare in both boys and girls. Human chorionic gonadotrophin (HCG) secreting tumours have been reported from chorio-epithelioma of ovary, testis or in the pineal region and mediastinal teratomas may secrete HCG-like hormones and these cases should be studied with sonography, CT and MRI if it is available. Likewise, the possibility of a gonadotrophin-secreting hepatoblastoma needs to be excluded in boys.

Specific syndromes. For true PP, specific syndromes such as McCune–Albright syndrome, Silver's syndrome, neurofibromatosis, tuberous sclerosis or hypothyroidism should be sought clinically and a skeletal radiograph performed as indicated.

SEXUAL AMBIGUITY

In cases of sexual ambiguity, demonstration of a normal uterus is important (Saenger, 1984). Sonography should be performed early and preferably before 2 months of age, with the role of outlining the internal anatomy where possible. A genitogram with injection of contrast into the lower genitourinary tract should also be performed (Figure 5). Combination of the two investi-

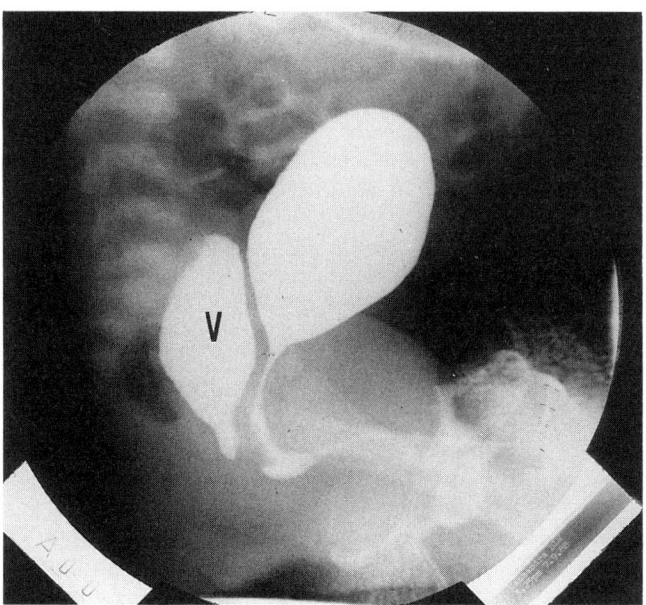

Figure 5. A 4-week-old infant with female karyotype and ambiguous genitalia showing a masculine phallus and a small apparent scrotum without palpable testes. Genitogram reveals a male-type urethra draining the bladder, but also fills a large cavity (V) between the bladder and the air-filled rectum. The appearance is compatible with a vagina. Sonography demonstrates a uterus at the top of this distended vagina.

gations can often delineate the internal structures for the urologists prior to proper gender assignment and appropriate planning for surgery. MRI with multiplanar views is sometimes used to investigate the complications of Mullerian duct anomalies. In cases of hermaphroditism, imaging often gives accurate assessment of the internal and external genitalia; and sonography may be used to localize the gonads for biopsy.

DETECTION OF GROWTH DISORDERS

Assessment of skeletal maturity is an essential component of the clinical practice of paediatric endocrinology. It complements the history and physical examination and although rarely diagnostic (except in Turner syndrome and pseudohypoparathyroidism), it helps to guide the clinician to the appropriate biochemical or organ imaging investigations. In children with disorders of growth and puberty, assessment of skeletal age provides important information on an individual's future height potential as the biological age of an individual is more closely reflected by their skeletal maturity than by their chronological age. Skeletal maturity is thus an important monitor of therapies for endocrine disorders such as hypothyroidism, growth hormone deficiency, precocious puberty and congenital adrenal hyperplasia.

Skeletal maturity assessment is based upon the appearance of the secondary ossification centres in the epiphyseal cartilages of the long bones. These centres nearly all appear after birth although there are standards available for the development of the epiphyseal ossification in the perinatal period (Kahus and Finnstrom, 1976). The rate of maturation is influenced by a variety of factors including race (black Americans mature more quickly than white Americans), sex (females mature earlier than males), socio-economic status (more mature in higher socio-economic status), nutrition, timing of puberty, as well as specific skeletal and endocrine disorders. Standards of skeletal maturity of the wrist have been developed for use in various geographical regions: North America, England, Sweden, Finland, Denmark, Germany, France, Japan, Spain and Poland. Standards are also available for other anatomical regions, e.g. the knee (Pyle and Hoerr, 1969). In practice the two most commonly used standards are the Greulich and Pyle Atlas (in North America) (Greulich and Pyle, 1959) and the Tanner–Whitehouse 2 atlas (in the United Kingdom) (Tanner et al, 1983).

The Greulich and Pyle (G & P) standards were developed from a series of radiographs performed longitudinally on 1000 white North American children between 1931 and 1942 (Brush Foundation Study). These children were referred by paediatricians for involvement in a study of growth and development and were above average in economic and educational status. Their skeletal maturity was advanced in relation to other children less fortunate. This selection bias in retrospect is fortuitous as it has made these standards applicable up to the present day despite the secular trend in increasing height and earlier development of puberty. The atlas contains a series of representative radiographs of the left hand at 31 different ages for males (0–19 years) and in 29 plates for females (0–50 years). Symmetry of left and right hand maturation has been examined by both the original Brush Foundation Study and Dreizen et al (1957). In the latter study, 435 comparisons were made: a significant maturity difference of greater than 3 months was found in 13% and a difference of greater than 6 months was found in only 1.5%.

The maturity is assessed by matching visually the radiograph of the individual to that closest to it in the atlas. Further assessment can be made by checking the accompanied text and drawings. The skeletal age (mean and standard deviation) expected for chronological age are provided for both sexes. The standard deviation is low in early childhood (2–8 months) and increases during the pubertal period (12–15 months) reflecting the variance in timing of puberty. Considerable interobserver difference is present because of the subjectivity of the method but, with practice, a single observer can be reproducible and even interpolate between the assigned ages. In some radiographs, considerable variation in maturity is found between the various epiphyseal centres. Garn et al (1963) commented that greater variation is seen in the carpal bones, which hence should be given less weighting.

The alternative method of assessment is by scoring each epiphysis on the basis of its size and shape. This method was first developed by Acheson (1954) using bones of the hands and knees. Tanner, Whitehouse and their colleagues subsequently developed a maturity score based on the epiphyses of the radius and ulna, first, third and fifth metacarpals, first, third and fifth proximal and distal phalanges, the third and fifth middle phalanges and the carpal bones. These radiographs had been collected on a random sample of children in the 1950s but many investigators have validated their application to today's children. The most recent version of this method (Tanner et al, 1983) allows either a score for the 13 epiphyses of the radius, ulna and short bones (RUS) or the sum of these bones and the seven carpals, totalling 20 bones (the TW2 method). The score is calculated after assigning a rating according to eight different configurations of each epiphysis matched against a radiograph and a line drawing in the TW2 atlas. This score with a range of 0–100 can be used to define a bone age or as a percentile of the maturity relative to an individual's chronological age. This method is less subjective and has been validated for use in children in various geographical locations. It generally assigns a higher skeletal age for an individual than the G & P method. It does however require considerably more time and thus has not enjoyed as wide an application as it may deserve.

Clinical applications

Estimation of final height

Fundamental to the management of growth or pubertal problems is an assessment of an individual's growth potential. Several methods have been developed to estimate final height based on an individual's height, chronological age and skeletal age. Bayley–Pinneau (B–P) tables (Bayley and

Pinneau, 1952) are based upon the percentage of final height that an individual has attained at an assigned skeletal age using the G & P atlas. There are three sets of tables: skeletal age delayed greater than 1 year, average, or advanced greater than 1 year, which allow for prediction of final height of girls with skeletal age greater than 6 years and boys greater than 7 years. The accuracy of height prediction increases with increasing skeletal age, being ± 3 cm in the pubertal years. These tables are applicable for use in tall and short children, including girls with Turner syndrome, and in children with advanced skeletal age (Zachmann et al, 1978).

Using the TW2 system, height prediction can be made using the RUS score along with their height, present age and growth velocity if available. Equations are available in the atlas and in girls accuracy is improved by accounting for the presence or absence of menarche. A similar method using regression equations, recumbent length and the TW2 skeletal maturity atlas was developed by Roche et al (1975) (RWT). Both the RWT and the TW2 methods are more accurate in estimating final height of normal children than the B–P method which tends to slightly overestimate. However, in several pathological conditions, e.g. Turner syndrome and precocious puberty, B–P provides the most accurate height prediction (Zachmann et al, 1978).

The accuracy of height prediction is limited by several factors including precision of the bone age assessment, precision of the height, the age and tempo of pubertal events, and the extent that the skeletal age varies from the chronological age. The greater the delay or advance in bone age, the less accurate will be the height predictions. The accuracy of height predictions is enhanced by serial examinations of skeletal age and height.

Growth disorders

Figure 6 shows an approach for the investigation of short children with particular reference to the use of radiology. The speed of investigation depends on the presence of other symptoms or signs and the degree of growth failure and growth deceleration.

Table 1. Causes of disorders of skeletal maturation.

Skeletal maturation		
Delayed	Average	Advanced

Constitutional delay in growth and puberty	Familial short stature
	Familial tall stature
	Premature menarche
		Obesity
		Premature adrenarche
		Sotos syndrome
		Sex steroid excess
		    Precocious puberty
		    Adrenal hyperplasia
		    Adrenal tumours

GH insufficiency Hypothyroidism Glucocorticoid excess		
Dysmorphic syndromes (i.e. Russell–Silver, Cornelia de Lange) Skeletal dysplasias		

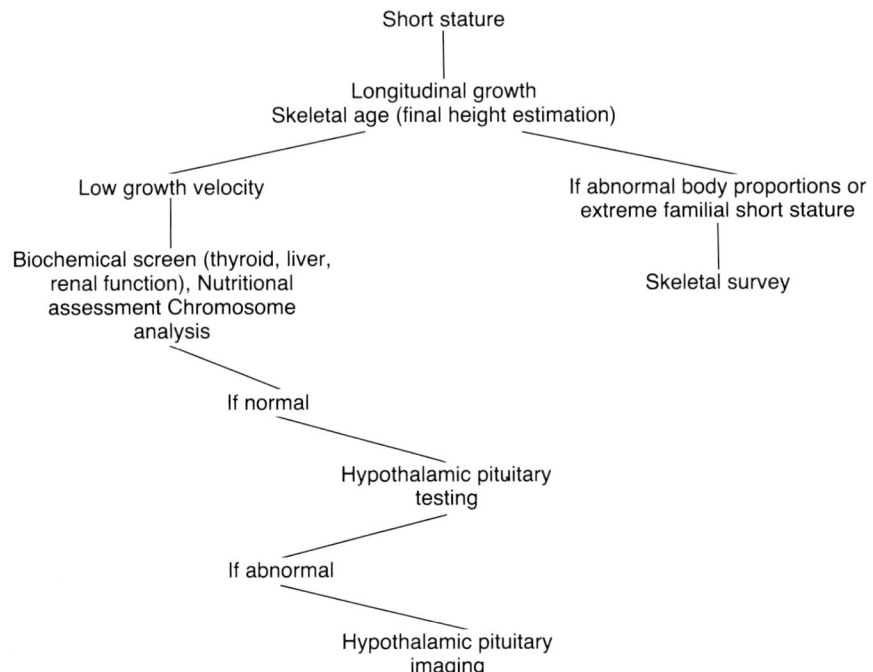

Figure 6. A flow chart outlining an approach to the investigation of short children, with particular reference to the application of medical imaging.

The skeletal age is used as an initial investigation to provide an assessment of growth potential. Occasionally it may be diagnostic such as in skeletal dysplasias, Turner syndrome (short 4th and 5th metacarpal) or pseudohypoparathyroidism (short 4th metacarpal). Delay in skeletal maturation is commonly seen in short children, the most common diagnosis being constitutional delay in growth and puberty. Other causes of skeletal delay, including endocrine disorders, are shown in Table 1. The degree of delay in skeletal maturation is not usually diagnostic except in primary hypothyroidism which may have severe delay and abnormal epiphyses. Large discrepancies however may be seen between chronological age and bone age (4–6 years) in children with constitutional delay in growth and growth hormone insufficiency. Further, hypothalamic–pituitary imaging may be required if either a skeletal dysplasia or an abnormality of growth hormone secretion is suspected.

Tall stature

The majority of children seen with tall stature are constitutional (familial). The radiological investigation required is a skeletal age and estimation of their final height. The other diagnoses which have to be considered include chromosomal disorders (47XXY, 47XXX), syndromal disorders (Marfan syndrome, homocystinuria, Sotos syndrome, Beckwith–Wiedemann syndrome) and other endocrine disorders (growth hormone excess, precocious puberty in a young child). In this latter group, further hypothalamic–pituitary imaging would be required. Hindmarsh et al (1986) used high resolution CT scans to evaluate pituitary gland in a group of constitutionally tall children. Interestingly they found morphological abnormalities suggesting microadenomas in 17 of 38 patients. These changes could have represented somatotroph hyperplasia or gonadotroph hyperplasia associated with the hormonal events of puberty. We would not recommend routine pituitary imaging for constitutionally tall children but rather reserve it for those with possible growth hormone excess, i.e. acromegalic features or an elevated level of insulin-like growth factor 1 (IGF-1) for their pubertal development.

Monitoring of therapies

Measurement of skeletal age is essential to the management of many paediatric endocrine disorders including precocious puberty, congenital adrenal hyperplasia, hypothyroidism and growth hormone insufficiency and with therapies to reduce final height in excessively tall children. The aim of therapies such as growth hormone in short children or GnRH analogues in precocious puberty is to show an increase in the estimated final height. Thus it is important to assess at regular intervals the change in bone age as compared to the change in height age and calculate the estimated final height. The B–P method or the TW2 (or RWT) method can be used for this purpose.

Interpretation of change in estimated final height in these conditions requires knowledge of expected change in normal children. Both methods using the TW2 atlas have been analysed (Greulich and Pyle, 1959; Roche and Chumlea, 1980). Using the RWT tables, annual height predictions vary by ± 2 cm (2 standard deviations) in boys below 12 years and girls below 10 years, and increase to 3–4 cm during the pubertal growth spurt for both sexes. The data are similar for the TW2 method with a variance of up to 5 cm seen in boys of 13–16 years of age. When assessing skeletal age during puberty, it is important to recognize that the skeletal maturity in normal children as assessed by TW2 method is slightly delayed prior to the growth spurt and accelerates rapidly during the growth spurt. The peak skeletal advancement reaches approximately 1.7 years per year of chronological age, coinciding with (Van Venrooij-Ysselmuiden and Van Ipenburg, 1978) or just prior to (Buckler, 1984) the peak height velocity.

HYPOTHALAMIC–PITUITARY IMAGING

Plain radiography

Plain radiographs and tomograms of the skull and pituitary fossa are of limited value in the investigation of endocrine disorders. The larger intrasellar masses may alter the shape and size of the sella, which may become rounded

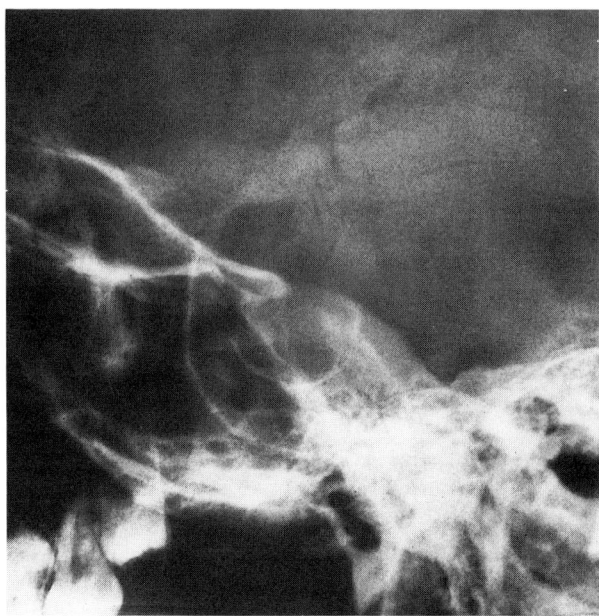

Figure 7. Adolescent patient with congenital hypothyroidism. Lateral skull radiograph shows that the sella is deepened and enlarged, giving it a rounded contour ('cherry sella').

('ballooned') or elongated ('J-shaped'). Suprasellar extension of intrasellar masses causes thinning and posterior displacement of the dorsum sellae. Downward expansion causes erosion of the sellar floor, and if asymmetric produces a double floor appearance on the lateral view. Large infrasellar extension may protrude into the sphenoid sinus or nasopharynx. Pituitary hyperplasia may cause pituitary enlargement as seen in the 'cherry sella' of primary hypothyroidism (Figure 7). Enlargement of the sella is also seen in hydrocephalus and in the 'empty sella syndrome'. Suprasellar masses extending into the sella (e.g. craniopharyngiomas, third ventricular enlargement in hydrocephalus) cause truncation of the dorsum sellae (Yock, 1984).

Suprasellar calcification is commonly seen in craniopharyngioma and may occur in the wall of the tumour or tumour cyst in a curvilinear distribution, or as floccular or nodular areas in the solid portions of the mass (Figure 8). Other suprasellar lesions such as astrocytomas, meningiomas and aneurysms, may also show calcification with erosion of the sella. Acromegalic patients show thickening of the skull vault, mandibular overgrowth and sinus enlargement. Changes of fibrous dysplasia are seen in children with precocious puberty in the McCune–Albright Syndrome.

Whilst physiological calcification of the pineal is not uncommonly seen in plain radiographs of the skull in older children (about 5% of those under 10 years of age) a pathological process (e.g. pinealoma or teratoma) should be suspected when the calcification is more than 1 cm in diameter. Calcification in this region is also seen in thrombosed malformations of the vein of Galen.

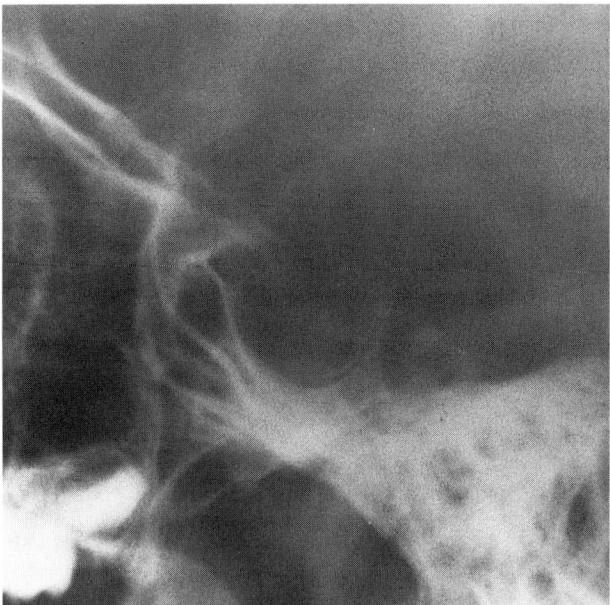

Figure 8. Enlarged sellar in craniopharyngioma. Crescentic calcification in the posterior cyst wall with thinning and elevation of the posterior clinoid process.

CT imaging

CT was the primary method of imaging the sellar and perisellar structures until the advent of MRI, and is still regularly performed. Direct coronal cuts are preferable, with 1.5 mm contiguous slices before and after intravenous contrast with a 512 matrix acquisition. Dynamic scanning provides better visualization of the enhanced pituitary and the vascular structures. The details of the CT techniques, the variation in the size and configuration of the pituitary and the anatomy of perisellar structures have been discussed in Chapter 2.

The calculated pituitary volume for adults ranges from 0.28 to 0.41 ml (Glaser et al, 1986), but no figures are yet available for children. The anterior lobe is 5–7 times larger than the posterior lobe and envelopes the posterior lobe with a small pars intermedia between them. The gland is of somewhat irregular CT density due to fibrous, glandular and neurovascular elements. The pars intermedia may appear to be of lower density than the rest of the gland and may be mistaken for a microadenoma. The contrast enhancement pattern is also non-uniform with the infundibulum and the anterior part of the posterior lobe enhancing more than the rest of the gland (Roppolo, 1985).

MR imaging

MRI provides clearer visualization of the hypothalamic–pituitary region than CT, needs no contrast agents and allows direct multiplanar imaging with ease. Contrast and spatial resolution are superior with MRI, and limited tissue characterization is possible using combinations of pulse sequences. Lack of ionizing radiation is an obvious advantage, especially with children. The anterior and posterior lobes of the pituitary gland have different signal characteristics to allow their differentiation (Fujisawa et al, 1987a). In T1-weighted images, the posterior pituitary gives a high signal similar in intensity to that of the fatty marrow in the clivus. In T2-weighted images, the high signal intensity of the posterior pituitary persists, while there is a reduced signal intensity from the fatty marrow. In addition, the fat marrow demonstrates a chemical shift artefact which is not produced by the posterior pituitary to allow further differentiation of the two. The observed behaviour of the posterior pituitary may be related to the concentration of neurosecretory granules which store vasopressin and oxytocin prior to their release (Fujisawa et al, 1987a). The signal intensity of the anterior pituitary parallels that of normal white matter in all pulse sequences.

The cerebrospinal fluid (CSF) in the suprasellar cistern and the third ventricle provides a natural contrast medium to enable exquisite visualization of the structures in this region. These structures are best seen in the T1-weighted sagittal and coronal sequences because the increased signal intensity of the CSF in T2-weighted images may obscure them. The diaphragma sella may be seen as a separate structure in long TR–short TE sequences. The inferior margin of the gland is well-defined due to lack of signal from the lamina dura. In coronal views, the cavernous sinus and associated structures are well delineated. The internal carotid arteries are also clearly seen due to the signal void produced by flowing blood. The interface between the anterior and posterior lobes of the pituitary can be convex forward, flat or convex backward in axial and sagittal images (Daniels et al, 1988).

Intravenous gadolinium-DTPA increases the signal intensity of the anterior pituitary by almost 60% in T1-weighted images. The enhancement of the cavernous sinuses is even greater, allowing differentiation of these structures. The carotid arteries show no signal increase (Daniels et al, 1988).

Embryology

Embryological aspects are helpful in understanding some of the MR features. The lobes of the pituitary develop from entirely different sources: the anterior lobe derives from Rathke's pouch, a diverticulum of the ectoderm of the stomodeum; posterior lobe is a downgrowth of the neuroectoderm of the diencephalon called the infundibulum. The two structures come into contact with each other by the 5th week of gestation. The Rathke's pouch passes between the chondral centres of the body of the sphenoid, and its stalk disappears by the 6th week (Figure 9). A remnant of the stalk may persist as the craniopharyngeal canal. Anterior lobe tissue may be seen anywhere along the path of regression of the stalk, giving rise to pharyngeal, intraosseous or intracranial accessory glands (Moore, 1982). Craniopharyngiomas are thought to arise from these remnants. The infun-

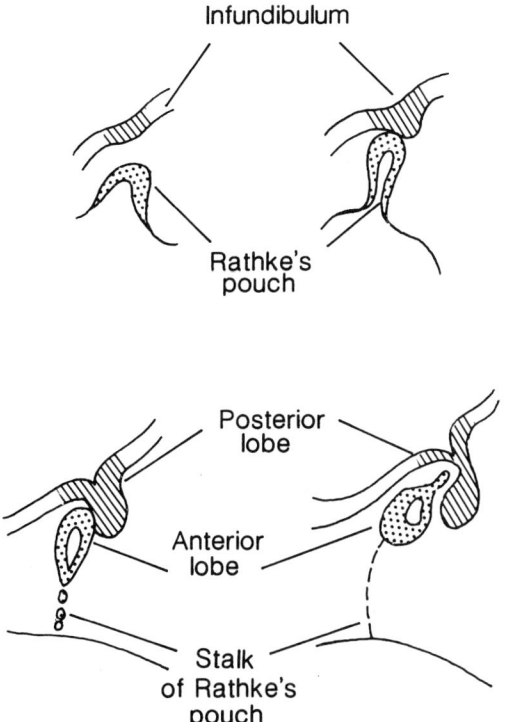

Figure 9. Diagrammatic illustration of the development of the pituitary gland. The anterior pituitary forms as an outgrowth of the stomadeum (Rathke's pouch) and the posterior pituitary arises as a bud from the floor of the forebrain. Rathke's pouch loses its connection with the oral cavity by 8 weeks. Adapted from Moore (1982), with permission.

dibulum gives rise to the median eminence on the floor of the third ventricle, the pituitary stalk, and the posterior pituitary gland. Nerve fibres from the hypothalamic area grow into the pituitary gland forming the hypothalamo–hypophyseal tract. Lack of descent of the infundibulum would result in hypoplasia or absence of the pituitary stalk and absence of the portal venous connection. It is postulated that this would result in anterior pituitary dysfunction (de Silva et al, 1987).

PITUITARY DISORDERS

Hyperfunction

Gland hyperplasia can be caused by excessive stimulation of the pituitary gland in end-organ failure e.g. primary hypothyroidism, primary hypo-gonadism (Okuno et al, 1980). Focal adenomatous areas may be seen in these conditions (Danzinger et al, 1979). The superior surface of the gland

becomes convex and the pituitary dimensions increase. Uniform enlargement of the pituitary gland is seen in cases of precocious puberty.

Adenomas of the anterior pituitary are mainly adult tumours and occur in
several histologic variants. *Microadenomas* are by definition less than 1 cm
in diameter. These are uncommon in childhood but can be seen in pituitary-
dependent Cushing's disease. On CT they are usually isodense compared to

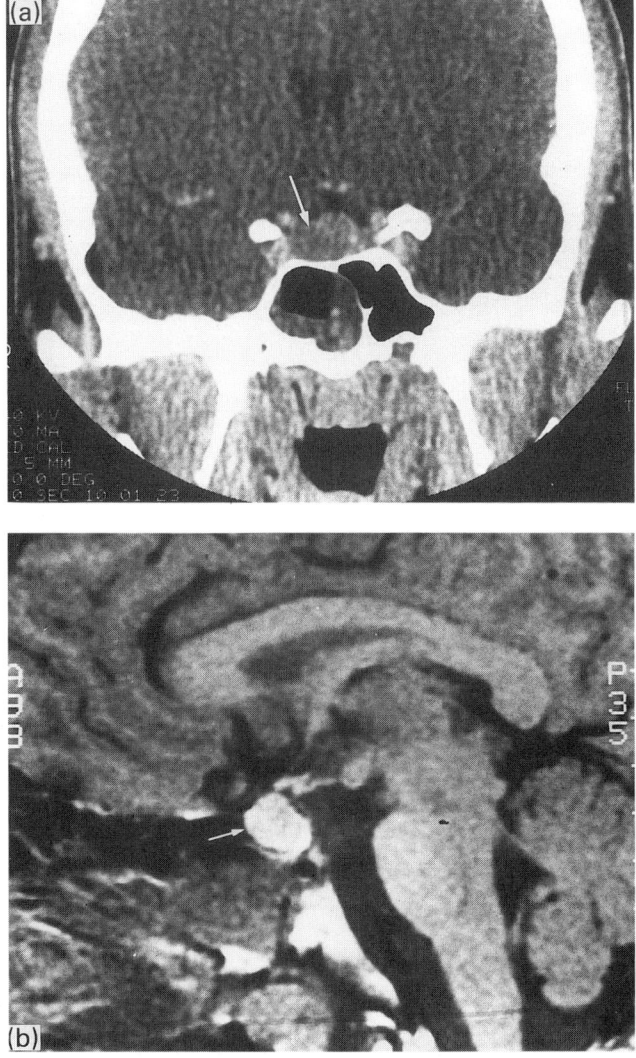

Figure 10. Macroadenoma of pituitary in a 13-year-old with tall stature; (a) coronal CT section
shows slight uniform contrast enhancement of a pituitary tumour (arrow); (b) MRI scan,
T1-weighted sagittal image, shows a rounded mass (arrow) with a slightly hyperintense uniform
signal.

brain. Their pattern of enhancement following contrast is variable, being hypodense, hyperdense or heterogeneous (Gardeur et al, 1981). There is no typical appearance on MRI: some show prolongation of T1 and T2 and others show shortening of T1 and T2. The reason for this is speculative and thought by some to be related to haemorrhage (Weissbuch, 1986). Intravenous gadolinium increases the signal intensity of these lesions, improving their visualization. Mild enlargement of the gland is usual.

Macroadenomas are usually hyperdense to brain on CT and show uniform or patchy contrast enhancement. A small number may show calcification causing confusion with craniopharyngioma. On MRI the tumour is seen as an ovoid mass with a uniform or inhomogeneous signal intensity in all

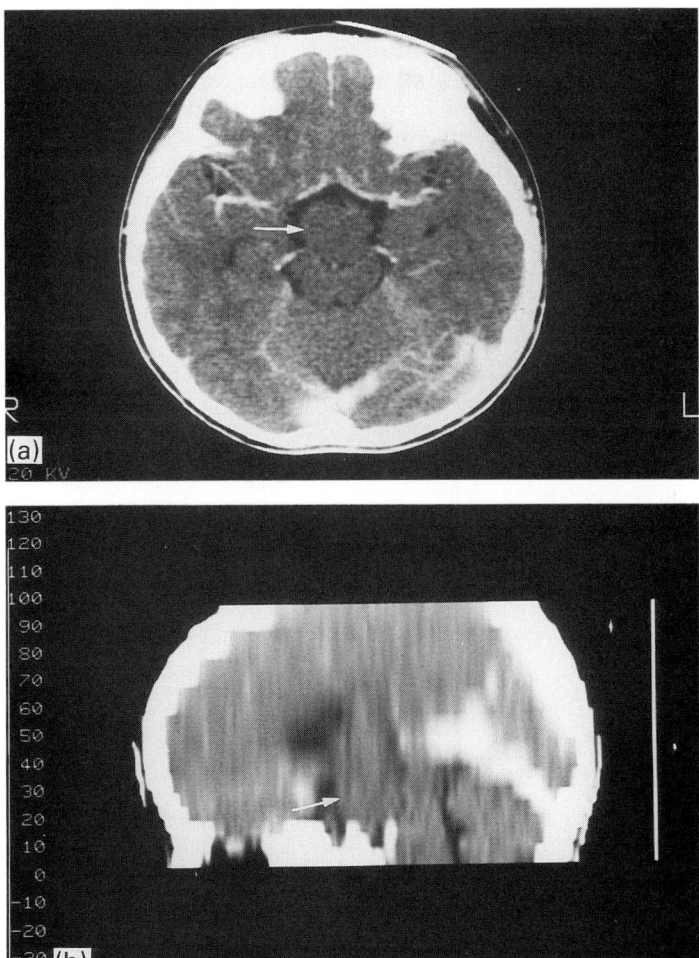

Figure 11. An 8-year-old boy with precocious puberty. CT (a) axial scan (b) sagittal reformation, shows a 1.5 cm hamartoma (arrow) of the tuber cinereum. Case provided by F. L. Chan, Hong Kong.

sequences. The inhomogeneity is the result of necrosis and/or haemorrhage in the tumour. Cystic areas have a signal intensity similar to CSF and haemorrhagic areas have a bright signal in the subacute stage. The tumour can extend superiorly into the suprasellar cistern, laterally into the cavernous sinuses obliterating Meckel's cave, or inferiorly into the sphenoid sinus. The diaphragma sella is obliterated with suprasellar extension, whereas it is preserved in cases of suprasellar meningioma (Daniels et al, 1986). Enhancement of the tumour with gadolinium-DTPA is variable. After bromocriptine therapy for prolactinoma (a rare lesion in children), cystic areas may appear with a signal intensity similar to CSF (Glaser et al, 1986). With large tumours, it is often difficult to separate the normal pituitary from the tumour. We have seen a 13-year old boy with pituitary gigantism due to a macroadenoma. This tumour was successfully removed by transphenoidal surgery with resolution of his symptoms (Figure 10).

Hypothalamic hamartoma is known to cause precocious puberty. They usually originate in the tuber cinereum and grow into the suprasellar cistern (Figure 11). They are of uniform CT density and isodense to brain both before and after intravenous contrast. On MR scans the lesions are iso-intense to grey matter on T1-weighted images and of high signal intensity in T2-weighted images (Hahn et al, 1988). Other *hypothalamic lesions* may also cause precocious puberty. Tumours commonly seen are optic nerve gliomas and hypothalamic astrocytomas with or without clinical findings of neurofibromatosis. The CT appearance is variable with solid, cystic and necrotic areas. Calcification is sometimes seen in astrocytoma. These tumours may also produce pituitary hypofunction. They are better demonstrated with MRI. *Pineal tumours* may also present with precocious puberty (Figure 12).

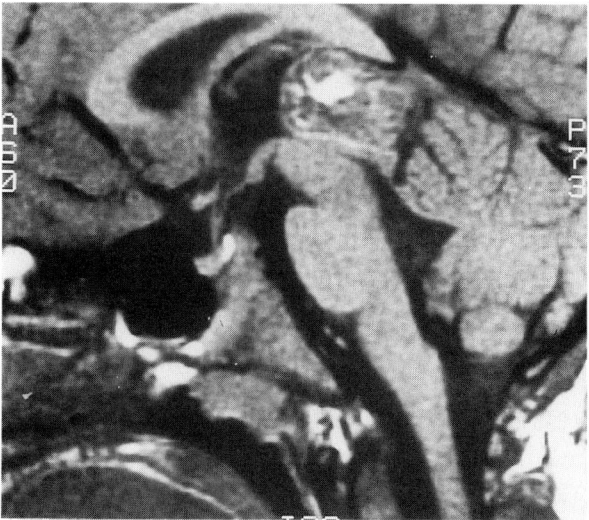

Figure 12. A pineal choriocarcinoma in an 8-year-old boy with pseudoprecocious puberty. On the T1-weighted sagittal MR image a mass with mixed signal intensities at the pineal region is causing aqueduct obstruction and hydrocephalus.

Hypofunction

Craniopharyngiomas account for 6–10% of intracranial neoplasms in childhood (Rubinstein, 1972). They usually occupy the sellar or suprasellar regions or both these areas. The majority occupy the suprasellar cistern and often cause obstructive hydrocephalus (Numaguchi et al, 1981).

Macroscopically, these tumours have soft tissue, calcific and cystic components. The calcific areas are not usually seen on MRI, and are best appreciated on CT scans or plain radiographs. On CT, the soft tissue component may show considerable contrast enhancement. The cysts usually have a density similar to CSF unless recent intracyst haemorrhage has occurred when they will become hyperdense. On MRI, the soft tissue component gives a signal intensity similar to that of normal brain. The fluid in the cysts behave like CSF, with a low signal intensity on T1-weighted images and a high signal on T2-weighted images. A bright intracyst signal on T1-weighted images corresponded to a high cholesterol level or presence of methaemoglobin following haemorrhage into the cyst (Pusey et al, 1987). Craniopharyngiomas often extend into the suprasellar cistern, elevating and compressing the third ventricle, causing hydrocephalus (Figure 13). Craniopharyngiomas which are predominantly intrasellar will cause enlargement of the pituitary fossa. The normal pituitary gland may or may not be demonstrable in intrasellar craniopharyngiomas. These patients may have mixed anterior and posterior pituitary hypofunction at presentation.

Other tumours encountered in the suprasellar and parasellar regions in childhood include *chiasmal gliomas*, *teratomas*, *haematomas* and *chordomas* (Karnaze et al, 1986). *Aneurysms* arising from the circle of Willis may present as a suprasellar mass. *Meningiomas* in this region are rare in childhood.

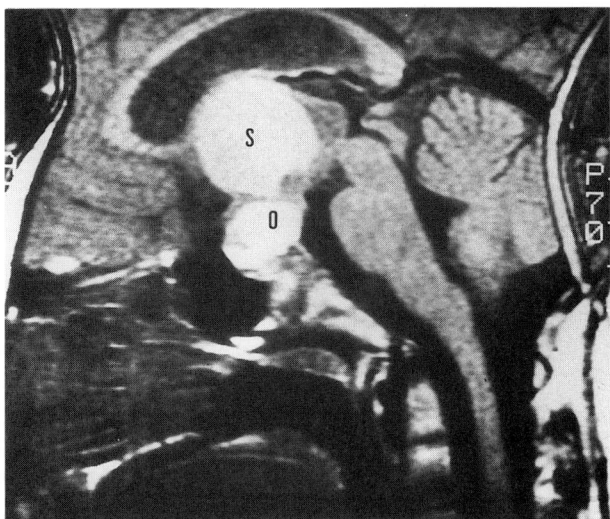

Figure 13. A craniopharyngioma with sella (O) and suprasellar (S) components. The high bright signal in the T1-weighted MR image was due to cholesterol in the cyst fluid. The mass compresses the third ventricle and causes hydrocephalus.

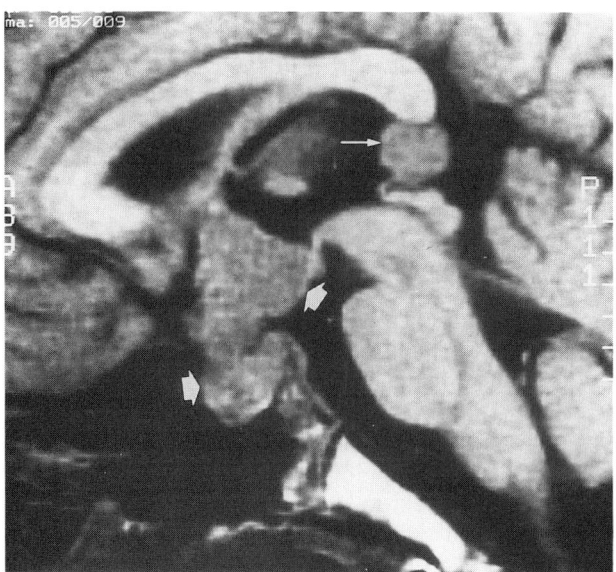

Figure 14. A pineal germinoma (small arrow) showing uniform signal intensity in a T1-weighted sagittal MR image. Suprasellar and intrasellar metastases (large arrows) with similar signal intensities are noted and are elevating the floor of the third ventricle.

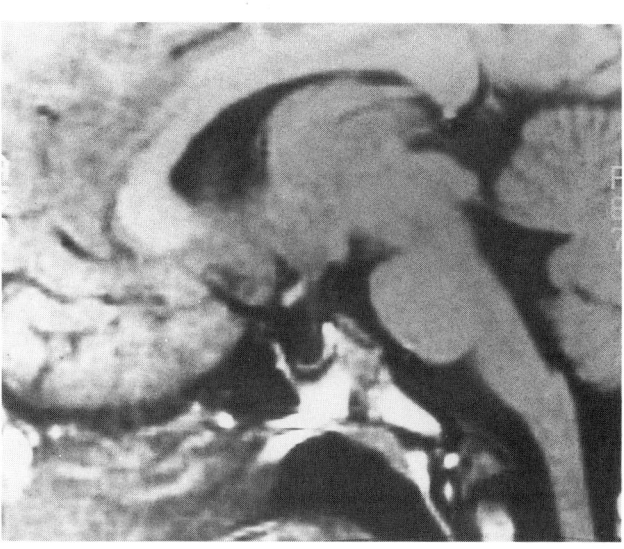

Figure 15. Sagittal MR image. Loss of pituitary gland with acquired 'empty sella' in an 8-year-old girl following cranial irradiation for leukaemia. She was growth retarded compared to her twin sister.

Metastases from pineal tumours may be encountered (Figure 14). Delayed or precocious puberty may be the presenting feature in children with *germinomas*.

In the *primary 'empty sella' syndrome*, the pituitary fossa is enlarged and filled with fluid resembling CSF (Gläser et al, 1986). This condition is readily diagnosed on coronal CT scans and T1-weighted sagittal and coronal MR scans. The pituitary gland is usually flattened inferiorly and posteriorly but its function usually remains normal. A *secondary 'empty sella' syndrome* is seen in patients treated with cranial irradiation (Figure 15). Such children often show evidence of growth hormone deficiency. 'Empty sella' may be seen in children with *congenital hypopituitarism* and can be mistaken for an intrasellar tumour on high resolution CT scanning. We have examined 11 children with congenital hypopituitarism and noted a failure of descent of the neurohypophysis in all but two (de Silva et al, 1987; Kelly et al, 1988). A rounded mass, measuring 2–5 mm in diameter, was noted in the floor of the third ventricle, just anterior to the mamillary bodies. The signal characteristics of this mass were similar to those seen in the posterior pituitary of normal subjects, and no posterior pituitary was noted in the usual location. The anterior pituitary was either small and in the usual location or absent. The infundibulum was either absent or small. The pituitary fossa appeared smaller than usual (Figure 16).

Lesions of *histiocytosis X* may be seen in the suprasellar region, and progression of these lesions following radiotherapy can be monitored using MR (Figure 17). These lesions appear to be associated with loss of the high intensity signal from the posterior pituitary gland, and is thought to reflect the

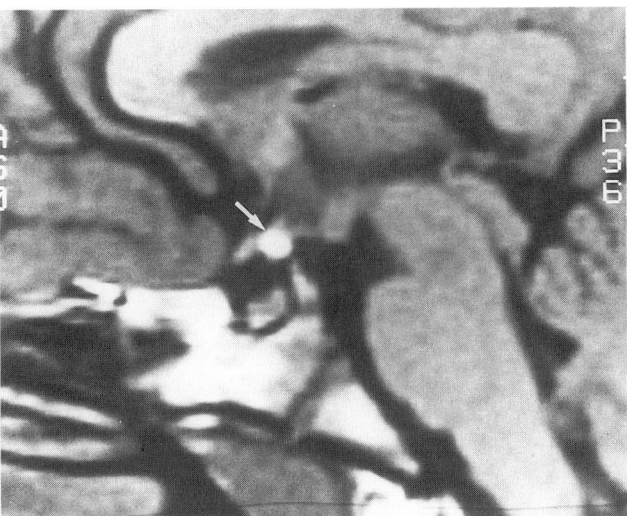

Figure 16. 'Undescended' posterior pituitary in a child with short stature. On the sagittal MR image, a rounded structure (arrow) measuring 3 mm in diameter is seen just anterior to the mamillary bodies. The bright signal corresponds to that of the posterior pituitary gland. No pituitary stalk is visualized and the anterior pituitary is in normal location.

reduction in neurotransmitter substances in the gland associated with diabetes insipidus seen with histiocytosis X. Lack of the normal high signal has been noted in cases of diabetes insipidus, resulting from other suprasellar tumours such as germinomas and teratomas, and in primary (idiopathic) diabetes insipidus (Figure 18) (Fujisawa et al, 1987b).

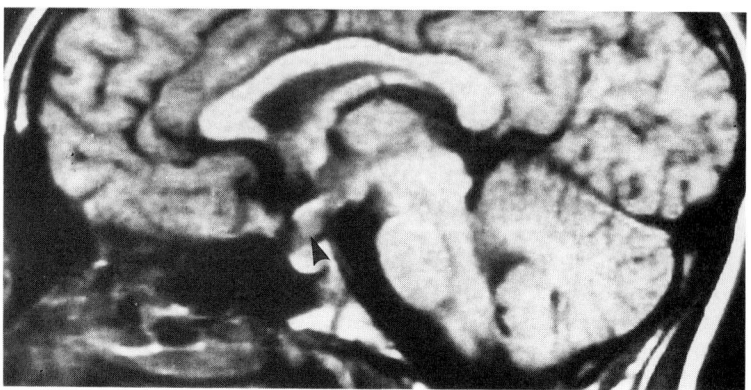

Figure 17. A rounded lesion (arrowhead) seen in the infundibular region in a child with an iliac bone lytic lesion. The bone lesion was proved by biopsy to be histiocytosis X. The mass has regressed following radiotherapy in a scan 2 months later.

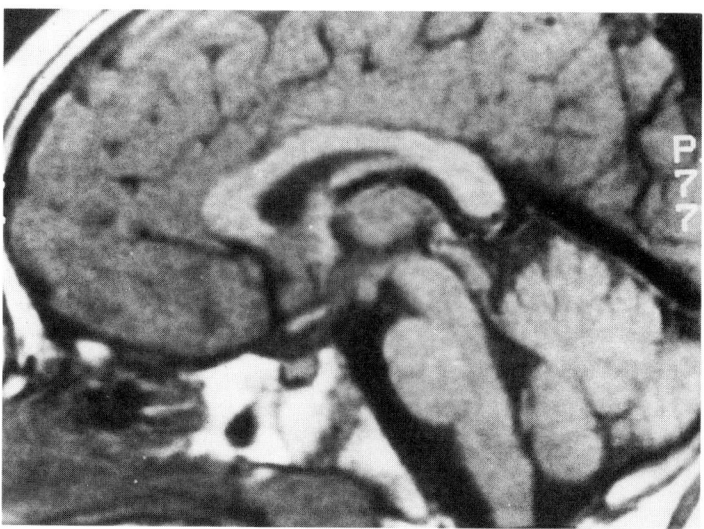

Figure 18. Absence of a posterior pituitary signal on MRI in a girl with idiopathic diabetes insipidus. The anterior pituitary appears normal.

THYROID DISORDERS

Radionuclide scanning remains the fundamental imaging modality in the diagnosis of thyroid disorders. It is essential however that their interpretation be made only with full knowledge of the appropriate thyroid function tests. Sonography may be used to supplement scintigraphy in certain well-defined areas. These include the differentiation of a solid from a cystic nodule and the differentiation of a diffuse goitre from a multinodular goitre.

In the paediatric age group the major isotope used is ^{99m}Tc because of the low radiation exposure. Iodine-123 is also used but is limited in its availability. Technetium-99m has a radiation exposure of 0.0008 rads/μCi and ^{123}I 0.038 rads/μCi. Localization of technetium in the thyroid gland occurs rapidly and is maximal by 20 min after intravenous injection. The radiation exposure of the thyroid gland depends upon the size of the gland and the percentage uptake of the radiopharmaceutical.

Gamma camera is the instrument of choice for thyroid scintigraphy. With the use of a pinhole collimator high resolution images can be obtained even in the neonatal period. Using a collimator aperture of 3–5 mm resolution of less than 4 mm can be achieved. Computer manipulation of images and background subtraction may also aid in improving visualization of poorly functioning areas of thyroid tissue.

Screening for congenital hypothyroidism

Neonatal screening programmes for congenital hypothyroidism have revealed an incidence of between 1:3000 and 1:5000. Thyroid scanning is valuable in these patients for genetic counselling as patients with dyshormonogenesis have an autosomal recessive disorder with a one in four chance of occurrence in subsequent siblings, whereas the other causes of congenital hypothyroidism are not inherited.

Common causes of congenital hypothyroidism are the ectopic thyroid (Figure 19) and athyreosis. The finding of ectopic glands is important because treated patients in this category often have best prognosis. In a large screening series of 127 newborn infants with hypothyroidism, ectopic thyroid was found in 23%, aplastic or hyperplastic glands in 63%, and a normal or enlarged thyroid gland in 14% (Fisher et al, 1979).

A normally sited hypofunctioning thyroid is caused usually by hypoplasia of the gland or secondary suppression by iodides or antithyroid drugs ingested by the mother. A normally placed enlarged thyroid gland that shows increased uptake of radiopharmaceutical represents dyshormonogenesis, i.e. an enzyme defect (Figure 20). A perchlorate discharge test using ^{131}I will confirm whether this is an organification defect.

Acquired hypothyroidism

Acquired hypothyroidism following surgery and irradiation is rare but thyroiditis is seen in prepubertal children, especially girls. The enlarged thyroid gland in chronic thyroiditis results in an irregular uptake of

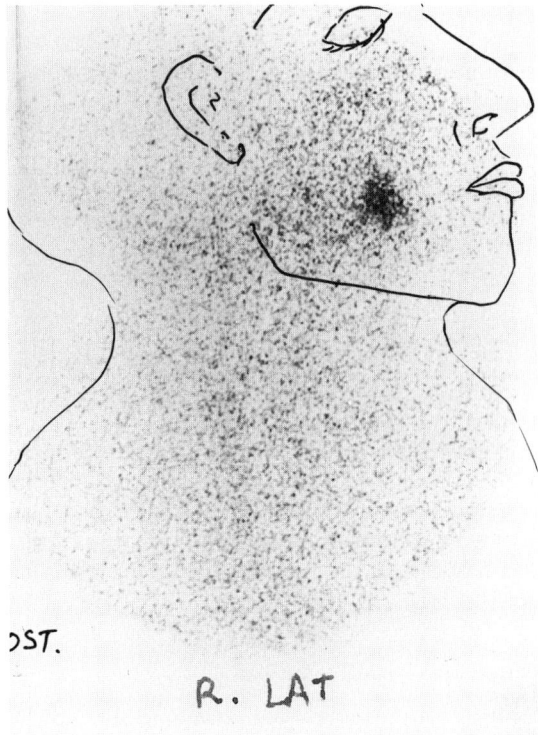

Figure 19. Ectopic lingual thyroid. A right lateral view of a radio-isotope thyroid scan. There is a small focus of radionuclide uptake at the posterior region of the tongue, with no functioning thyroid in the region of the thyroid cartilage.

radiopharmaceutical. Occasionally this may have a multinodular appearance or have a focal cold area on the scan.

Neck masses

In children with a neck mass it may be necessary to ensure that this area does not contain functioning thyroid tissue especially if surgery is considered necessary. It is often difficult to distinguish ectopic functioning thyroid tissue from a thyroglossal cyst. The thyroid scan enables areas of functioning tissue to be determined. Occasionally a unilateral enlargement of the thyroid gland is due to hemiagenesis of the contralateral lobe.

Thyroid nodules

Nodules in the thyroid gland are not common in the paediatric population and the differential diagnosis includes adenoma, cyst, focal hyperplasia and carcinoma. In general, carcinoma causes a focal decrease or cold area on the scan. These focal cold areas should be evaluated with ultrasound to determine

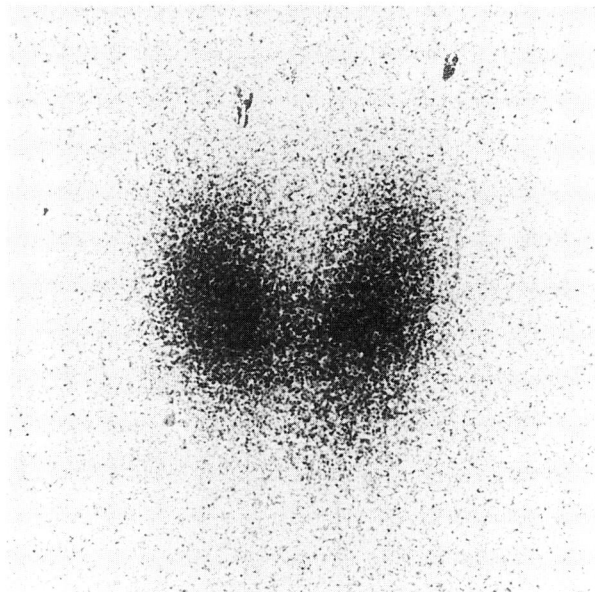

Figure 20. Dyshormonogenesis of the thyroid. Technetate thyroid scan shows enlarged gland with avid trapping of the tracer (20-min uptake measured at 17%, normal being 1–5%). The patient was clinically hypothyroid.

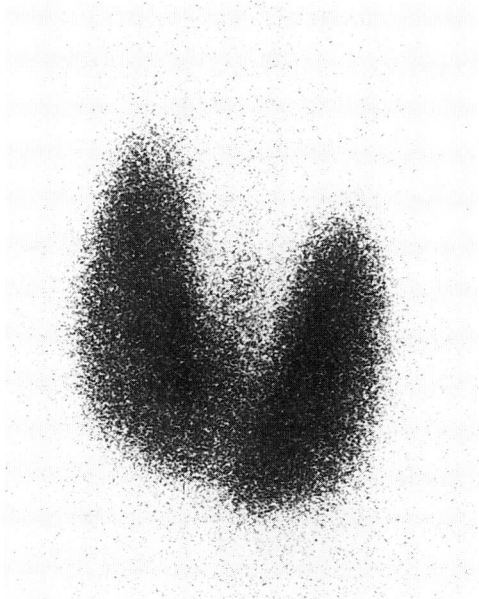

Figure 21. Diffuse toxic goitre in a 14-year-old girl. The gland is diffusely enlarged with a uniform uptake of tracer. The 20-min uptake is 32%.

whether they are composed of solid or cystic material or a combination of solid and cystic elements. Solitary nodules are rare in children. Hung et al (1982) described 39 children with solitary nodules of which 35 were surgically removed. Twenty-seven of the 39 were cold on the thyroid scan. The commonest cause was a non-functioning follicular adenoma. Five of the 27 children had a malignancy in the thyroid gland. No malignant nodules were found in warm or hot nodules. Focal solid cold nodules have been described in focal thyroiditis. Hot nodules may represent autonomous thyroid tissue where there has been suppression of the remainder of the gland. Hot nodules are rare in children.

Hyperthyroidism

The thyroid scan is valuable in differentiating the diffuse goitre (Figure 21) associated with Graves' disease from a toxic nodular goitre and an autonomous nodule, which are usually due to a toxic adenoma. However, very rarely an autonomous nodule may be due to a toxic functional carcinoma.

DISORDERS OF THE PARATHYROID GLANDS

Secondary hyperparathyroidism is the most common parathyroid disorder in the paediatric population. In developed countries this is usually due to chronic renal failure or one of the renal tubular disorders. Primary disorders are less common, with primary hypoparathyroidism and pseudohypoparathyroidism together being more common than primary hyperparathyroidism in children. The diagnosis of a parathyroid disorder is best made or confirmed from the biochemical and hormone profile.

Hypoparathyroidism

Primary idiopathic hypoparathyroidism may be familial or sporadic. It is usually diagnosed in childhood and may be associated with Addison disease, pernicious anaemia, ovarian dysgenesis, hypothyroidism and mucocutaneous candidiasis. Congenital absence of the parathyroid glands occurs in the Di George syndrome together with absence of the thymus.

The most common plain radiographic feature, although occurring in only about 20%, is generalized or focal osteosclerosis (Resnick and Niwayama, 1981), particularly in the calvarium, pelvis and proximal femora. There is thickening of the cranial vault and facial bones. Increased intracranial pressure with sutural diastasis may occur. Abnormal tooth development with delayed eruption and hypoplasia of enamel and dentine (Resnick and Niwayama, 1981), or aplastic or supernumerary teeth may be seen (Destouet and Murphy, 1987). Hypoparathyroidism is one of the causes of premature fusion of the epiphyses. Dense metaphyseal bands may also be seen.

Soft tissue calcification may be found in the subcutaneous tissues, tendons and spinal ligaments. The latter may resemble ankylosing spondylitis or diffuse idiopathic skeletal hyperostosis. Basal ganglia calcification is seen as a late manifestation.

Pseudohypoparathyroidism

Pseudohypoparathyroidism (PHP) is a heritable disorder usually diagnosed in late childhood. The parathyroid glands are structurally normal or hyperplastic and are biologically active. There is an end-organ resistance to parathyroid hormone. This can be classified into three major groups (Frame et al, 1972; Burnstein et al, 1985).

In the first group there is renal resistance and skeletal resistance only at the osteocyte level. There is hypocalcaemia and hyperphosphataemia with no response in the cyclic AMP or urinary phosphorous levels to the parenteral injection of parathyroid hormone. The skeleton will display the changes of hyperparathyroidism in addition to the features of classic PHP, although the latter may be absent in some cases. The second group is the classic form with renal resistance and skeletal resistance at the osteocyte and osteoclast level. There is hypocalcaemia, hyperphosphataemia and high plasma parathyroid hormone levels. These patients may exhibit the typical radiographic features of PHP without the changes of hyperparathyroid bone disease. In the third group, there is skeletal resistance only, with a normal

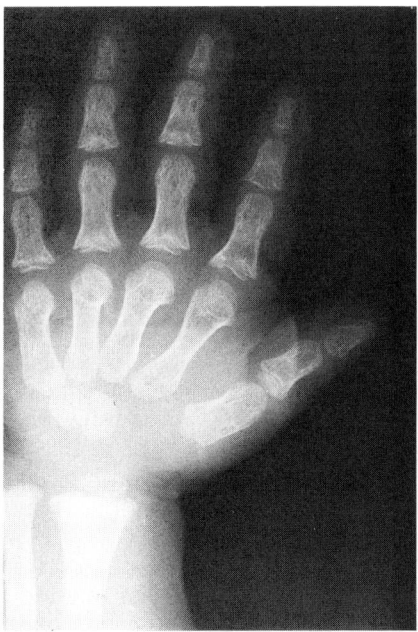

Figure 22. A 3-year-old girl with pseudohypoparathyroidism. The hand shows short metacarpals and phalanges with cone-shaped epiphyses. An identical appearance is seen in acrodysostosis.

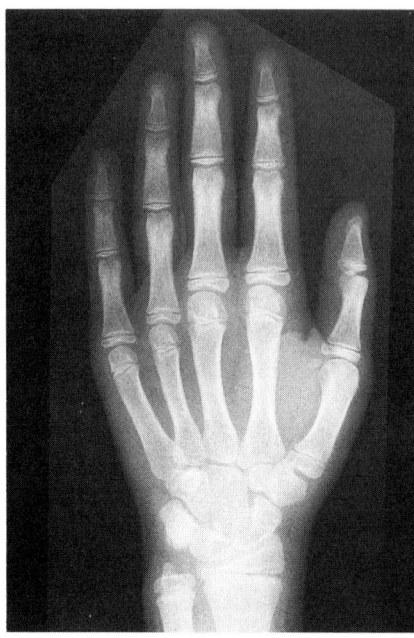

Figure 23. Girl aged 11 years with pseudohypoparathyroidism showing shortened 4th meta-carpal. A line drawn tangential to the heads of the 3rd and 5th metacarpals passes beyond the head of the 4th metacarpal. This sign is also found in Turner syndrome.

renal response to parathyroid hormone. The serum calcium is decreased and the serum phosphate is normal or decreased. The skeletal changes of classic PHP may be present.

Pseudopseudohypoparathyroidism (PPHP) is the normocalcaemic form of pseudohypoparathyroidism (PHP).

A typical plain radiographic feature is shortening of one or more of the metacarpals or metatarsals probably due to premature fusion of the growth plates (Figures 22 and 23), most commonly affecting the 4th or 5th digits. This is present in the hands in 75% of cases of PHP and in 90% of cases of PPHP. In the feet it is present in 70% of cases of PHP and 99% PPHP (Destouet and Murphy, 1987). Other skeletal changes include diaphyseal exostoses, coxa vara or coxa valgus, bowed long bones, cone-shaped epiphyses and accelerated skeletal maturity. There may be abnormal dentition. Cases have been described which present the clinical phenotypic and radiographic features of acrodysostosis (Figure 22) but which also have the metabolic abnormalities of PHP or PPHP (Ablow et al, 1977).

Soft tissue calcification is seen in 40–55% of cases. It may occur in the skin, subcutaneous tissues, fascial planes, ligaments and in the tendons particularly in the periarticular regions of the hands and feet. In the brain, calcification of the basal ganglia (Figure 24) and dentate nucleus, best demonstrated on CT scan, is seen in late childhood or early adulthood in about 45% of cases of PHP and 8% of PPHP.

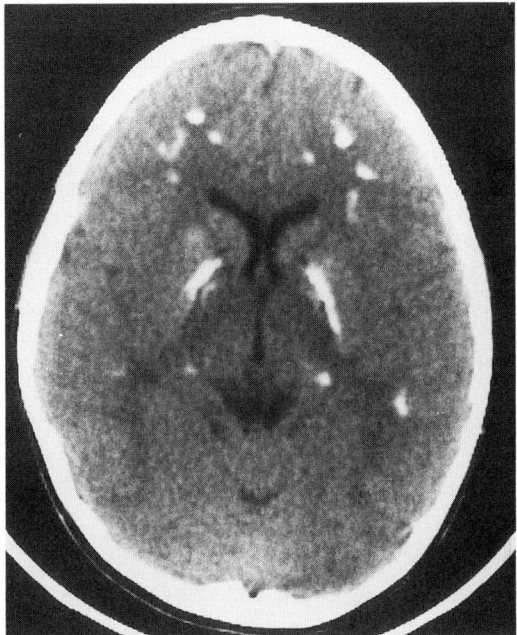

Figure 24. Boy aged 6 years with pseudohypoparathyroidism. CT scan shows high density changes in the basal ganglia and at the grey–white junctions, showing calcification.

Hyperparathyroidism

Primary hyperparathyroidism may rarely occur in infants and children. Congenital hyperparathyroidism demonstrates an autosomal recessive inheritance. Transient hyperparathyroidism of the neonate occurs in infants of hypoparathyroid mothers. This is self-limited and resolves rapidly although fractures and hypocalcaemia may occur (Resnick and Niwayama, 1981). Acquired primary hyperparathyroidism of the adult type rarely occurs in children. Its management and diagnosis would be the same as that for adults. Secondary hyperparathyroidism is of course common in children with renal failure.

In older children, the plain radiographic features include reduced bone density with a coarsened trabecular pattern, subperiosteal erosions or cortical tunnelling particularly well seen in the hands. Larger areas of bone erosion may be seen particularly at the medial side of the femoral neck, the lateral ends of the clavicles and the proximal ends of the tibias. Metastatic soft tissue calcification may develop in vessels, the viscera and in the subcutaneous and periarticular soft tissues. Chondrocalcinosis may occur. Slipped epiphyses, genu valgum and fractures may be secondary consequences. With secondary renal involvement due to nephrocalcinosis, rickets-like changes will occur at the metaphyses and growth plates.

In infants there is severe bone disease with subperiosteal bone resorption, florid periosteal new bone formation, reduced trabecular pattern, erosions of tubular bones and fractures.

SUMMARY

Disorders of growth and development, including delayed and precocious puberty may be idiopathic, constitutional or due to a disorder of one of several endocrine systems including the hypothalamic–pituitary system, the adrenal and the thyroid. Sonography is of great importance in the classification of precocious puberty in children. Skeletal maturation assessment is useful to evaluate the severity of the growth disorder and to monitor subsequent therapy. Magnetic resonance imaging and computed tomography are essential in the study of the pituitary and central nervous system. MRI has special advantages in the imaging of the hypothalamic–pituitary region.

The thyroid gland and its function are still best imaged with radionuclide scintigraphy. Sonography can play a complementary though less important role.

Hypoparathyroidism, pseudohypoparathyroidism and pseudopseudo-hypoparathyroidism although rare are more common in children than primary hyperparathyroidism. Valuable clues as to the presence of these conditions can be gained by examination of the plain radiographs. Confirmation of their diagnosis still rests with the biochemical and endocrine profile.

REFERENCES

Ablow RC, Hsia YE & Brandt IK (1977) Acrodysostosis coinciding with pseudohypoparathyroidism and pseudopseudohypoparathyroidism. *American Journal of Roentgenology* **128:** 95–99.

Acheson RM (1954) A method of assessing skeletal maturity from radiographs. A report from the Oxford Child Health Survey. *Journal of Anatomy* **88:** 498–508.

Bayley N & Pinneau SR (1952) Tables for predicting adult height from skeletal age: Revised for use with the Greulich–Pyle hand standards. *Journal of Pediatrics* **40:** 423–441.

Buckler JMH (1984) Skeletal age changes in puberty. *Archives of Disease in Childhood* **59:** 115–119.

Burnstein MI, Kottamasu SR, Pettifor JM et al (1985) Metabolic bone disease in pseudohypoparathyroidism: radiologic features. *Radiology* **155:** 351–356.

Daniels DL, Pojunas KW, Kilgore DP et al (1986) MR imaging of the diaphragma sella. *American Journal of Neuroradiology* **7:** 765–769.

Daniels DL, Haughton VM & Czervionke LF (1988) Skull base. In Stark DD & Bradley WG Jr (eds) *Magnetic Resonance Imaging*, pp 532–539. St Louis: CV Mosby.

Danzinger J, Wallace S, Handel S et al (1979) The sella tursica in primary end organ failure. *Radiology* **131:** 111.

Davies RP & Lam AH (1987) Adrenocortical neoplasm in children: Ultrasound appearance. *Journal of Ultrasound in Medicine* **6:** 325–328.

Destouet JM & Murphy WA (1987) Parathyroid disease. In Taveras JM & Ferrucci JT (eds) *Radiology*, vol. 5. Philadelphia: JB Lippincott.

Dreizen S, Snodgrasse RM, Webb-Peploe H et al (1957) Bilateral symmetry of skeletal maturation in the human hand and wrist. *American Journal of Diseases of Children* **93:** 122–127.

Fisher DA, Dussault JH, Foley TP et al (1979) Screening for congenital hypothyroidism: results of screening one million North American infants. *Journal of Pediatrics* **94:** 700–705.

Frame B, Hanson CA, Frost HM, Block MA & Arnstein AR (1972) *American Journal of Medicine* **52:** 311–321.

Fujisawa I, Asato R, Nishimura K et al (1987a) Anterior and posterior lobes of the pituitary gland: Assessment by 1.5 T MR imaging. *Journal of Computer Assisted Tomography* **11**(2): 214–220.

Fujisawa I, Nishimura K, Asato R et al (1987b) Posterior lobe of the pituitary in diabetes insipidus: MR findings. *Journal of Computer Assisted Tomography* **11**(2): 221–225.

Gardeur D, Naidich TP & Metzger J (1981) CT analysis of intrasellar pituitary adenomas with emphasis on patterns of contrast enhancement. *Neuroradiology* **20:** 241.

Garn SM, Rohmann CG & Davis AA (1963) Genetic of hand–wrist ossification. *American Journal of Physical Anthropology* **21:** 33–40.

Glaser B, Sheinfeld M, Benmair J & Kaplan N (1986) Magnetic resonance imaging of the pituitary gland. *Clinical Radiology* **37:** 9–14.

Greulich WW & Pyle SI (1959) *Radiographic atlas of skeletal development of the hand and wrist*, 2nd edn. Stanford, California: Stanford University Press.

Hahn FJ, Leibrock LG, Huseman CA & Makos MM (1988) The MR appearances of hypothalamic hamartoma. *Neuroradiology* **30:** 65–68.

Hindmarsh PC, Stanhope R, Kendall BE & Brook CG (1986) Tall stature: a clinical, endocrinological and radiological study. *Clinical Endocrinology* **25:** 223–231.

Hung W, August GP, Randolph JG et al (1982) Solitary thyroid nodules in children and adolescents. *Journal of Paediatric Surgery* **17:** 225–229.

Ivarsson SA, Nilsson KO & Persson PH (1983) Ultrasonography of pelvic organ in prepubertal and post-pubertal girl. *Archives of Disease in Childhood* **58:** 353–354.

Kahus LR & Finnstrom O (1976) New standards of ossification of the newborn. *Radiology* **119:** 655–660.

Karnaze MG, Sartor K, Winthrop JD, Gado MH & Hodges III FJ (1986) Suprasellar lesions: evaluation with MR imaging. *Radiology* **161:** 77–82.

Kelly WM, Kucharczyk W, Kucharczyk J et al (1988) Posterior pituitary ectopia: A MR feature of pituitary dwarfism. *American Journal of Neuroradiology* **9:** 453–460.

Moore KL (1982) *The Developing Human*, 3rd edn, pp. 396–398. Philadelphia: WB Saunders.

Numaguchi Y, Kishikawa T, Ikeda J et al (1981) Neuroradiological manifestations of suprasellar pituitary adenomas, meningiomas and craniopharyngiomas. *Neuroradiology* **21:** 67.

Okuno T, Sado M, Momoi T et al (1980) Pituitary hyperplasia due to hypothyroidism. *Journal of Computer Assisted Tomography* **5:** 600.

Orsini LF, Salardi S, Pilu G, Bovicelli L & Cacciari E (1984) Pelvic organs in premenstrual girls: realtime ultrasonography. *Radiology* **153:** 113–116.

Peters H, Himelstein-Braw R & Faber M (1976) The normal development of ovary in childhood. *Acta Endocrinologica* **82:** 617–630.

Pusey E, Kortman KE, Flannigan BE et al (1987) MR of Craniopharyngiomas: Tumor delineation and characterization. *American Journal of Neuroradiology* **8:** 439–444.

Pyle SI & Hoerr NL (1969) *A radiographic standard of reference for the growing knee*, 2nd edn, Springfield: Charles C. Thomas.

Rayner PHW (1981) Early puberty. In Brook CGD *Clinical paediatric endocrinology*, p 224. Oxford: Blackwell Scientific.

Resnick D & Niwayama G (1981) Parathyroid disorders and renal osteodystrophy. In Resnick D & Niwayama G *Diagnosis of Bone and Joint Disorders*, pp 1802–1859. Philadelphia: WB Saunders.

Rieth KG, Comite F, Dwyer AJ et al (1987) CT of cerebral abnormalities in precocious puberty. *American Journal of Neuroradiology* **8:** 283–290.

Roche AF & Chumlea WC (1980) Serial changes in predicted adult statures for individuals. *Human Biology* **52:** 507–514.

Roche AF, Wainer H & Thissen D (1975) Predicting adult stature for individuals. *Monographs in Paediatrics* **3:** 1–114.

Roppolo HMN (1985) Normal intrasellar and parasellar anatomy. In Latchaw RE (ed.) *Computed Tomography of the Head, Neck and Spine*, pp 305–319. Chicago: Year Book Medical.

Rubinstein LJ (1972) Tumours of the central nervous system. *Armed Forces Institute of*

Pathology, Washington DC, pp 292–294.

Saenger P (1984) Abnormal sex differentiation. *Journal of Pediatrics* **104:** 1–17.

Salardi S, Orsini LF, Cacciari E, Bovicelli P, Tassoni P & Reggiani A (1985) Pelvic ultrasonography in premenstrual girls: Relation to puberty and sex hormone concentration. *Archives of Disease on Childhood* **60:** 120–125.

Salardi S, Orsini LF, Cacciari E et al (1988) Pelvic ultrasonography in girls with precocious puberty, congenital adrenal hyperplasia, obesity, or hirsutism. *Journal of Paediatrics* **112:** 880–887.

Sample WF, Lippes BM & Gyepes MT (1977) Gray-scale ultrasonography of the ovary of normal female pelvis. *Radiology* **125:** 477–483.

Shawker TH, Comite F, Reith KG, Dwyer AJ, Cutler GB & Loriaux DL (1984) Ultrasound evaluation of iso-sexual precocious puberty. *Journal of Ultrasound in Medicine* **3:** 309–316.

de Silva M, Wong H, Cowell C et al (1987) *Proceedings of the Royal Australasian College of Radiology—Annual Meeting*, Sydney.

Stanhope R, Adams J, Jacobs HS & Brook CGD (1985) Ovarian ultrasound assessment in normal children, idiopathic precocious puberty, and during low dose pulsatile gonadotrophin releasing hormone treatment of hypogonadotrophic hypogonadism. *Archives of Disease in Childhood* **60:** 116–119.

Tanner JM, Whitehouse RH, Cameron N, Marshall WA, Healy MJR & Goldstein H (1983) *Assessment of skeletal maturity and prediction of adult height (TW2 method)*, 2nd edn. London: Academic Press.

Van Venrooij-Ysselmuiden ME & Van Ipenburg A (1978) Mixed longitudinal data on skeletal age from a group of Dutch children living in Utrecht and surroundings. *Annals of Human Biology* **5:** 359–380.

Weissbuch SS (1986) Explanation and implication of MR signal changes after bromocriptine therapy. *American Journal of Neuroradiology* **7:** 214–216.

Yock DH Jr (1984) Techniques in imaging of the brain. In Rosenberg RN (ed.) *The Clinical Neurosciences*, vol. 4, pp 24–28. New York: Churchill Livingstone.

Zachmann M, Sobradillo B, Frank M, Frisch H & Prader A (1978) Bayley–Pinneau, Roche–Wainer–Thissen and Tanner height predictions in normal children and in patients with various pathological conditions. *Journal of Paediatrics* **93:** 749–755.

Index

225